ACUTE PANCREATITIS

Edited by **Luis Rodrigo**

Acute Pancreatitis
Edited by Luis Rodrigo

Published by InTech
Janeza Trdine 9, 51000 Rijeka, Croatia

Publishing Process Manager Vedran Greblo

Technical Editor Teodora Smiljanic

Cover Designer InTech Design Team

Additional hard copies can be obtained from orders@intechopen.com

Acute Pancreatitis, Edited by Luis Rodrigo
p. cm.
978-953-307-984-4

For EU product safety concerns:
IN TECH d.o.o., Prolaz Marije Krucifikse Kozulić 3, 51000 Rijeka, Croatia,
info@intechopen.com or visit our website at intechopen.com.

Meet the editor

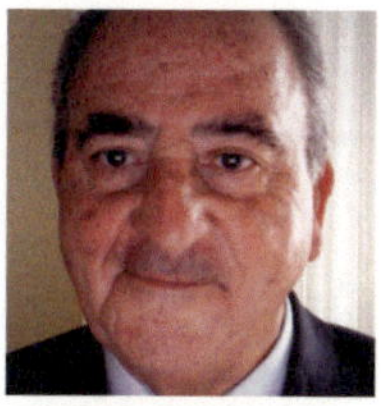

Luis Rodrigo PhD is 67 years old and was born in Vitoria, Spain. He studied in the Medical School at the Central University of Madrid from 1962 to 1967, graduating as Licensee in Medicine and Surgery. Dr Rodrigo obtained his PhD in Medicine in Oviedo in 1975. He is currently Professor of Medicine at the University of Oviedo – a positon he has held since 1983, and has served as the Chief of Gastroenterology at the University Hospital Center of Asturias, Spain since 1996. He is a Member of the National Program of Fellowship along with around 100 Specialists in Gastroenterology and the main author or co-author of 178 scientific papers written in English and 254 in Spanish. He has written a total of 55 chapters of books on Gastroenterology, and 5 books about treatment of Gastroenterological diseases.

Contents

Preface XI

Part 1 Etiology 1

Chapter 1 **Acute Biliary Pancreatitis 3**
Mehmet Ilhan and Halil Alıs

Chapter 2 **Acute Pancreatitis Induced by Drugs 17**
Karel Urbánek, Ilona Vinklerová,
Ondřej Krystyník and Vlastimil Procházka

Chapter 3 **Obesity and Acute Pancreatitis 35**
Davor Štimac and Neven Franjić

Chapter 4 **Acute Pancreatitis During Pregnancy 47**
Tea Štimac and Davor Štimac

Chapter 5 **Pancreatitis in Children 55**
Alfredo Larrosa-Haro, Carmen A. Sánchez-Ramírez
and Mariana Gómez-Nájera

Chapter 6 **Pancreatitis in Cystic Fibrosis and CFTR-Related Disorder 67**
Michael J. Coffey and Chee Y. Ooi

Chapter 7 **Diabetes or Diabetes Drugs:**
A Cause for Acute Pancreatitis 91
Leann Olansky

Part 2 Pathogenesis 99

Chapter 8 **Role of Peritoneal Macrophages on Local and Systemic**
Inflammatory Response in Acute Pancreatitis 101
Marcel Cerqueira Cesar Machado
and Ana Maria Mendonça Coelho

Chapter 9 **Molecular Biology of Acute Pancreatitis 109**
Francisco Soriano and Ester C.S. Rios

Chapter 10 **Oxidative Stress and Antioxidative Status in the Acute Pancreatitis 117**
Andrzej Lewandowski, Krystyna Markocka-Mączka, Maciej Garbień, Dorota Diakowska and Renata Taboła

Chapter 11 **Microcirculatory Disturbances in the Pathogenesis of Acute Pancreatitis 141**
Dirk Uhlmann

Part 3 Diagnosis 171

Chapter 12 **Endoscopic Retrograde Cholangiopancreatography-Related Acute Pancreatitis – Identification, Prophylaxis and Treatment 173**
Alejandro González-Ojeda, Carlos Dávalos-Cobian, Elizabeth Andalón-Dueñas, Mariana Chávez-Tostado, Arturo Espinosa-Partida and Clotilde Fuentes-Orozco

Chapter 13 **Endoscopic Retrograde Cholangiopancreatography (ERCP) Related Acute Pancreatitis 197**
Zoltán Döbrönte

Chapter 14 **Nutrition Assessment and Therapy in Acute Pancreatitis 215**
Vanessa Fuchs-Tarlovsky and Krishnan Sriram

Part 4 Treatment 233

Chapter 15 **Changes in the Management of Treatment in Acute Pancreatitis Patients 235**
Juraj Bober, Jana Kaťuchová and Jozef Radoňak

Chapter 16 **Hypertriglyceride Induced Acute Pancreatitis 259**
Joshua Lebenson and Thomas Oliver

Chapter 17 **The Role of Percutaneous Drainage in the Treatment of Severe Acute Pancreatitis on the Basis of the Modified Atlanta Classification 279**
Zsolt Szentkereszty, Róbert Kotán and Péter Sápy

Preface

It is a great pleasure r to be the editor of this interesting book about Acute Pancreatitis, written by an international group of experts, doctors, university professors, and investigators, experienced in this field.

Acute pancreatitis is one of the more commonly encountered etiologies in the emergency setting and its incidence is rising. Presentations range from a mildself-limiting condition which usually responds to conservative management,to one with significant morbidity and mortality in its most severe forms. While clinical criteria are necessary to make the initial diagnosis, contrast-enhanced CT is the mainstay of imaging and has a vital role in assessing the extent and evolution of the disease and its associated complications.

Disease severity is best predicted from a number of clinical scoring systems which can be applied at diagnosis in association with repeated clinical assessment, measurement of acute inflammatory markers, and CT.

Establishing a biliary etiology in acute pancreatitis is clinically important because of the potential need for invasive treatment, such as endoscopic retrograde cholangiopancreatography. The etiology of acute biliary pancreatitis (ABP) is multifactorial and complex. Passage of small gallbladder stones or biliary sludge through the ampulla of vater. seems to be important in the pathogenesis of ABP. Other factors such as, anatomical variations associated with an increased biliopancreatic reflux, bile and pancreatic juice exclusion from the duodenum, and genetic factors, might contribute to the development of ABP. A diagnosis of a biliary etiology in acute pancreatitis is supported by both laboratory and imaging investigations. An increased serum level of alanine aminotransferase (>1.0 microkat/l) is associated with a high probability of gallstone pancreatitis (positive predictive value 80-90%). Confirmation of choledocholithiasis is most accurately obtained using endoscopic ultrasonography or magnetic resonance cholangiopancreatography.

Prophylactic antibiotics are not effective in reducing the incidence of (peri)-pancreatic infection in patients with severe disease (or even documented necrotizing pancreatitis). The only rational indication for antibiotics is documented infection.

Recurrent acute pancreatitis is a common clinical problem. Most cases of pancreatitis are identified by a careful history and physical examination. Despite advanced evaluation, the cause is not apparent in about 10% of cases. The etiology of recurrent acute pancreatitis appears to be multifactorial, with genetic and environmental influences playing a significant role. The strength of evidence for certain etiologies is highly variable, and natural history data is limited. Controversy exists regarding the most appropriate diagnostic and therapeutic approach. Recurrent acute pancreatitis often represents a continuum with chronic pancreatitis.

Although most cases of acute pancreatitis are uncomplicated and resolve spontaneously, the presence of complications has significant prognostic importance. Necrosis, hemorrhage, and infection convey up to 25%, 52%, and 80% mortality, respectively. Other complications such as pseudocyst formation, pseudoaneurysm formation, or venous thrombosis, increase morbidity and mortality to a lesser degree.

Luis Rodrigo PhD
HUCA,
Spain

Part 1

Etiology

1

Acute Biliary Pancreatitis

Mehmet Ilhan and Halil Alıs
Ministry of Health Bakırkoy, Dr Sadi Konuk Training and Research Hospital General Surgery, Istanbul, Turkey

1. Introduction

Acute pancreatitis is an inflammatory disease of the pancreas. The etiology and pathogenesis of acute pancreatitis have been intensively investigated for centuries worldwide. It can be initiated by several factors, including gallstones, alcohol, trauma, infections and hereditary factors. About 75% of pancreatitis is caused by gallstones or alcohol. In this chapter we discuss the causes, diagnosis, imaging findings, therapy, and complications of acute biliary pancreatitis.

2. Anatomy and physiology

The pancreas is perhaps the most unforgiving organ in the human body, leading most surgeons to avoid even palpating it unless necessary. Situated deep in the center of the abdomen, the pancreas is surrounded by numerous important structures and major blood vessels. Surgeons that choose to undertake surgery on the pancreas require a thorough knowledge of its anatomy. However, knowledge of the relationships of the pancreas and surrounding structures is also critically important for all surgeons to ensure that pancreatic injury is avoided during surgery on other structures.

The pancreas is a retroperitoneal organ that lies in an oblique position, sloping upward from the C-loop of the duodenum to the splenic hilum. In an adult, the pancreas weighs 75 to 100 g and is about 15 to 20 cm long. The fact that the pancreas is situated so deeply in the abdomen and is sealed in the retroperitoneum explains the poorly localized and sometimes ill-defined nature with which pancreatic pathology presents.

Surgeons typically describe the location of pathology within the pancreas in relation to four regions: the head, neck, body, and tail. The head of the pancreas is nestled in the C-loop of the duodenum and is posterior to the transverse mesocolon.

Most of the pancreas drains through the duct of Wirsung, or main pancreatic duct, into the common channel formed from the bile duct and pancreatic duct. (Figure 1) The length of the common channel is variable. In about one third of patients, the bile duct and pancreatic duct remain distinct to the end of the papilla, the two ducts merge at the end of the papilla in another one third, and in the remaining one third, a true common channel is present for a distance of several millimeters.

The main pancreatic duct is usually only 2 to 3 mm in diameter and runs midway between the superior and inferior borders of the pancreas, usually closer to the posterior than to the anterior surface. Pressure inside the pancreatic duct is about twice that in the common bile duct, which is thought to prevent reflux of bile into the pancreatic duct. The main pancreatic duct joins with the common bile duct and empties at the ampulla of Vater or major papilla, which is located on the medial aspect of the second portion of the duodenum. The muscle fibers around the ampulla form the sphincter of Oddi, which controls the flow of pancreatic and biliary secretions into the duodenum. Contraction and relaxation of the sphincter is regulated by complex neural and hormonal factors.

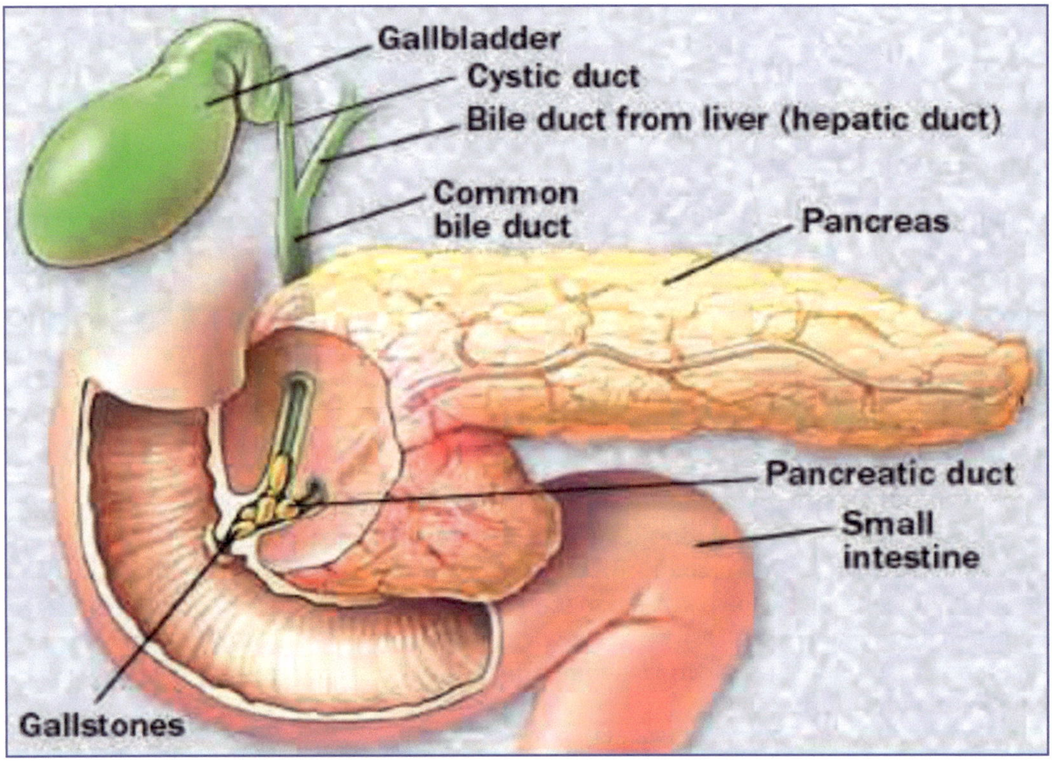

Fig. 1. Pancreas and biliary system anatomy

The exocrine pancreas accounts for about 85% of the pancreatic mass; 10% of the gland is accounted for by extracellular matrix, and 4% by blood vessels and the major ducts, whereas only 2% of the gland is comprised of endocrine tissue.

The pancreas secretes approximately 500 to 800 mL per day of colorless, odorless, alkaline, isosmotic pancreatic juice. Pancreatic juice is a combination of acinar cell and duct cell secretions. The acinar cells secrete amylase, proteases, and lipases, enzymes responsible for the digestion of all three food types: carbohydrate, protein, and fat. The acinar cells are pyramid-shaped, with their apices facing the lumen of the acinus. Near the apex of each cell are numerous enzyme-containing zymogen granules that fuse with the apical cell membrane.

Pancreatic amylase is secreted in its active form and completes the digestive process already begun by salivary amylase. Amylase is the only pancreatic enzyme secreted in its active form, and it hydrolyzes starch and glycogen to glucose, maltose, maltotriose, and dextrins.

These simple sugars are transported across the brush border of the intestinal epithelial cells by active transport mechanisms. Gastric hydrolysis of protein yields peptides that enter the intestine and stimulate intestinal endocrine cells to release cholecystokinin (CCK)-releasing peptide, CCK, and secretin, which then stimulate the pancreas to secrete enzymes and bicarbonate into the intestine.

The proteolytic enzymes are secreted as proenzymes that require activation. Trypsinogen is converted to its active form, trypsin, by another enzyme, enterokinase, which is produced by the duodenal mucosal cells. Trypsin, in turn, activates the other proteolytic enzymes. Trypsinogen activation within the pancreas is prevented by the presence of inhibitors that are also secreted by the acinar cells. Chymotrypsinogen is activated to form chymotrypsin. Elastase, carboxypeptidase A and B, and phospholipase are also activated by trypsin. Trypsin, chymotrypsin, and elastase cleave bonds between amino acids within a target peptide chain, and carboxypeptidase A and B cleave amino acids at the end of peptide chains. Individual amino acids and small dipeptides are then actively transported into the intestinal epithelial cells. Pancreatic lipase hydrolyzes triglycerides to 2-monoglyceride and fatty acid. Pancreatic lipase is secreted in an active form. Colipase is also secreted by the pancreas and binds to lipase, changing its molecular configuration and increasing its activity. Phospholipase A2 is secreted by the pancreas as a proenzyme that becomes activated by trypsin. Phospholipase A2 hydrolyzes phospholipids and, as with all lipases, requires bile salts for its action. Carboxylic ester hydrolase and cholesterol esterase hydrolyze neutral lipid substrates like esters of cholesterol, fat-soluble vitamins, and triglycerides. The hydrolyzed fat is then packaged into micelles for transport into the intestinal epithelial cells, where the fatty acids are reassembled and packaged inside chylomicrons for transport through the lymphatic system into the bloodstream.

The centroacinar and intercalated duct cells secrete the water and electrolytes present in the pancreatic juice. About 40 acinar cells are arranged into a spherical unit called an *acinus*. Centroacinar cells are located near the center of the acinus and are responsible for fluid and electrolyte secretion. These cells contain the enzyme carbonic anhydrase, which is needed for bicarbonate secretion.

The acinar cells release pancreatic enzymes from their zymogen granules into the lumen of the acinus, and these proteins combine with the water and bicarbonate secretions of the centroacinar cells. The pancreatic juice then travels into small intercalated ducts. Several small intercalated ducts join to form an interlobular duct. Cells in the interlobular ducts continue to contribute fluid and electrolytes to adjust the final concentrations of the pancreatic fluid. Interlobular ducts then join to form about 20 secondary ducts that empty into the main pancreatic duct. Destruction of the branching ductal tree from recurrent inflammation, scarring, and deposition of stones eventually contributes to destruction of the exocrine pancreas and exocrine pancreatic insufficiency.

There are nearly 1 million islets of Langerhans in the normal adult pancreas. Alpha cells that secrete glucagon, Beta cells that secrete insulin, Delta cells that secrete somatostatin, Epsilon cells that secrete ghrelin, and PP cells that secrete PP.[1]

3. Incidence

Acute pancreatitis is a relatively common disease that affects about 300,000 patients per annum in America with a mortality of about 7%. Acute pancreatitis is mild and resolves itself without serious complications in 80% of patients, but it has complications and a substantial mortality in up to 20% of patients despite the agressive intervention[1]. The incidence of alcoholic pancreatitis is higher in male, and the risk of developing acute pancreatitis in patients with gallstones is greater in male. However, more women develop this disorder since gallstones occur with increased frequency in women[2].

4. Etiology and pathophysiology

The pathogenesis of acute pancreatitis has not been fully understood. The general belief today is that pancreatitis begins with the activation of digestive enzymes inside acinar cells, which cause acinar cell injury. The Factors in Acute Pancreatitis can be classified as:

Metabolic

Alcoholism
Hyperlipoproteinemia
Hypercalcemia
Drugs (e.g., thiazide diuretics)
Genetic
Scorpion poison

Mechanical

Trauma
Gallstones
Iatrogenic injury
Perioperative injury
Endoscopic procedures with dye injection
Pancreas divisium
Pancreatic duct obstruction(tumors, ascariasis, ampullar stenosis)
Pancreatic duct bleeding
Duodenal obstruction

Vascular

Shock
Atheroembolism
Vasculitis (Polyarteritis nodosa)

Infectious

Viral

Mumps
Coxsackievirus
EBV
HIV (Human Immunodeficiency Virus)

Bacterial

Mycoplasma pneumonia
Campylobacter
Legionella

Parasites

Ascaris
Clonorchis sinensis

Of note, 10% to 20% of patients with acute pancreatitis have no known associated processes. Although this condition is currently termed idiopathic.

The underlying reason of gallstone disease and other conditions causing acute pancreatitis is ductal hypertension resulting from ongoing exocrine secretion into an obstructed pancreatic duct. Elevated intraductal pressure, due to ongoing exocrine secretion, causes rupture of the smaller ductules and leakage of pancreatic juice into the parenchyma. Pancreatic tissue favors activation of proteases when transductal extravasation of fluid occurs.

In the normal pancreas, the inactive digestive zymogens and the lysosomal hydrolases are found separately in discrete organelles. However, in response to ductal obstruction, hypersecretion, or a cellular insult, these two classes of substances become improperly colocalized in a vacuolar structure within the pancreatic acinar cell. Coalescence of zymogen granules with lysosome vacuoles resulting in intrapancreatic activation of proteolytic enzymes. Small amounts of trypsin can be countered by endogenous pancreatic trypsin inhibitor. However, large amounts of trypsin release can overwhelm the serological defense mechanism (α-1-antitrypsin and α-2-macroglobulin) and activate other enzymes resulting in destruction of acinar cells, local and systemic complications commonly seen in the course of the disease. Activation of the enzyme phospolipase A2 has important consequences like destruction of pulmonary surfactant that can result in ARDS and liberation of prostaglandins and leucotriens that may be important in the pathogenesis of the systemic inflammatory response which can lead to multi organ failure. More than that, inflammatory mediators may be used as predictors of disease severity in the near future. Also, trypsin activates and complements kinin, kallikrein, possibly playing a part in disseminated intravascular coagulation, shock, renal failure and vascular instability. [3], [4].

5. Diagnosis

A detailed history and careful physical examination are the first step towards making the diagnosis. The diagnosis of gallstone pancreatitis should be suspected if the patient has a prior history of biliary colic. [5], [6] Acute pancreatitis typically presents with severe upper abdominal pain which may radiate through to the back and be associated with nausea and vomiting.

On physical examination, the patient may show tachycardia, tachypnea, hypotension, and hyperthermia. The temperature is usually only mildly elevated in uncomplicated pancreatitis. Voluntary and involuntary guarding can be seen over the epigastric region. The bowel sounds are decreased or absent. There are usually no palpable masses. The abdomen may be distended with intraperitoneal fluid. There may be pleural effusion, particularly on the left side. With increasing severity of disease, the intravascular fluid loss may become life-threatening as a result of sequestration of edematous fluid in the retroperitoneum.

6. Biochemical markers

Due to the destruction of acinar cells, the levels of the enzymes that they contain (e.g., amylase, lipase, trypsinogen, and elastase) are found elevated in the serum of most pancreatitis patients. Serum amylase concentration increases almost immediately with the onset of disease and peaks within several hours. It remains elevated for 3 to 5 days before returning to normal. There is no significant correlation between the magnitude of serum amylase elevation and severity of pancreatitis. [7,8]

Lipase is more specific for pancreatitis. Serum lipase has a longer half life than amylase and therefore tends to remain elevated for longer.

Urinary clearance of pancreatic enzymes from the circulation increases during pancreatitis; therefore, urinary levels may be more sensitive than serum levels.

Several tests can help differentiate biliary pancreatitis from other causes of pancreatitis. Aspartate aminotransferase (AST), alanine aminotransferase (ALT), gamma-glutamyl Transpeptidase (GGT), alkaline phosphatase and serum bilirubin are the so-called liver function tests; they should be reviewed before making a confident diagnosis.

Several recent research studies have suggested additional markers that may have prognostic value, including C-reactive protein (CRP), alpha$_2$-macroglobulin, polymorphonuclear neutrophil–elastase, alpha1-antitrypsin, and phospholipase A2. [9],[10] Although CRP measurement is commonly available, many of the others are not. Therefore, at this time, CRP seems to be the marker of choice in clinical settings. The measurement of IL-6 has recently been shown to distinguish patients with mild or severe forms of the disease. Another prognostic marker under evaluation is urinary–trypsinogen activation peptide (TAP). It has a good correlation between the severity of pancreatitis and concentrations of TAP in urine.

Currently, these new markers have limited clinical availability, but there is significant interest in better understanding markers of immune response and pancreatic injury because these could be valuable tools for reliably predicting the severity of acute pancreatitis and supplementing imaging modalities. [10],[11],[12]

7. Radiologic imaging

Ultrasound: Abdominal ultrasound (US) examination is the best way to confirm the presence of gallstones in suspected biliary pancreatitis. It also can detect extrapancreatic ductal dilations and reveal pancreatic edema, swelling, and peripancreatic fluid collections. But abdominal ultrasonography seldom visualizes the pancreas in patients with acute pancreatitis due to air in the distended loops of the small bowel. [13] (**Figure 2**)

Computed Tomography Scan (CT): A CT allows identification of pancreatic edema, fluid or cysts, and the severity of pancreatitis to be graded, detects complications including development of pseudocysts, abscess, necrosis, hemorrhage, and vascular occlusion. The finding of gallstones and dilatation of the extra-hepatic biliary tree on cross-sectional abdominal imaging further support to the diagnosis of gallstone pancreatitis. [14]

Currently the best method to stage the acute pancreatitis is CT. Specific CT findings can be categorized into pancreatic and peripancreatic changes. Pancreatic changes include diffuse or focal parenchymal enlargement, edema, or necrosis with liquefaction. Peripancreatic involvement includes blurring or thickening of the surrounding tissue planes. An approximate correlation exists between the degree of CT abnormalities and the clinical course and severity of acute pancreatitis.

An early discrimination between mild edematous and severe necrotizing forms of the disease is of the utmost importance to provide optimal care to the patient. CT has become the gold standard for detecting and assessing the severity of pancreatitis. Although clinically mild pancreatitis is usually associated with interstitial edema, severe pancreatitis is associated with necrosis. The presence of air bubbles on a CT scan is an indication of infected necrosis or pancreatic abscess. [15]

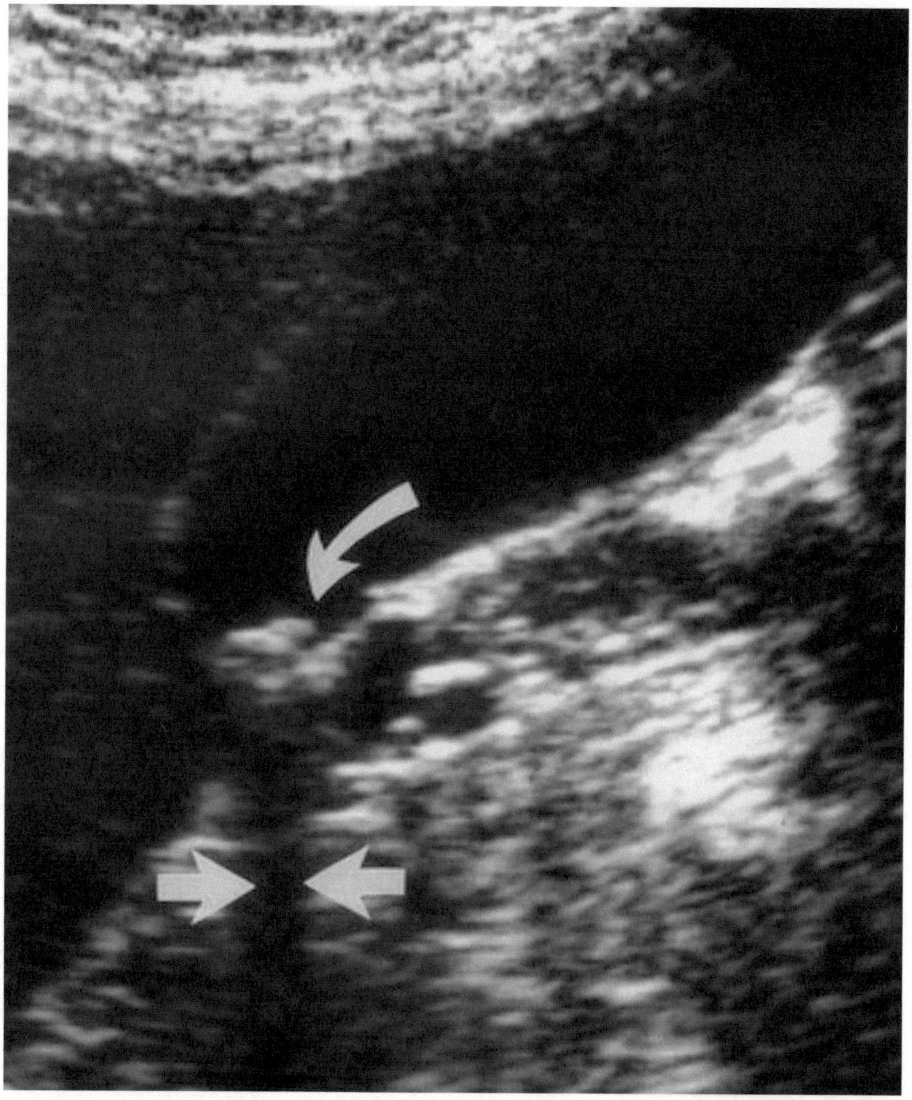

Fig. 2. Ultrasound image of the gallbladder demonstrates multiple dependent gallstones (curved arrow) with acustic shadowing (straight arrows). The patient had elevated pancreatic enzyme levels and underwent cholecystectomy because of gallstone pancreatitis.

Magnetic Resonance Cholangiopancreatography (MRCP): MRCP has been found to be as accurate as contrast-enhanced CT in predicting the severity of pancreatitis and identifying pancreatic necrosis but is less sensitive for detection of small stones.

Endoscopic Ultrasonography: It is useful in obese patients and patients with ileus, and can help determine which patients with acute pancreatitis would benefit most from therapeutic ERCP. [16], [17]

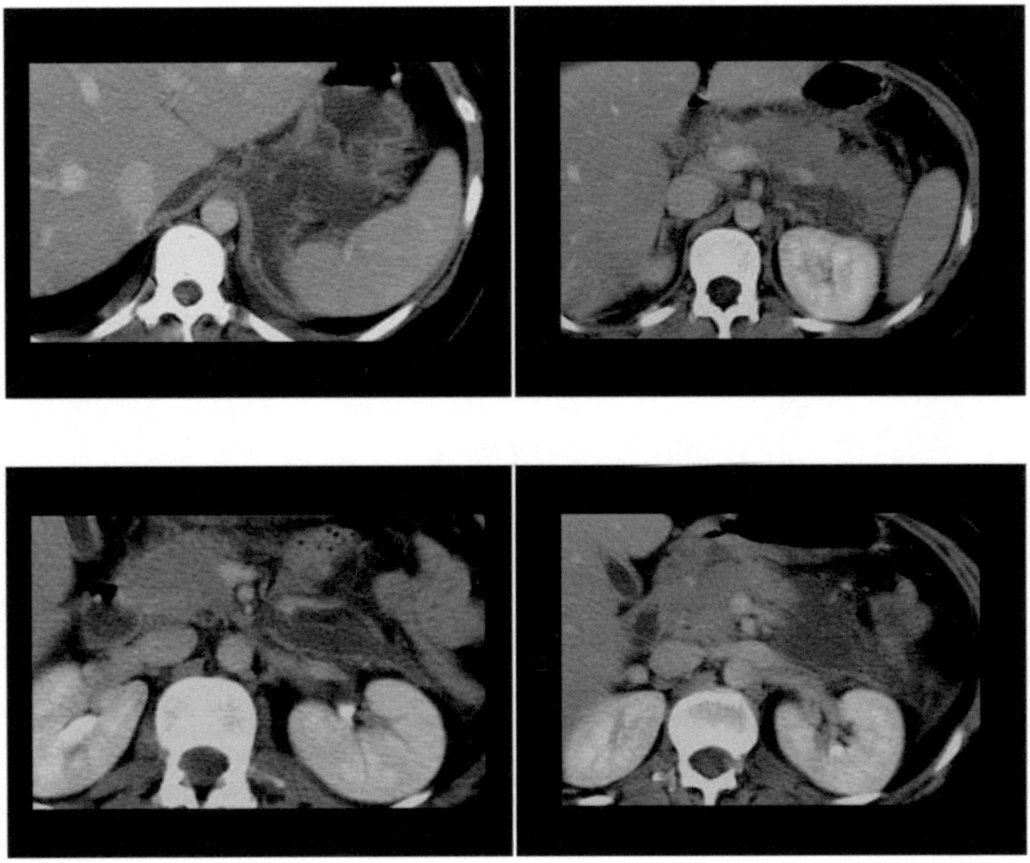

Fig. 3. Acute biliary pancreatitis with a thickened pancreas and an effusion around the pancreatic tail and around the spleen - CT scan

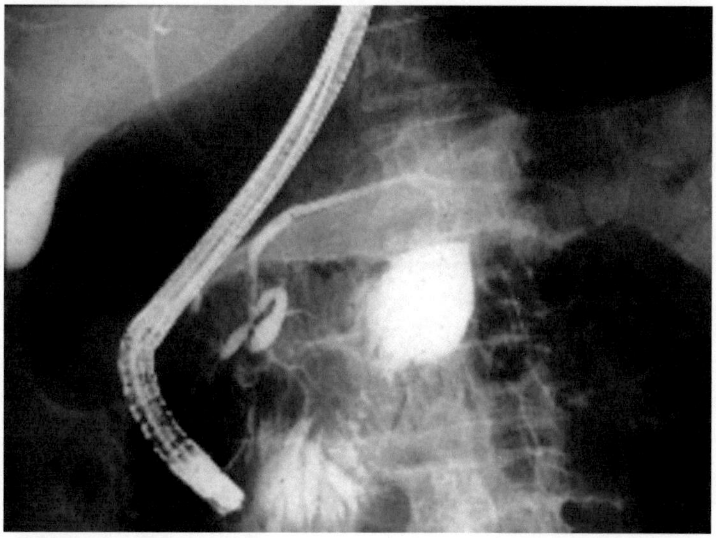

Fig. 4. Sigmoid configuration of the main pancreatic duct with distal dilation of both main and dorsal ducts, suggesting the presence of an obstructive condition at the level of both major and minor papillae.

ADMISSION	INITIAL 48 HOURS
Gallstone Pancreatitis	
Age > 70 yr	Hct fall >10
WBC >18,000/mm^3	BUN elevation >2 mg/100 mL
Glucose > 220 mg/100 mL	Ca^{2+} <8 mg/100 mL
LDH >400 IU/L	Base deficit >5 mEq/L
AST >250U/100 mL	Fluid sequestration >4 L
Nongallstone Pancreatitis	
Age >55 yr	Hct fall >10
WBC >16,000/mm^3	BUN elevation >5 mg/100 mL
Glucose >200 mg/100 mL	Ca^{2+} <8 mg/100 mL
LDH >350 IU/L	PaO_2 <55 mm Hg
AST >250U/100 mL	Base deficit >4 mEq/L
	Fluid sequestration >6 L

Adapted from Ranson JHC, Rifkind KM, Roses DF, et al: Prognostic signs and the role of operative management in acute pancreatitis. Surg Gynecol Obstet 139:69-81, 1974; and Ranson JHC: Etiological and prognostic factors in human acute pancreatitis: A review. Am J Gastroenterol 77:633, 1982. (AST, aspartate transaminase; BUN, blood urea nitrogen; Ca^{2+}, calcium; Hct, hematocrit; LDH, lactic dehydrogenase; PaO_2, arterial oxygen; WBC, white blood cell count.)

8. Scoring systems in acute pancreatitis

A variety of scoring systems have been proposed for accurate assessment of the severity of acute pancreatitis. These include the clinical scoring scales as Ranson criteria, Glasgow scales, simplified acute physiology (SAP), score and acute physiology and chronic health evaluation II (APACHE II) score. The CT severity index (CTSI) derived by Balthazar grading of pancreatitis and the extent of pancreatic necrosis is now widely used in describing CT findings of acute pancreatitis and serves as the radiological scoring system. [18]

Ranson identified a series of prognostic signs for early identification of patients with severe pancreatitis. Out of these 11 objective parameters, five are measured at the time of admission, whereas the remaining six are measured within 48 hours of admission. Morbidity and mortality of the disease are directly related to the number of signs present. It is important to realize that Ranson's prognostic signs are best used within the initial 48 hours of hospitalization and have not been validated for later time intervals.

Another set of criteria often used to assess the severity of pancreatitis is the *a*cute *p*hysiology *a*nd *c*hronic *h*ealth *e*valuation (APACHE-II) score. This grading system assesses severity on the basis of quantitative measures of abnormalities of multiple variables, including vital signs and specific laboratory parameters, coupled with the age and chronic health status of the patient. The main advantage of the APACHE-II scoring system is the immediate assessment of the severity of pancreatitis. A score of eight or more at admission is usually considered indicative of severe disease. APACHE II, although complicated, ensures the highest positive predictive value up to 69%. [19]

The risk of severe acute pancreatitis is increased at Glasgow's or Ranson's score ≥3 in 48 hours, APACHE II on admission ≥8, Balthazar's score ≥4.

In 1985, Balthazar and colleagues introduced a scoring system based on radiological findings by means of a 5- grade scale: the presence of pancreatic and peripancreatic inflammation and fluid accumulation. [20].

Grade CT findings:

Grade A Normal pancreas

Grade B Pancreatic enlargement

Grade C Pancreatic inflammation and/or peripancreatic fat

Grade D Single peripancreatic fluid collection

Grade E Two or more fluid collections and/or retroperitoneal air.

A correlation was shown between the grade on CT performed within 10 days of admission and the clinical follow-up finding, morbidity, and mortality. Therefore, CT was appreciated as a useful prognostic indicator for outcome in Acute pancreatitis. The study showed a morbidity of only 4% and no mortality in patients with Acute pancreatitis and a CT grade of A, B, or C. In patients with CT grade D or E, the morbidity rate was 54% and the mortality 14%. The Balthazar radiological prognostic score was easy to assign without the need of contrast-enhanced CT. Unfortunately, this score did not assign any value to pancreatic necrosis as a prognostic parameter and did not make the distinction between Acute fluid collections and pseudocysts vs. post-necrotic fluid collections and walled-off pancreatic necrosis. With the introduction of newer CT-based scoring systems, some authors question the value of Balthazar's score in predicting prognosis and severity in Acute Pancreatitis [21].

9. Treatment

Gallstones are the most common cause of acute pancreatitis worldwide. According to the physical examination, radiological findings and labarotory results the etiology of the acute pancreatitis is diagnosed as biliary or non-biliary. The most important initial treatment of biliary pancreatitis is conservative intensive care with the goals of oral food and fluid restriction, replacement of fluids and electrolytes parenterally as assessed by central venous pressure and urinary excretion, and control of pain. [22], [23]

After stabilizing the patient, specific treatment and timing of the intervention have to be planned. The issue of when to intervene for clearance of gallstones is controversial. General consensus is either urgent intervention (cholecystectomy) within the first 48 to 72 hours of admission, or briefly delayed intervention (after 72 hours, but during the initial hospitalization) to give an inflamed pancreas time to recover. Cholecystectomy and common duct clearance is the best treatment of biliary acute pancreatitis. Patients who have persistent impacted stone in the distal common bile duct or ampulla should have confirmation by radiologic imaging (CT, magnetic resonance cholangiopancreatography, or endoscopic ultrasonography) before intervention. If common duct stone are diagnosed, stones are cleared and endoscopic sphincterotomy is done by ERCP and then laparoscopic cholecystectomy is performed.[24]

Routine ERCP for examination of the bile duct is discouraged in cases of biliary pancreatitis, as the probability of finding residual stones is low, and the risk of ERCP-induced pancreatitis is significant. But in the case of acute biliary pancreatitis in which analytical studies suggest that the obstruction persists after 24 hours of observation, emergency ERCP has to be done to prevent biliary sepsis.

Although ERCP with Endoscopic Sphincterotomy (ES) and stone extraction has been shown to be useful for early treatment of severe biliary pancreatitis, the incidence of bile duct stones at elective surgery is low and most of these ERCP are unnecessary. For this reason accurate predictors of common bile duct stones are required; studies have shown that the sensitivity of preoperative abdominal US for predicting common bile duct stones is 42% and specificity is 86% [25]. Furthermore, an endoscopic approach is unable to fully resolve the patient's biliary pathology with one procedure and one anesthesia. This adds substantial risk of morbidity and even mortality. Concern remains also regarding the potential long-term risks of ES. Although the immediate complications of ES are well documented, the long-term effects are less defined. Stricture formation and stone recurrence account for nearly all longterm complications. Although most of the authors prefer the endoscopic to the surgical treatment of CBD stones, there is still some minor discussion on it[26].

Timing of laparoscopic surgery in acute biliary pancreatitis depends upon the severity of the disease. In the case of mild pancreatitis it doesn't matter when, within 1 week, laparoscopic cholecystectomy is performed. However, in patients with severe pancreatitis, laparoscopic cholecystectomy, when performed within the 1st week after the onset of symptoms, as other authors have observed [27], places patients at increased risk of operative morbidity and technical complications. In these patients, the management of complications of pancreatitis is strongly advisable before cholecystectomy.

Delaying surgery for more than a week after hospitalization, in our experience, does not adversely affect technical difficulty. Delaying surgery for several weeks in severe acute pancreatitis allows acute inflammation to settle down and might allow stones in the

common bile duct to clear spontaneously. However, studies showed that approximately one-quarter of patients have symptomatic recurrence within 6 weeks if gallstones are untreated, and it increases with time [28], [29]
Cholangiogram of good quality during laparoscopic cholecystectomy, since the risk of common bile duct stones is 14–20% . [30] This strategy minimizes the need for common bile duct exploration and still achieves the goal of a limited hospital stay and the prevention of recurrence of pancreatitis. If common bile duct stones are found at cholangiogram they should be treated laparoscopically if at all possible. In most instances, it should be possible to retrieve the stones via the cystic duct, since acute pancreatitis is usually caused by the migration of small stones. If this is not feasible, one alternative is to perform a laparoscopic choledochotomy. These cases have a rather long hospital stay and delayed return to work, but their level of pain is diminished. Our current impression is that this procedure is possible though technically demanding. In case of failure, traditional exploration is mandatory.
In severe acute pancreatitis, or when signs of infection are present, most experts recommend broad-spectrum antibiotics (e.g., imipenem) and careful surveillance for complications of the disease.

10. Complications of acute pancreatitis

Acute pancreatitis complications may be divided as systemic and local. Pancreatic phlegmon, pancreatic abscess, pancreatic pseudocyst, pancreatic ascites and involvement of adjacent organs, with hemorrhage, thrombosis, bowel infarction, obstructive jaundice, fistula formation, or mechanical obstruction are local complications. Systemic complications are classified as hematologic (Hemoconcentration, Disseminated intravascular coagulopathy), cardiovascular (Hypotension, Hypovolemia, Sudden death, Nonspecific ST-T wave changes, Pericardial effusion), pulmonary (Pneumonia, atelectasis, Acute respiratory distress syndrome, Pleural effusion), renal (Oliguria, Azotemia, renal artery/vein thrombosis), metabolic (Hyperglycemia, Hypocalcemia, Hypertriglyceridemia, Encephalopathy, Sudden blindness (Purtscher's retinopathy), central nervous system (Psychosis, Fat emboli, Alcohol withdrawal syndrome), gastro intestinal system (Peptic ulcer, Erosive gastritis, Portal vein or splenic vein thrombosis with varices)

11. References

[1] F.Charles Brunicardi, D. K. Andersen, Timothy R. Billiar, D. Dunn, J. Hunter, J. Matthews, R. Pollock Schwartz's Principles of surgery, 2005; 33:1265-73
[2] Eland IA, Sturkenboom MJ, Wilson JH, Stricker BH. Incidence and mortality of acute pancreatitis between 1985 and 1995". Scand J Gastroenterol 2000;35:1110-6.
[3] Reila A,Zeinthmeister AR,Milton Lj. Etiology,incidence and survival of acute pancreatitis in olmested county, Minnosota. Gastroentrology 1991. p. 100-A269.
[4] Banerjee, A.K.; Galloway, S.W.; Kingsnorth, A.N.: Experimental models of acute pancreatitis. Br J Surg 1994;81:1093-106.
[5] Formela LJ, Galloway SW, Kingsnorth AN. Inflamatory mediators in acute pancreatitis. Br J Surg 1995;82:6-13.

[6] Acosta JM, Ledesma CL. Gallstone migration as a cause of acute pancreatitis. N Engl J Med 1974;290:484-7.
[7] Kelly TR. Gallstone pancreatitis: the timing of surgery. Surgery 1980;88:345-50.
[8] Moody FG, Senninger N, Runkel N. Another challenge to the Opie's theory. Gastroenterology 1993;104:927-31.
[9] Crunkel N, Moody F, Mueller W. Experimental evidence against Opie's common channel bile reflux theory. Digestion 1992;52:67-67.
[10] Smotkin J, Tenner S. Laboratory diagnostic tests in acute pancreatitis. J Clin Gastroenterol 2002;34:459-62.
[11] Clavien PA, Burgan S, Moossa AR. Serum enzymes and other laboratory tests in acute pancreatitis. Br J Surg 1989;76:1234-43.
[12] Neoptolemos JP, Kemppainen EA, Mayer JM, Fitzpatrick JM, Raraty MG, Slavin J, *et al* . Early prediction of severity in acute pancreatitis by urinary trypsinogen activation peptide: a multicentre study. Lancet 2000;355:1955-60.
[13] Tenner S. Initial management of acute pancreatitis: critical issues during the first 72 hours. Am J Gastroenterol 2004;99:2489-94.
[14] Chak A, Hawes RH, Cooper GS, Hoffman B, Catalano MF, Wong RC, *et al* . Prospective assessment of the utility of EUS in the evaluation of gallstone pancreatitis. Gastrointest Endosc 1999;49:599-604.
[15] Baron RL, Stanley RJ, Lee JK, Koehler RE, Levitt RG. Computed tomographic features of biliary obstruction. AJR Am J Roentgenol 1983;140:1173-8.
[16] Kemppainen E, Sainio V, Haapiainen R, Kivisaari L, Kivilaakso E, Puolakkainen P. Early localization of necrosis by contrast-enhanced computed tomography can predict outcome in severe pancreatitis. Br J Surg 1996;83:924-9.
[17] Makary MA, Duncan MD, Harmon JW, Freeswick PD, Bender JS, Bohlman M, *et al* . The role of magnetic resonance cholangiography in the management of patients with gallstone pancreatitis. Ann Surg 2005;241:119-24
[18] Norton SA, Alderson D. Endoscopic ultrasonography in the evaluation of idiopathic acute pancreatitis. Br J Surg 2000;87:1650-5.
[19] Wahab S, Khan RA. Imaging and clinical prognostic indicators of acute pancreatitis: a comparative insight. 2010 Sep;40(3):283-7.
[20] Gravante G, Garcea G, Ong SL, Metcalfe MS, Berry DP, Lloyd DM, et al. Prediction of mortality in acute pancreatitis: asystematic review of the published evidence. Pancreatology 2009;9:601-614.
[21] Balthazar EJ, Ranson JHC, Naidich DP, et al. (1985) Acute-pancreatitis—prognostic value of CT. Radiology 3:767–772
[22] Ju S, Chen F, Liu S, Zheng K, Teng G (2006) Value of CT and clinical criteria in assessment of patients with acute pancreatitis. Eur J Radiol 1:102–107
[23] Neoptolemos JP, Carr-Locke DL, London NJ, Bailey IA, James D, Fossard DP. Controlled trial of urgent endoscopic retrograde cholangiopancreatography and endoscopic sphincterotomy versus conservative treatment for acute pancreatitis due to gallstones. Lancet 1988;2:979-83.
[24] Carroll BJ, Phillips EH. The early treatment of acute biliary pancreatitis [letter; comment]. N Engl J Med 1993;329:58-9.

[25] Uhl W, Müller CA, Krδhenbühl L, Schmid SW, Schφlzel S, Büchler MW. Acute gallstone pancreatitis: timing of laparoscopic cholecystectomy in mild and severe disease.
[26] Soper NJ, Brunt ML, Callery MP, Edmundowicz SA, Aliperti G (1994) Role of laparoscopic cholecystectomy in the management of acute biliary pancreatitis. Am J Surg 167: 42–51
[27] Graham SM, Flowers JL, Scott TR et al. (1993) Laparoscopic cholecystectomy and common bile duct stones. Ann Surg 218: 61–67
[28] Tang E, Stain SC, Tang G, Froes E, Berne TV (1995) Timing of laparoscopic surger in gallstones pancreatitis. Arch Surg 130: 496–500
[29] Patti MG, Pellegrini CA (1990) Gallstone pancreatitis. Surg Clin North Am 70: 1277 1295
[30] Pellegrini CA (1993) Surgery for gallstone pancreatitis. Am J Surg 165: 515–518
[31] Acosta JM, Rossi R, Galli MR, Pellegrini CA, Skinner DB (1978) Early surgery for acute gallstone pancreatitis: evaluation of a systemic approach. Surgery 83: 367–370

2

Acute Pancreatitis Induced by Drugs

Karel Urbánek[1], Ilona Vinklerová[2],
Ondřej Krystyník[2] and Vlastimil Procházka[2]
[1]Department of Pharmacology,
[2]Department of Internal Medicine II – Gastroenterology and Hepatology ,
Faculty of Medicine, Palacký University and University Hospital, Olomouc,
Czech Republic

1. Introduction

Drug-induced acute pancreatitis (DIP) is generally considered to be a rare disease. Indeed, the incidence of cases caused by medication use is much lower than of those caused by biliary disorder or alcohol. On the other hand, the total incidence of acute pancreatitis in developed countries continues to rise as does the exposition of general population to medication. The disease was almost unknown before the 1960s. Probably the first two cases were reported in the late 1950s: by Zion *et al.* in 1955 and Johnston & Cornish in 1959. From that time, the number of reported cases has increased steadily until these days. A further increase in the incidence of drug-induced acute pancreatitis may be expected and seems to be actually present in recent scientific papers on the topic.

For a proper understanding of the disease, we must regard it not simply as one of many other types of acute pancreatitis, but primarily as an adverse drug reaction (ADR). A recent definition describes an ADR as "an appreciably harmful or unpleasant reaction, resulting from an intervention related to the use of a medicinal product, which predicts hazard from future administration and warrants prevention or specific treatment, or alteration of the dosage regimen, or withdrawal of the product" (Edwards & Aronson, 2000).

Type of ADR	Mnemonic	Dose dependence / Predictability	Characteristics
A	Augmented	Dose-related, predictable	Most usual; frequent
B	Bizarre	Dose-unrelated, unpredictable	Immunity-mediated reactions or idiosyncrasies; rare
C	Continuous	Related to a cumulative dose and time	Effect of chronic use, late toxicity
D	Delayed	Related to time	Long time from drug cessation
E	End of use	Related to drug withdrawal	Immediately after withdrawal

Table 1. Types of adverse drug reactions

The vast majority of the reported DIP cases seem to have an idiosyncratic character (see Table 1). This also means that it is nearly impossible to obtain sufficiently large cohorts with similar patient characteristics. From that point of view, every case of drug-induced pancreatitis should be documented as well as possible, and also reported to a pharmacovigilance system for further evaluation.

2. Epidemiology

It is usually estimated that drug use accounts for 2% of all the causes of acute pancreatitis. It must be pointed out that the diagnosis might be underestimated, particularly for the difficulties in diagnosing this etiology. The overall incidence varies in different studies from 0.1 to 2% with a tendency to increase over time (Balani *et al*, 2008).

There are three sources of information on the DIP incidence: data from clinical studies on acute pancreatitis, individual or serial case reports published in medical journals, and data on spontaneous reports from pharmacovigilance databases. Another possible source - data from clinical testing of new drugs - is not very useful because of an idiosyncratic character of DIP. The B-type of adverse drug reactions occurs with a frequency lower than 1:10,000, so their record in the first three phases of clinical drug investigation is almost impossible.

The number of cases reported to pharmacovigilance databases and of published case reports is increasing so rapidly that any number will be obsolete by the time it manages to be printed. According to Lancashire *et al.*, the WHO database of ADRs listed 2,479 episodes suspected of being caused by 529 different drugs from 1968 to 1993. An analysis of the DIP cases reported to the Danish Committee on Adverse Drug Reactions from 1968 to 1999 (Andersen *et al.*, 2001) showed an increasing number of reports in time and a predominance of women, but estimating the proportion of DIP in total acute pancreatitis incidence is clearly improper. The mortality of 9% among the cases analyzed shows a tendency to report the most severe cases, whilst the majority of mild-to-moderate cases remain unreported. On the other hand, an information bias, due to more frequent notification of a drug already known to cause a specific ADR, is limiting the validity of spontaneous reporting. A Medline search of the English literature revealed 1,214 case reports with 120 suspected drugs between 1955 and 2006 (Badalov *et al.*, 2007). The weakness of estimating DIP incidence from these sources is in preferential publication of the case reports describing ADRs of new - therefore more "attractive" - agents rather than of older ones in which the risk is considered to be well-known.

In a multicenter study by Gullo *et al.*, published 2002, in which the etiology and mortality of acute pancreatitis were studied, the proportion of drug injury was almost negligible: only 0.2% (2 patients) out of 1,068 cases. It is worth noting that three out of the seven centers involved in this study (providing 581 AP cases for the study) were surgical departments; moreover, 139 (13%) cases of acute pancreatitis in this study were classified as idiopathic. We believe that the incidence of DIP in this study may be somewhat underestimated. As will be discussed below, establishing the diagnosis of DIP often requires a re-evaluation and knowledge of the patient's post-episode history.

On the other hand, at least two published studies showed a significantly higher incidence of DIP in retrospective analysis. A study by Mennecier *et al.*, published 2007, found an incidence of drug-induced cases of 8.3 % among a total of 108 acute pancreatitis cases hospitalized in hepatogastroenterology and intensive care units of a French hospital over a 9-year period. Our study, published in 2010, included 170 acute pancreatitis cases hospitalized in a tertiary hospital during a period of two years. The proportion of DIP in this cohort was 5.3% (Vinklerová *et al.*, 2010). Obviously, the incidence found in these studies is higher than in the general population. If DIP occurrence depends on the use of specific drugs, in tertiary hospitals as centers for the treatment of specific diseases (e.g. Crohn's disease or malignancies) it must be higher.

The discrepancy in the published results demonstrates, in particular, the fact that the importance of drug-induced pancreatic injury will be different in the general population than among the cases reported in surgical or medical departments. It is also clearly improper to suppose that this disease can have similar incidence in all countries because of its dependence on the consumption of causative drugs and, secondarily, the dependence on the incidence of diseases treated with these medications.

Studies with very low report of DIP are usually characterized by a high number of idiopathic acute pancreatitis cases. Clinicians sometimes forget that there is no such thing as an "idiopathic" disease. The word "idiopathic" means that we are not able to establish the actual cause of the disease - and a not insignificant number of idiopathic cases of acute pancreatitis might be caused by xenobiotics, including medication. The only way how to determine the real incidence of drug-induced acute pancreatitis is to perform prospective multicenter studies targeted at the etiology of non-alcoholic, non-biliary acute pancreatitis.

3. Etiology

The pathogenesis of acute pancreatitis is probably very uniform differing only by the initial injury mechanism. It consists of three steps: (i) premature activation of trypsin in acinar cells; (ii) intrapancreatic inflammation; and (iii) extrapancreatic inflammation (Banks & Freeman, 2006). The mechanisms by which drugs initiate a cascade of damaging events remain shrouded in mystery. However, it should be borne in mind that the same is true for the vast majority of responses independent of drug dose.

3.1 Mechanisms of injury

Mechanism of medication's action against pancreas remains unknown. Two possible mechanisms of pancreatic injury caused by drugs are usually recognized, but in our opinion, at least three more possible mechanisms should be also mentioned:

a. Direct toxic effect on pancreatic tissue;
b. Idiosyncratic reaction;
c. Influence of medication on the bile flow;
d. Amplification of direct toxic effect of ethanol on pancreatic tissue;
e. Secondary pancreatic damage.

Simple direct toxic injury of pancreatic tissue, similar to the hepatic injury caused by some drugs or their metabolites (e.g. paracetamol), seems very unlikely in the majority of reported DIP cases. This (A-type) pattern of ADR is dose-dependent, irrespective of the patient's response, reproducible and usually occurs in much higher numbers than usual in DIP. Although acute pancreatitis sometimes develops under the condition of an overdose of some drugs, its incidence remains so rare that an underlying predisposition must play a role in these cases. Genetic differences in metabolism are usually supposed to be the most probable predisposing factor here. Only several drugs are reported as causing DIP by overdose: paracetamol (or acetaminophen), erythromycin and carbamazepine. We had an opportunity to describe DIP in a patient overdosed on mycophenolate (Vinklerová *et al.*, 2001). Some kind of cumulative dose-dependent effect of toxic metabolites is also sometimes hypothesized in drugs showing a consistent long latency (more than 30 days) at the onset of the first episode of DIP. It is supposed mainly in valproate, but possibly also in didanosine, tamoxifen, chlorothiazide and estrogens. This would correspond to the C-type (continuous) of ADR, but other mechanisms can also explain the late onset of DIP in these agents.

The definition of an idiosyncratic adverse drug reaction (B-type) best matches the actual characteristics of DIP. A strong correlation with some immune disorders (mainly Crohn's disease and HIV infections) implicates an immune-mediated reaction as a chief causative factor of the disease. Often, the latency between initiation of the drug and the onset of DIP is one week to one month, but later rechallenge led to a second episode in one to three days. The frequently mentioned lack of hypersensitivity symptoms (rash, fever, lymphadenopathy and eosinophilia) is of no major importance as it is rare in the majority of immune-mediated organ damage and cannot be considered pathognomic. An immune-mediated process is undoubtedly the pathogenetic nature of many rare ADRs also connected with the drugs mentioned here, such as drug-induced pericarditis, lupus-like syndrome and, moreover, some types of drug-induced liver injury. It is possible that all these reactions have a common immune-mediated nature and the specific organ is injured in fact "accidentally" as a current *locus minoris resistentiae*. Unfortunately, there is as little evidence available for this hypothesis as there is for the others. This should lead us to study these rare ADRs more in terms of patient characteristics than those of individual drugs.

The latter three mechanisms may not be as irrelevant as it might seem. Several drugs involved in acute pancreatitis have been implicated as causing cholestatic liver injury, e.g. azathioprine, cytarabine, estrogens and erythromycin. Codeine, morphine and possibly some other drugs can cause spasm of sphincter of Oddi. An interesting relationship between rofecoxib-induced cholestatic hepatitis and acute pancreatitis was observed (Sato *et al*, 2006). Human leukocyte antigen haplotype HLA-A33/B44/DR6 is involved in both these reactions reported simultaneously in several patients. Cholestatic hepatitis caused by this haplotype may induce secondary pancreatitis. Also, the occurrence of drug-induced pancreatitis in alcoholic patients has been described, but this issue has not been given much attention. Secondary (off-target) injury of pancreatic tissue is also possible in some drugs. Known potential indirect effects of drugs on the pancreas comprise ischemia (azathioprine, diuretics), hypercalcemia (thiazide diuretics), thrombosis of pancreatic blood vessels (estrogens), and an increase in pancreatic juice viscosity (diuretics, pentamidine).

3.2 Predispositions

Several populations at higher risk have been identified during research in drug-induced pancreatitis. Predisposing demographic characteristics are female gender and younger age. The male-to-female ratio is inversed in comparison to other acute pancreatitis types, at least to 1:1.3. DIP is also more commonly reported in younger patients, not exceptionally in children. An increased risk in older patients with polypharmacy seems to be a bias: the risk is in the use of many drugs by a large segment of this population rather than old age itself.

Three types of diseases were recognized as the most frequent predisposing health factors: inflammatory bowel diseases, HIV infection and cancer treated by combined chemotherapy. In patients with advanced HIV infection (CD4 counts < 200 cells/mm^3), treated with antiretroviral drugs, an incidence of 14% was found, but incidence of up to 40% is also mentioned (Trivedi *et al.*, 2005). In an anticancer chemotherapy, the risk is also higher, but sometimes it is difficult to decide which of the multiple medications have caused the disease. The use of dexamethasone or cytarabine seems to be of the highest risk.

The etiology of acute pancreatitis in patients with Crohn's disease was evaluated in a targeted study (Moolsintong *et al.*, 2005). Among the 48 patients treated for Crohn's disease who had acute pancreatitis between 1976 and 2001, an ADR was the cause in 17% of cases with the vast majority being caused by purine analogs - azathioprine and 6-mercaptopurine. The most common etiologies of AP - biliary and alcoholic - were found only in 21% and 15%, respectively. A higher risk of induction of AP in Crohn's disease was also proven by evidence in a study by Weersma *et al.* in which the risk was significantly higher in patients treated for Crohn's disease compared to the risk of those treated for autoimmune diseases or organ transplant. Also, a similar study performed by Bajaj *et al.* supports these findings. In ulcerative colitis, the risk is probably increased, but lower than in Crohn's disease. On the other hand, in a Danish population-based case-control study (1,590 incident cases of acute pancreatitis and 10 controls per case), a nearly four-fold increased risk of acute pancreatitis in patients with Crohn's disease and a 1.5-fold increased risk for ulcerative colitis were found, but the use of mesalazine or sulfasalazine was not associated with an increased risk (Munk *et al.*, 2004). We suppose that this can be explained by the low proportion of DIP in the etiology of acute pancreatitis. In the population with a significantly increased risk, the number of medication-associated cases cannot influence the total risk.

3.3 Experimental findings

The obvious aim of experimental models is to mimic as closely as possible the conditions in an organism suffering from acute pancreatitis. Some of those models were based on the systemic administration of an exogenous substance. They are not considered to be best available for many reasons, but they can help in further research on DIP pathophysiology.

Cerulein is a ten amino acid oligopeptide, similar to cholecystokinin, that stimulates gastric, biliary, and pancreatic secretion and also contraction of certain smooth muscles. It has been used by intravenous (as well as intraperitoneal or subcutaneous) route to cause acute pancreatitis in mice, rats, hamsters and dogs. Within one hour from application, cerulein causes pancreatic interstitial edema reaching a maximum in 12 hours. The supposed mechanism of action is the upregulation of NF-κB (nuclear factor κ-light-chain-enhancer of activated B cells) leading to activation of ICAM-1 protein and promotion neutrophil adhesion onto pancreatic acinar cells. An increase in digestive enzyme production and activation of NADPH oxidase could be supporting mechanisms. Pancreatitis caused by cerulein is mild, with negligible mortality (Su *et al.*, 2006).

L-arginine is one of the most common natural amino acids. If administered intraperitoneally, it causes acute pancreatitis in mice and rats. Significantly increased plasma amylase levels, pancreatic MPO activity, trypsin activation, and histological changes including accumulation of fluid, disruption of histoarchitecture, acinar cell vacuolization, extensive acinar cell necrosis, and neutrophilic infiltration have been described. It is believed that nitric oxide synthase (NOS), present in acinar cells and metabolizing L-arginine, might play a role in the initiation of pancreatitis. Induction of NOS by L-arginine leads to an interaction of NO and superoxide radicals, which can generate peroxynitrite radicals causing cell injury (Dawra *et al.*, 2007). Effects are dose dependent and a higher dose can lead to acute pancreatitis within a few hours.

It is worth noting that some drugs known to cause human DIP (e.g. azathioprine) are able to successfully suppress the development of acute pancreatitis in various experimental models. This supports the opinion that host factors (most probably the immune system) are more important for the development of DIP than the pharmacodynamic properties of causative agents.

4. Causative drugs

Several hundreds of chemical substances have been reported to cause acute pancreatitis in humans. The majority of these reports remain single with a limited level of evidence. Drugs causing pancreatic injury more frequently have been listed in several reviews, some of which tried to quantify the risk of individual agents. A comparison of the ability to cause drug-induced pancreatitis is very difficult as the probability of an adverse effect is conditioned by many population or individual risk factors.
An interesting attempt to estimate the potential of individual drugs to cause DIP by pharmacoepidemiological methods was performed by Lancashire *et al.* in 2003. They examined the data held in the General Practitioner Research Database and compared the frequency of intake of different drugs by individuals with and without acute pancreatitis (3,673 cases of pancreatitis, 3 controls for each case). Odds ratios were calculated for recent (1–90 days before the episode), past (91–360 days before the episode) or continuing (prescription in both periods) use. A nine-fold increased risk in recent takers of mesalazine was found as well as a ten-fold increased risk in ever-takers of azathioprine in comparison to never-takers. Only a moderate risk was found for captopril and valproate. Strikingly increased odds ratios were found for recent takers of acid inhibitory drugs without having a peptic ulcer diagnosed. Although these drugs can certainly cause DIP, this is clearly a bias because their prescription is related to abdominal pain and other GIT symptoms preceding the diagnosis of acute pancreatitis. This result also shows the limitation of a study performed by using this method - no data on the etiology of acute pancreatitis were used. Estimating the risk of drugs to cause a rare ADR also requires a much greater population. There is no doubt that some diseases may predispose to the occurrence of acute pancreatitis in themselves. To distinguish the impact of this predisposition from the influence of medication, it will be necessary to carry out such studies in much larger cohorts. Therefore, a classification system based on the number of DIP reports appears to be the most appropriate way to assess the risk potential of a drug.

4.1 Classification systems

Because the risk potential of individual drugs is difficult to establish, it is generally estimated from the absolute numbers of published cases. In earlier critical reviews, the potential of a drug to induce AP was evaluated as definite, probable or possible (Mallory & Kern, 1980; McArthur, 1996). The current knowledge has recently been summarized and used to propose classification systems in papers published by Trivedi and Pitchumoni in 2005 and Badalov *et al.* in 2007.
Trivedi & Pitchumoni classified risk drugs on the basis of the search of the reported cases in the National Library of Medicine/Pubmed from 1966 to 2004. Drugs were indexed into Classes I-III: Class I drugs were medications implicated in greater than 20 reported cases of acute pancreatitis with at least one documented case following re-exposure; Class II

involved medications implicated in more than ten cases of acute pancreatitis; and Class III drugs were all other medications reported to be associated with pancreatitis.

Also, Badalov *et al.* reviewed Medline reports of drug-induced AP from 1955 to 2006. The authors classified reported medications into four classes based on the published weight of evidence for each agent and the pattern of clinical presentation. Class I included medications in which at least one case was proven by a re-challenge with the drug. Class II included drugs with a consistent latency in 75% or more of the reported cases. Class III included drugs that had two or more case reports published, but neither a re-challenge nor a consistent latency period. Class IV drugs were similar to class III drugs, but only one case report had been found.

An apparent weakness of all existing drug classifications is the lack of the knowledge on the relationship between the incidence of drug-induced AP and population exposure to the causative drugs. Quantifying this relationship is a challenge for pharmacoepidemiology. In addition, regular updating of existing classifications appears necessary because every year new cases of DIP occur, which may result in a reclassification of the drugs included.

4.2 Drugs commonly associated with drug-induced pancreatitis

Among several hundreds of drugs reported as causative for drug-induced pancreatitis, only a few have a sufficiently strong evidence base to be clearly associated with this rare adverse drug reaction. These agents are listed in Table 2. At least some of them also deserve more detailed mention, which can be found in following sections..

4.2.1 Azathioprine

Azathioprine is a purine analog used in low doses as immunosuppressant. It is a pro-drug metabolized into the active 6-mercaptopurine, itself a purine synthesis inhibitor. Enzyme thiopurine S-methyltransferase (TPMT) deactivates 6-mercaptopurine. The most severe adverse effect of azathioprine is bone marrow suppression, especially in TPMT genetic polymorphism. Its adverse effects on the pancreas are well documented, so it is classified into class I according to the risk of induction of DIP by both classification systems. A significantly higher risk of azathioprine-induced acute pancreatitis was demonstrated in patients with Crohn's disease compared to all the others, including those with ulcerative colitis. Consistent latency of the DIP onset with an average of 25 days has been found. This adverse effect is neither dose related nor associated with myelotoxicity or the defect of TPMT. It is believed that the cause may be an immune-mediated response based on a genetic predisposition common to that predisposing to Crohn's disease.

4.2.2 Mesalazine

Mesalazine (mesalamine, 5-aminosalicylic acid) is an anti-inflammatory drug used to treat the inflammation of the digestive tract in ulcerative colitis and Crohn's disease. The mechanism of action remains unknown, but is limited to the intestine as the agent is not absorbed systemically in significant amounts. Therefore, systemic adverse reactions, e.g. interstitial nephritis and lupus-like syndrome, are uncommon and immune-mediated. Mesalazine belongs to drugs with the best documented association (Class I) with drug-induced acute pancreatitis. Acute pancreatitis induced by mesalazine usually occurs during the first days or weeks of treatment; however, an occurrence following prolonged use has also been sporadically reported. No dose dependence has been observed and the symptoms usually disappear within 10 days after drug withdrawal.

Drug class	Drug name	Risk class Trivedi	Risk class Badalov	Usual onset latency
Analgesics	codeine*	I	Ia	1 day
	paracetamol	II	II	1 day
	sulindac	I	Ia	> 30 days
Anesthetics	propofol	III	II	1 day
Antidiabetics	exenatide*	-	-	
	sitaglipin*	-	-	
Anti-infectives				
Antivirals	didanosine	I	II	> 30 days
	lamivudine	II	Ib	
Antibacterials	cotrimoxazole	I	Ia	1 - 30 days
	erythromycin	II	II	1 day
	tetracycline	I	Ia	
Antiparazitic agents	pentamidine	I	Ib	1 - 30 days
	stibogluconate*	I	Ia	1 - 30 days
Anticonvulsants	valproate	I	I and II	> 30 days
Antineoplastic agents	asparaginase	I	II	1 - 30 days
	cytarabine	I	Ib	1 - 30 days
Cardiovascular drugs				
ACE inhibitors*	enalapril	II	Ia	> 30 days
Diuretics	furosemide	I	Ib	
Statins*	pravastatin	III	Ia	> 30 days
Gastrointestinal drugs	mesalazine	I	Ia	1 - 30 days
	omeprazole	III	Ib	> 30 days
Steroid hormones	estrogens*	I	Ib	> 30 days
	glucocorticoids*	I	Ib	1 - 30 days
Immunosuppressants	azathioprine	I	Ib and II	1 - 30 days
	sulfasalazine	I	Ia	1 - 30 days

Table 2. Drugs commonly associated with drug-induced pancreatitis (* class effect probable)

4.2.3 Valproate

Valproic acid is an anticonvulsant, acting as an inhibitor of GABA transaminase in the CNS and blocking the neuronal voltage-gated sodium channels and T-type calcium channels. Tens of DIP cases caused by its use have been reported, with 75% of them being observed in children. There is a long latency of the first episode onset (3–17 months) and a short one in rechallenge (6–12 weeks). Although usually mild, valproate-induced pancreatitis may have a severe course with associated complications such as necrosis or even death.

4.2.4 Propofol

Propofol is an intravenously administered general anesthetic with several proposed mechanisms of action, mainly the potentiation of $GABA_A$ receptor activity and blockade of neuronal sodium channels. The nature of an agent used as an anesthetic results in an immediate onset of drug-induced pancreatitis following a single use. At least 20 cases of propofol-associated acute pancreatitis have been reported in the literature with subsequent discussions on the possible role of drug formulation in the oil-in-water emulsion. Elevated serum lipids do not seem to be a reason for this ADR; the rarity of the ADR suggests an idiosyncratic nature (Jawaid *et al.*, 2002).

4.2.5 Enalapril and other ACE inhibitors

ACE inhibitors belong to the most widely used and most effective cardiovascular drugs. In contrast to their wide use, the occurrence of acute pancreatitis caused by these agents is rare. The number of reported cases clearly depends on the time from introduction of the specific agent and its widespread use; thus, enalapril is the most commonly reported agent (Class II, Trivedi; Class Ia, Badalov). Some cases of a second episode of DIP caused by another drug with a similar mechanism of action suggest the class effect. The risk of acute pancreatitis in patients using cardiovascular drugs has been extensively studied in the European study on drug-induced acute pancreatitis. The use of ACE inhibitors has been associated with an increased risk of acute pancreatitis (adjusted odds ratio 1.5). The risk increased with higher daily doses and was highest in the first six months of therapy (Eland *et al.*, 2006).

4.2.6 Statins

HMG-CoA reductase inhibitors are currently the most popular hypolipidemic agents. The number of DIP reports related to this drug class exceeded 50, most often concerning simvastatin and pravastatin. An odds ratio of 1.41 was found for the risk of acute pancreatitis in patients with a past history of exposure to statins (Singh & Loke, 2006). The risk appears to increase with the duration of treatment. The ability to cause pancreatitis is believed to be a class effect.

4.3 Controversial issues: Acid-suppressing drugs

The relationship between drugs suppressing the secretion of gastric acid and acute pancreatitis is a frequently discussed issue. Histamine H_2 receptor antagonists cimetidine and ranitidine have been reported to cause drug-induced pancreatitis in several case reports without an evidence of rechallenge or a consistent latency. Some experimental findings also indicate the possible causative relationship, whilst others deny it. Also, in much more effective drugs with a similar effect, the proton pump inhibitors (PPIs, namely omeprazole), the risk of inducing pancreatitis has been described. In the above-mentioned study by

Lancashire *et al.*, the odds ratios were extremely high for both H_2-receptor inhibitors and PPIs. On the other hand, a previous, much larger and better designed study brought no evidence for this suspicion (Eland *et al.*, 2000). We therefore believe that the relationship of these drugs with DIP is overestimated, perhaps with the exception of cimetidine.

4.4 Controversial issues: Incretin-related antidiabetics

Soon after the introduction of a new class of oral antidiabetic agents, stimulating receptors for glucagon-like peptide 1 (GLP-1), reports on acute pancreatitis caused by their use began to emerge. In a subgroup of direct GLP-1 receptor agonists, eight cases during clinical development and 36 cases in postmarketing surveillance were reported for exenatide (the first-of-class agent) and another four cases were reported for liraglutide (Anderson & Trujillo, 2010). This phenomenon was probably even more pronounced in a newer group of agents with similar effects, dipeptidyl peptidase-4 inhibitors. At least 88 cases of acute pancreatitis in patients using sitagliptin were reported to FDA until 2010 (Olansky, 2010).

A considerable effort has been made to refute this connection, which is, of course, in the interest of the manufacturers. It has been found that the risk of acute pancreatitis is significantly higher in the diabetic compared to the non-diabetic population and that the use of drugs affecting the GLP-1 system does not further increase this risk (Garg *et al.*, 2010). Here is yet another example of a negative result in a pharmacoepidemiological study. Again, the probable reason lies in an extremely small proportion of drug-induced cases in total numbers of acute pancreatitis, which of course cannot influence the overall risk in high-risk populations. Nevertheless, the number of DIP cases reported in these medications is exceptional and supports the hypothesis of an association between the use of these drugs and DIP. Only the future will reveal whether this new group of drugs will be more beneficial for the treatment of diabetes or for studying the pathogenesis of DIP.

4.5 Toxins and illicit agents

Acute pancreatitis caused by animal toxin poisoning has been sporadically described in the literature. Probably the best known are the effects of scorpion venom. Available clinical case reports or series are usually too outdated to rely on the information contained (Bartholomew, 1970), but experimental studies on the effects of scorpion toxin are very interesting. Concurrent stimulation of pancreatic secretion and contraction of the sphincter of Oddi have been demonstrated in the late 1970s. Recently, it has been proven that the venom from the Brazilian scorpion *Tityus serrulatus* and a purified fraction selectively cleave essential SNARE proteins within exocrine pancreatic tissue (Fletcher et al., 2010). Rare reports on pancreatitis caused by adder bite (venom containing neurotoxic phospholipase A_2) or even blue-ringed octopus bite (venom containing tetrodotoxin) have been published.

Aside from alcohol, another addictive substance often mentioned in association with acute pancreatitis is marijuana, abused by smoking. A smaller series of marijuana-induced pancreatitis cases was reported by Wargo *et al.* in 2007. The authors suggest a dose-related mechanism of pancreatic injury. Cannabinoid receptors CB1 and CB2 were found in the pancreas, so their stimulation might be a trigger of the proinflammatory cascade there. Interestingly, stimulation of cannabinoid receptors was found to be a protective mechanism during experimental pancreatitis. This is yet another example of ambivalent behavior of some xenobiotics towards the pancreatic tissue. The importance of smoking, as a route of THC administration, for the initiation of pancreatitis has not yet been reviewed.

5. Diagnostics, disease course and management

Among the reasons why the real incidence of drug-induced acute pancreatitis is still not known, the difficulties in diagnosis are probably most important. Milder cases of pancreatic injury are often missed because serum amylase and lipase estimations are not part of the metabolic profile obtained during a routine health checkup and abdominal pain is often attributed to underlying diseases. Many cases of DIP are also erroneously classified as alcoholic or biliary in etiology often by default, whether they are causal or innocent bystanders. If acute pancreatitis is diagnosed, the treatment invariably includes exclusion of oral intake and, thus, also abolishment of causative oral medication and thereby the opportunity to diagnose DIP is missed (Trivedi & Pitchumoni, 2005).

5.1 Diagnosis

As is usual with the vast majority of idiosyncratic adverse drug reactions, no specific test for establishing the diagnosis of drug-induced pancreatitis is available. Therefore, the diagnosis is usually based on the following criteria:

a. Acute pancreatitis occurs during the administration of a drug;
b. All other common causes are excluded;
c. Symptoms of acute pancreatitis disappear after drug withdrawal;
d. Symptoms recur after a re-challenge of the suspected drug.

These criteria bring some problems in all ADRs, not only in such a difficult one as DIP. The first criterion seems to be easy to achieve until we remember that monotherapy in our patients becomes more and more scarce. If DIP occurs in the later course of the pharmacotherapy, the decision which drug is most suspicious is not easy. Use of the classification systems mentioned above may be very useful for that purpose.

Excluding all other causes of the disease is also not so straightforward in many cases of acute pancreatitis. However, modern diagnostic methods have led to a great progress in this area. The validity of diagnosis may depend on the equipment available and even more on the experience of the medical staff. From this point of view, previously published DIP case reports should also be considered since the possibilities of excluding other causes of acute pancreatitis are quite different now than they were in the 1970s.

Disappearance of symptoms following drug withdrawal is also sometimes misleading. Discontinuation of oral therapy is a natural part of any management of acute pancreatitis. In patients treated by multiple pharmacotherapy, it is impossible to decide which medication withdrawal led to a resolution of the symptoms and laboratory findings. A similar problem occurs in drugs administered at once, e.g. general anesthetics or anticancer chemotherapeutics. In these cases, acute pancreatitis is usually diagnosed within several days from drug administration.

Due to the character of the disease and ethical considerations, deliberate, repeated administration of suspect drug to induce a new episode of acute pancreatitis is not possible. Re-challenge is usually unintended, mainly if the cause of the first AP episode was not properly recognized. An exception is the use of essential drugs in cases where the benefits outweigh the risks. In such cases, the patient's written informed consent should be obtained.

A simplified algorithm for diagnosing drug-induced pancreatitis is given in Figure 1. The suspected drug etiology should be considered after the exclusion of more common causes of illness. For the above reasons, it seems obvious that it is not always possible to establish a definitive diagnosis of drug-induced AP immediately. A "second-look" with the knowledge of the subsequent patient's history may often be necessary. For that purpose, a proper documentation of each case is needed. A detailed medication history documentation is obvious as well as the determination of suspicious substances. We strongly recommend the use of scoring system of ADR probability and classification of suspicious drugs according to the DIP risk in the patient's files.

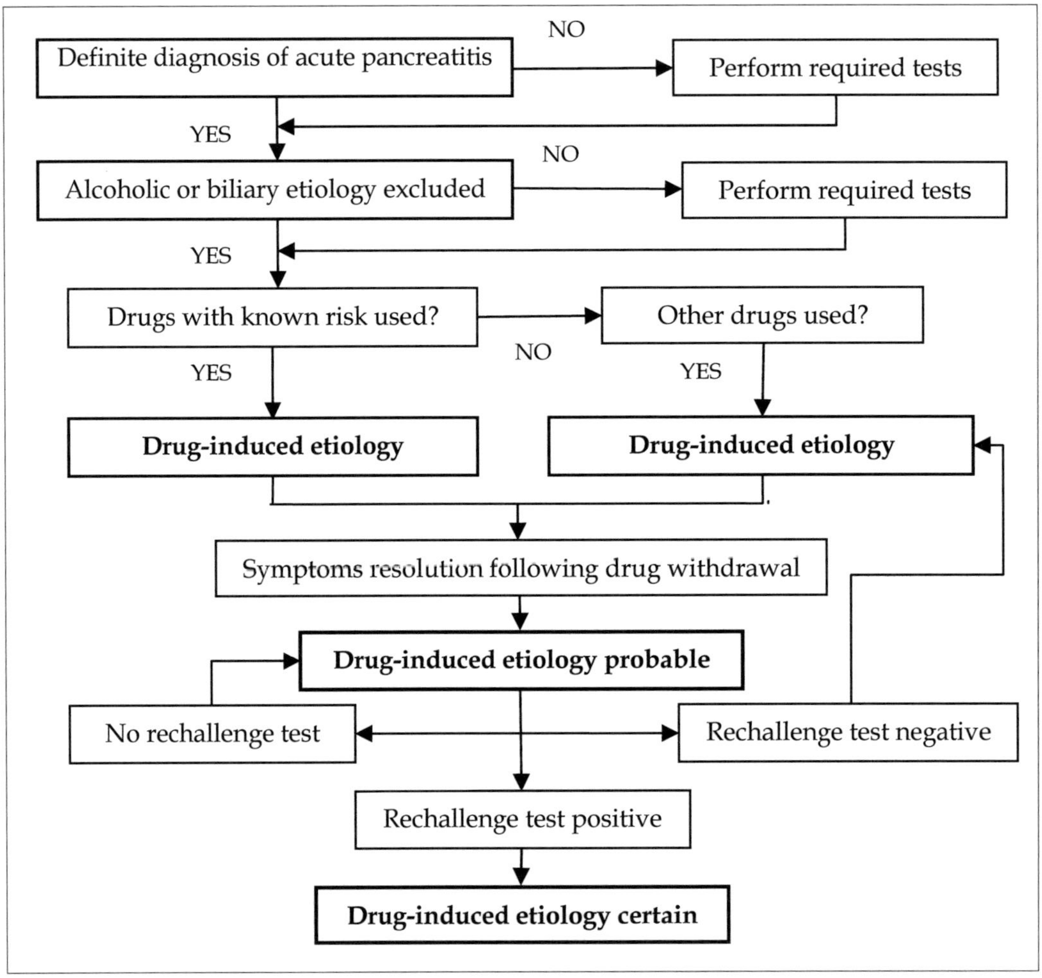

Fig. 1. Algorithm for diagnosing drug-induced acute pancreatitis

5.2 Probability scoring

For the purposes of future re-evaluation of each DIP case, it is very useful to classify drugs involved in the event by the above classification systems. There is no evidence for preferring one of these systems, so it is possible to use both, mainly if there is a difference between them in classifying a specific suspicious agent. Assigning probability of causation to a suspected adverse drug reaction can be best done by using the WHO scoring system (see Table 3). Of course, the diagnosis of DIP comes into consideration only in the first three degrees of probability: certain, probable or possible.

It is therefore appropriate that a record of the event in the patient's documentation should be written as follows: "Acute pancreatitis, drug induced; probability level: probable according to WHO scoring system; causative agent: azathioprine, class I according to Badalov". Using these classification systems may improve the quality of information for further patient treatment and further processing of the event for scientific or pharmacovigilance purposes.

Level of probability	Characteristics
Certain	A clinical event, including a laboratory test abnormality, that occurs in a plausible time relation to drug administration, and which cannot be explained by concurrent disease or other drugs or chemicals The response to withdrawal of the drug (dechallenge) should be clinically plausible The event must be definitive pharmacologically or phenomenologically using a satisfactory rechallenge procedure if necessary
Probable	A clinical event, including a laboratory test abnormality, with a reasonable time relation to administration of the drug, unlikely to be attributed to concurrent disease or other drugs or chemicals, and which follows a clinically reasonable response on withdrawal (dechallenge) Rechallenge information is not required to fulfill this definition
Possible	A clinical event, including a laboratory test abnormality, with a reasonable time relation to administration of the drug, but which could also be explained by concurrent disease or other drugs or chemicals Information on drug withdrawal may be lacking or unclear
Unlikely	A clinical event, including a laboratory test abnormality, with a temporal relation to administration of the drug, which makes a causal relation improbable, and in which other drugs, chemicals, or underlying disease provide plausible explanations
Conditional / unclassified	A clinical event, including a laboratory test abnormality, reported as an adverse reaction, about which more data are essential for a proper assessment or the additional data are being examined
Unassessable / unclassifiable	A report suggesting an adverse reaction that cannot be judged, because information is insufficient or contradictory and cannot be supplemented or verified

Table 3. Causality assessment of suspected ADRs (Edwards & Aronson, 2000)

5.3 Disease severity, management and secondary prevention

It is believed that drug-induced pancreatitis usually has a mild course. Lankisch *et al.* in 1995 showed that the disease course was usually favorable in patients with drug-induced AP, but more recent greater studies strongly suggest that the etiology of acute pancreatitis generally does not determine the severity (Gullo *et al.*, 2002). Also, a number of deaths from DIP were reported, for example, in a Danish analysis of spontaneous reports, four (9%) out of 47 DIP episodes led to death (Andersen *et al.*, 2001). Of course, severe cases tend to be more often reported both in the literature and in spontaneous pharmacovigilance reports. Sometimes it may be rather difficult to decide to what extent DIP contributed to the death, especially in the presence of a severe, often end-stage underlying disease such as HIV infection or disseminated tuberculosis (Ksiądzyna, 2001).

In the disease management, there are no specific issues concerning drug-induced pancreatitis, with an exception of an immediate withdrawal of the suspected drug. The treatment does not differ from other types of acute pancreatitis. A difficult question is how to reintroduce medication if the causative agent is not unambiguously identified. We recommend not introducing all withdrawn drugs at the same time to distinguish the cause of a possible flare-up. An agent with the lowest risk should be reintroduced first. The most suspected drugs should be substituted by their analogs with a different chemical structure. Secondary prevention consists of avoiding the drug which caused the episode of acute pancreatitis. Rechallenge of such an agent is justified only if its benefits outweigh the risks, as discussed above.

The relationship between acute DIP and chronic pancreatitis is not known. Trivedi & Pitchumoni in their above cited paper hypothesized – on the basis of a known sequence in the pathogenesis of chronic pancreatitis – that prolonged use of a causative drug in a patient who experienced an episode of DIP may lead to chronic pancreatitis by causing repeated clinical or subclinical episodes of DIP but no evidence is available for this suggestion to date.

6. Future research

Given how inadequate the current state of knowledge on drug-induced pancreatic injury is, the area for further research in this field is remarkably wide. The majority of the knowledge on the topic has been obtained from case reports or their series. These will remain a major source of information, so it is necessary to improve their informative value substantially. The following recommendations for processing case reports on DIP were proposed by Balani & Grendell in 2008. Published case reports should:

a. Provide the age and sex of the patient, along with the indication for treatment with a drug; provide the dose and frequency of medication;
b. Document a definite case of pancreatitis based on current diagnostic guidelines;
c. Provide information on the time course between initiation of drug and onset of pancreatitis;
d. Exclude the most common causes of pancreatitis; document a positive response to withdrawal of medication;
e. Provide the response to a rechallenge, if available.

Higher level of knowledge may be obtained by performing multicenter studies targeted at the etiology of non-alcoholic, non-biliary pancreatitis. Several thousands of acute pancreatitis cases must be involved in these studies to reveal the actual occurrence of drug-induced pancreatitis. Better cooperation between gastroenterologists and pharmacoepidemiologists is also needed to assess the actual risk of DIP for individual drugs. Any new pharmacoepidemiological study on this topic would be useful, but to improve the validity of its outcomes, substantially better input data are required. For this purpose, it would be optimal that each single case of acute pancreatitis included in such a study be documented according to the above principles.

Integration of the research in different disciplines would also be very useful for studying the causes of DIP. An obvious field for this research is the issue of diseases with a high incidence of this disorder. Identifying the genetic differences predisposing to pancreatic injury caused by medication in patients suffering from Crohn's disease or AIDS would be the most axiomatic target. Another issue is the experimental pharmacological research of mechanisms by which xenobiotics can damage the pancreatic tissue as well as the common mechanisms of immune-mediated tissue injury caused by drugs. Any substantial progress in this research can contribute to a progress in two scientific challenges: recognizing the nature of more frequent causes of acute pancreatitis and also recognizing the cause and pathogenesis of idiosyncratic adverse drug reaction.

7. Conclusion

Drug-induced injury is a rare cause of acute pancreatitis. Epidemiological studies show a very wide range of its incidence, but at least the absolute number of its cases is undoubtedly increasing. We are able to identify the drugs with the greatest risk and populations at risk, but the absolute risk for medication users is still very low. On the other hand, the pathogenesis of the disease remains completely unknown. A better understanding of drug-mediated pancreatic injury can also help to understand the etiology of more common types of acute pancreatitis. Research in drug-induced acute pancreatitis is both a challenge and an opportunity to improve the collaboration of gastroenterology and clinical pharmacology.

8. Acknowledgment

Supported by grants IGA UPOL LF_2011_005 and MSM 6198959216.

9. References

Andersen, V; Sonne, J. & Andersen, M. (2001) Spontaneous reports on drug-induced pancreatitis in Denmark from 1968 to 1999. *European Journal of Clinical Pharmacology*, Vol. 57, No. 6-7, (September 2001), pp. 517-21, ISSN 0031-6970.

Anderson, S.L. & Trujillo, J.M. (2010) Association of pancreatitis with glucagon-like peptide-1 agonist use. The Annals of Pharmacotherapy, Vol. 44, No. 5, (May 2010), pp. 904-909, ISSN 1060-0280.

Badalov, N.; Baradarian, R.; Iswara, K.; Li, J.; Steinberg, W. & Tenner, S. (2007) Drug-induced acute pancreatitis: an evidence-based review. *Clinical gastroenterology and hepatology*, Vol. 5, No. 6, (June 2007), 648-61. ISSN 1542-3565.

Bajaj, J.S; Saeian, K; Varma, R.R; Franco, J; Knox J.F; Podoll, J; Emmons, J; Levy, M. & Binion, D.G. (2005) Increased rates of early adverse reaction to azathioprine in patients with Crohn's disease compared to autoimmune hepatitis: a tertiary referral center experience. *The American Journal of Gastroenterology*; Vol. 100, No. 5, (May 2005), pp. 1121-5, ISSN 0002-9270.

Balani, A.R. & Grendell, J.H. (2008) Drug-Induced Pancreatitis. Incidence, Management and Prevention. *Drug Safety*, Vol. 31, No. 10, (October 2008), pp. 823-37, ISSN 0114-5916.

Banks, P.A. & Freeman, M.L. (2006) Practice Parameters Committee of the American College of Gastroenterology. Practice guidelines in acute pancreatitis. *The*

American Journal of Gastroenterology, Vol. 101, No. 10 (October 2006), pp. 2379-400, ISSN 0002-9270.

Bartholomew C. (1970) Acute scorpion pancreatitis in Trinidad. *British Medical Journal*, Vol. 5697, No. 1, (March 1970), pp. 666-8, ISSN 0007-1447.

Dawra, R; Sharif, R; Phillips, P; Dudeja, V; Dhaulakhandi, D. & Saluja, A.K. (2007) Development of a new mouse model of acute pancreatitis induced by administration of L-arginine. *American journal of physiology. Gastrointestinal and liver physiology*, Vol. 292, No. 4, (April 2007), G1009-18, ISSN 0193-1857.

Edwards, I.R. & Aronson, J.K. (2000) Adverse drug reactions: definitions, diagnosis, and management. *Lancet*, Vol. 356, No. 9237 (October 2000), pp. 1255-9, ISSN 0140-6736.

Eland I.A; Alvarez C.H; Stricker B.H. & Rodríguez, L.A. (2000) The risk of acute pancreatitis associated with acid-suppressing drugs. *British Journal of Clinical Pharmacology*, Vol. 49, No. 5, (May 2000), pp. 473-478, ISSN 0306-5251.

Eland, I.A; Sundström, A; Velo, G.P; Andersen. M; Sturkenboom, M.C; Langman, M.J; Stricker, B.H. & Wiholm, B. (2006) Antihypertensive medication and the risk of acute pancreatitis: the European case-control study on drug-induced acute pancreatitis (EDIP). Scandinavian Journal of Gastroenterology, Vol. 41, No. 12, (December 2006), pp-1484-1490, ISSN:0036-5521.

Fletcher, P.L.Jr; Fletcher, M.D; Weninger, K; Anderson, T.E. & Martin, B.M. (2010) Vesicle-associated membrane protein (VAMP) cleavage by a new metalloprotease from the Brazilian scorpion *Tityus serrulatus*. *The Journal of Biological Chemistry*, Vol. 285, No. 10, (March 2010), pp. 7405-16, ISSN 0021-9258.

Garg, R; Chen, W. & Pendergrass, M. (2010) Acute pancreatitis in type 2 diabetes treated with exenatide or sitagliptin: a retrospective observational pharmacy claims analysis. *Diabetes Care*, Vol. 33, No. 11, (November 2010), pp. 2349-2354, ISSN 0149-5992.

Gullo, L; Migliori, M; Oláh, A; Farkas, G; Levy, P; Arvanitakis, C; Lankisch, P. & Beger, H. (2002) Acute pancreatitis in five European countries: etiology and mortality. *Pancreas*, Vol. 24, No. 3, (April 2002), pp. 223-7, ISSN 0885-3177.

Jawaid, Q; Presti, M.E; Neuschwander-Tetri, B.A. & Burton F.R. (2002) Acute pancreatitis after single-dose exposure to propofol: a case report and review of literature. *Digestive Diseases and Sciences*; Vol. 47, No.3, (March 2002), pp. 614-8, ISSN 0163-2116.

Johnston, D.H. & Cornish, A.L. (1959) Acute pancreatitis in patients receiving chlorothiazide. *Journal of the American Medical Association*, Vol. 170, No. 17 (August 1959), pp. 2054-6, ISSN 0002-9955.

Księdzyna, D. (2011) Drug-induced acute pancreatitis related to medications commonly used in gastroenterology. European Journal of Internal Medicine, Vol. 22, No. 1, (February 2011), pp. 20-25, ISSN 0953-6205.

Lancashire, R.J; Cheng, K. & Langman, M.J. (2003) Discrepancies between population-based data and adverse reaction reports in assessing drugs as causes of acute pancreatitis. *Alimentary Pharmacology and Therapeutics*, Vol. 17, No. 7, (April 2003), pp. 887-93, ISSN 0269-2813.

Lankisch, P.G; Droge, M. & Gottesleben, F. (1995) Drug induced acute pancreatitis: incidence and severity. *Gut*, Vol. 37, No. 4, (October 1995), pp. 565-7, ISSN:0017-5749.

Mallory, A. & Kern, F. Jr. (1980). Drug-induced pancreatitis: a critical review. *Gastroenterology*, Vol.78, No.4, (April 1980), pp. 813-20, ISSN 0016-5085.

McArthur, K.E. (1996). Review article: drug-induced pancreatitis. *Alimentary Pharmacology and Therapeutics*, Vol.10, No.1, (February 1996), pp. 23-38. ISSN 0269-2813.

Mennecier, D; Pons, F; Arvers, P; Corberand, D; Sinayoko, L., Harnois, F.; Moulin, O; Thiolet, C; Nizou, C & Farret, O. (2007) Incidence and severity of non alcoholic and non biliary pancreatitis in a gastroenterology department. *Gastroentérologie clinique et biologique*; Vol. 31, No. 8-9, (August-September 2007), pp. 664-667, ISSN 0399-8320.

Moolsintong, P; Loftus, E.V., Jr; Chari, S.T, Egan, L,J; Tremaine, W.J. & Sandborn, W.J. (2005) Acute pancreatitis in patients with Crohn's disease: clinical features and outcomes. *Inflammatory Bowel Diseases*, Vol. 11, No. 12, (December 2005), pp. 1080-1084, ISSN 1078-0998.

Munk, E.M; Pedersen, L; Floyd, A; Nørgård, B; Rasmussen, H.H. & Sørensen, H.T. (2004) Inflammatory bowel diseases, 5-aminosalicylic acid and sulfasalazine treatment and risk of acute pancreatitis: a population-based case-control study. *The American Journal of Gastroenterology*, Vol. 99, No. 5, (May 2004), pp. 884-888, ISSN 0002-9270.

Olansky, L. (2010) Do incretin-based therapies cause acute pancreatitis? Journal of Diabetes Science and Technology, Vol. 4, No. 1, (January 2010), pp. 228-229, ISSN 1932-2968.

Sato, K; Yamada, E; Uehara, Y; Takagi, H. & Mori M. (2006) Possible role for human leukocyte antigen haplotype in rofecoxib-associated acute pancreatitis and cholestatic hepatitis. *Clinical Pharmacology and Therapeutics*, Vol. 80, No. 5, (November 2006), pp. 554-555, ISSN 0009-9236.

Singh, S. & Loke, Y.K. (2006) Statins and pancreatitis: a systematic review of observational studies and spontaneous case reports. *Drug Safety*, Vol. 29, No. 12, (December 2006), pp. 1123-1132, ISSN 0114-5916.

Su, K.H; Cuthbertson, C. & Christophi. C. (2006) Review of experimental animal models of acute pancreatitis. *HPB: the official journal of the International Hepato-Pancreato-Biliary Association*, Vol. 8, No. 4, (2006), pp. 264-86, ISSN 1365-182X.

Trivedi, C.D. & Pitchumoni, C.S. (2005) Drug-induced pancreatitis: an update. *Journal of Clinical Gastroenterology*; Vol. 39, No. 8, (September 2005), pp. 709-716. ISSN 0192-0790.

Vinklerová, I; Procházka, M; Procházka, V. & Urbánek, K. (2010) Incidence, severity, and etiology of drug-induced acute pancreatitis. *Digestive Diseases and Sciences*, Vol. 55, No. 10 (October 2010), pp. 2977-81, ISSN 0163-2116.

Wargo, K.A; Geveden, B.N. & McConnell, V.J. (2007) Cannabinoid-induced pancreatitis: a case series. *Journal of the Pancreas*, Vol. 8, No. 5, (September 2007), pp. 579-83, ISSN 1590-8577.

Weersma R.K; Peters F.T; Oostenbrug L.E; van den Berg A.P; van Haastert M; Ploeg R.J; Posthumus M.D; Homan van der Heide J.J; Jansen, P.L. & van Dullemen, H.M.

(2004) Increased incidence of azathioprine-induced pancreatitis in Crohn's disease compared with other diseases. *Alimentary Pharmacology and Therapeutics*, Vol. 20, No. 8, (October 2004), pp. 843-50, ISSN 0269-2813.

Zion, M.M; Goldman, B. & Suzman, M.M. (1955) Corticotrophin and cortisone in the treatment of scleroderma. *The Quarterly Journal of Medicine*, Vol. 24, No. 95, (July 1955), pp. 215-27, ISSN 0033-5622.

3

Obesity and Acute Pancreatitis

Davor Štimac and Neven Franjić
Division of Gastroenterology, Department of Internal Medicine, University Hospital Rijeka, Rijeka, Croatia

1. Introduction

Evidence accumulated for the past two decades leads to the conclusion that obesity enhances the development of acute pancreatitis and worsens its clinical course. Is this true? We will try to give an answer to this issue by presenting the scientific data accumulated thus far.

"Obesity is a medical condition in which excess body fat has accumulated to the extent that it may have an adverse effect on health, leading to reduced life expectancy and/or increased health problems." (World Health Organization, 2000) The main problem with obesity is determining the best (and easiest) way to measure it. According to the definition, one should calculate the total amount of body fat a person has and deduct the "normal" amount of fat from it. Several methods have been developed, each with its strengths and weaknesses. (Kamel et al, 2000; Browning et al, 2011)

Body mass index or BMI is the basic method used to determine obesity. It is a measure obtained by dividing the patient's weight (in kilograms) with the square of his/her height (in meters); obesity is defined as BMI > 30 kg/m^2. The method is based on the presumption that a person's excess weight predominantly consists of fat. The advantage of this method is its application simplicity, namely the lack of complicated procedures needed to determine it as well as the fact that it has been globally accepted. The disadvantages are the consequences of the above mentioned presumption namely that a person's excess weight predominantly consists of fat as well as the lack of body composition in the equation: a person who gains weight due to a component other than fat will have a falsely increased BMI, e.g. athletes have muscle hypertrophy; patients with ascites (liver cirrhosis) and peripheral edema (renal failure, heart failure) accumulate water, etc.

Other methods used to determine obesity measure the amount of subcutaneous fat tissue. These methods are based on the fact that the amount of subcutaneous fat tissue correlates well with the amount of excess fat tissue. The methods include the measurement of skin fold thickness, waist diameter and waist-to-hip ratio. As is the case for BMI, these methods are simple, requiring only a meter or a simple measuring instrument and the results are easily interpreted. The limiting factor for these methods is the presence of edema in the investigated areas (liver cirrhosis, heart and kidney diseases).

The method that is not affected by the presence of excess water is dual-energy X-ray absorptiometry (DEXA). It is used to measure body composition based on the difference in the absorption of X-rays in different types of tissues (bone, fat, muscle, water). Compared to other methods, DEXA is rather expensive, requires radiological equipment and a radiology specialist to interpret the results; also, it uses radiation (X-rays), which makes it potentially harmful for the patients.

After two decades of tedious work in finding the best method for estimating the amount of body fat in acute pancreatitis, scientists offer no clear answers. Although some data suggest that waist diameter and waist-to-hip ratio have the best correlation with the occurrence of complications in acute pancreatitis, BMI is still widely used as the standard procedure. The following sections offer a detailed insight into the best methods for estimating the amount of body fat in acute pancreatitis.

2. Epidemiology, etiology and pathogenesis

2.1 Epidemiology and etiology

The epidemiology of acute pancreatitis indicates that the incidence of acute pancreatitis during the last decades has been increasing. (Satoh et al, 2011) Although definitive data are not available, the authors suspect that the main reasons for this are linked to the rise of the underlying causes of pancreatitis - increased alcohol consumption and gallstones. Each cause is responsible for approximately 40% of cases of acute pancreatitis. (Lowenfels et al, 2009; Spanier et al, 2008; Goldacre & Roberts, 2004)

Whether obesity has direct consequence on the increased incidence of acute pancreatitis is not clear. Only few epidemiological studies have tried to establish a direct link between obesity and the onset of acute pancreatitis, but the studies' findings are contradictory. (Blomgren et al, 2002; Lowenfels et al, 2005, 2009) The main problem with this theory is the fact that obesity is a well-known risk factor for biliary calculi and consequently for acute biliary pancreatitis. Therefore, it is hard to determine whether or not obesity has a direct impact on the onset of acute pancreatitis.

Another factor taken into consideration when analyzing obesity's effect on the onset of acute pancreatitis is weight distribution. Analyses show that there is no difference in the weight distribution of patients suffering acute pancreatitis and the general population. The reason for this lies in the fact that while patients with biliary pancreatitis tend to be overweight (as obesity is a risk factor for biliary stones), patients suffering alcoholic pancreatitis tend to be lean or even malnourished.

2.2 Pathogenesis

The increased interest in obesity is the consequence of the epidemiological boom of obese people and children in post-industrial societies. Since obesity is linked to acute pancreatitis, there have been many speculations about the pathogenetic links between the two. (Bastard et al, 2006; Fuentes et al, 2010; Frossard et al, 2009)

Ever since the discovery of adipokines, hormones synthesized and excreted by the cells residing in the adipose tissue, the endocrine function of adipose tissue has become even more intricate. Adipokines once included only biologically-active substances secreted by the adipocytes, but today they refer to all biologically-active substances produced by the adipose tissue.

The principal anti-inflammatory substance secreted by the adipocytes is adiponectin. It is a 30-kDa protein with plasma levels ranging from 5 to 30 mg/L in lean subjects. Adiponectin has many potentially beneficial effects in acute pancreatitis (Zyromski et al, 2008): it enhances insulin-sensitivity (Yamauchi et al, 2002), modulates endothelial adhesion molecules (Ouchi et al, 1999), alters macrophage and lymphocyte action (Ouchi et al, 2001; Wolf et al, 2004) and modulates the balance of cytokines in favor of anti-inflammatory cytokines (Ouchi et al, 2000; Huang et al, 2008; Masaki et al, 2004)

Leptin, a pro-inflammatory adipokine synthesized in the adipocytes, is on the opposite side of the spectrum. Leptin acts pro-inflammatory by regulating cytokine production in favor of pro-inflammatory cytokines (Fantuzzi & Faggioni, 2000; Santosa et al, 2007) and by enhancing leukocyte activity (Loffreda et al, 1998; Lord et al, 1998). On the other hand, a study performed by Matyjek et al. showed an inhibitory effect of leptin on cholecystokinin-related secretion of pancreatic enzymes. (Matyjek et al, 2003)

Resistin is another adipokine, a 12.5 kDa protein produced mainly by monocytes and macrophages. Its effects include increased insulin resistance and dyslipidemia. (Steppan et al, 2001; Trayhurn & Wood, 2004)

According to modern conceptions, obese people are in a state of chronic inflammation. Studies have shown that excess adipose tissue generates more leptin and resistin, and less adiponectin. This, in turn, leads to the prevalence of pro-inflammatory over anti-inflammatory cytokines, resulting in a state of constant inflammation of the adipose tissue. (Frossard et al, 2009) The residing macrophages are affected as well. Normal fat tissue contains a balance of the so-called M1 or pro-inflammatory macrophages and the so-called M2 or anti-inflammatory macrophages. In obesity, the scale is tipped in favor of M1 macrophages; the net-result is a constant over-production of various pro-inflammatory cytokines, like interleukin-1 (IL-1), interleukin-6 (IL-6) or tumor necrosis factor-alpha (TNF-alpha).

The pro-inflammatory effect of excess adipose tissue varies throughout the body and depends on the place where excess fat is stored. The worst place it can be stored is the intraabdominal compartment; visceral adipose tissue is metabolically the most active adipose tissue and the most "pro-inflammatory oriented". (Clement & Langin, 2007) Because the veins of the visceral adipose tissue drain into the portal system, the hormonal products and free-fatty acids (FFAs) produced by the visceral adipose tissue directly influence the liver and cause central insulin resistance. This is the pathogenetic pathway by which the central obesity causes cardiovascular diseases as well as diabetes. Free-fatty acids, however, act through toll-like receptors (TLRs) inducing an inflammatory response in macrophages, adipocytes and muscle-cells.

The central dogma of the acute pancreatitis etiopathogenesis is the uncontrolled intrapancreatic conversion of trypsinogen into trypsin. In theory, it is rather easy to imagine how an altered pro-inflammatory cytokine milieu could trigger the activation of trypsinogen, leading to the onset of acute pancreatitis. Clinical data are, however, inconclusive. Therefore, we must be overlooking some important factors in the development of acute pancreatitis.

3. Clinical course

The clinical course of acute pancreatitis follows two discrete patterns. It can be a mild disease, resulting in edematous interstitial inflammation of the pancreas and resolving without consequences within a week. On the other hand, it can be a severe, debilitating disease, manifested by pancreatic and peripancreatic necroses and resulting, in turn, in local and systemic complications. Can obesity influence the course of the disease?

Obesity is a chronic subclinical inflammatory disorder that, in theory, can influence the clinical course of acute pancreatitis. There is evidence that obese patients have elevated levels of pro-inflammatory cytokines circulating in their blood. (Clement & Langin, 2007) This, in turn, can affect the course of the disease by enhancing inflammation and increasing the chance of necrosis.

The second way excess fat can influence the course of acute pancreatitis is by increasing the risk of pancreatic infection and the severity of inflammation. In the course of acute pancreatitis, the inflammation affects peri-pancreatic adipose tissue as well. The risk of complications is proportional to the amount of excess fat tissue in the peri-pancreatic area, which is a component of the visceral adipose tissue. (Frossard et al, 2009) On the other hand, excess peripancreatic fat could be a protective factor by separating the pancreatic tissue from the retroperitoneal structures thus localizing the necrotizing process.

The third, and often neglected problem in obese patients with acute pancreatitis is (chronic) insulin resistance. It is a common denominator of obesity and carries the burden of type II diabetes development. Insulin resistance is a system-wide problem which affects both the vasculature and the immune system and can give rise to microcirculatory problems which can cause pancreatic ischemia. (Mentula et al, 2007) Insulin resistance (acute) is actually a physiological reaction accompanying acute immune reactions and stress. The body needs energy and nutrients, i.e. glucose, amino-acids and free-fatty acids. In order to meet its needs, the body must inhibit nutrient uptake and reverse the process: cells which are not needed degrade its proteins, carbohydrates and lipids in order to produce the above-mentioned nutrients. That way the body fuels up the immune reactions and makes healing possible. When the healing (reconvalescence period) is complete, the body lowers insulin resistance to normal levels. The problem is when this state persists for a long time, as in the case of obesity. As a result, the body is not able to adequately react to the traumatic experience (acute pancreatitis) and prolonged healing follows.

Although all the proposed mechanisms seem logical, clinical data have failed us once again. Some of the studies do show a statistical significance in the outcomes of obese and non-obese pancreatitis patients; however, other studies do not confirm these findings. Even in some studies, which support the idea that obese patients tend to have a more complicated course of acute pancreatitis, the confidence interval is rather wide, indicating possibly biased data. A possible explanation is that the measure of obesity used in the studies is not the real measure of obesity.

Unfortunately, as with many other topics covering acute pancreatitis, we still await an unequivocal conclusion.

4. Obesity measures

Various obesity measurements are used in everyday practice. However, modern tendencies are to simplify disease management and at the same time be cost-effective. Complex measurements are performed in high-volume hospitals and university hospitals; smaller hospitals employ simplified methods more suited to smaller budgets. Body-mass index (BMI) and waist diameter are the methods which fulfill the mentioned criteria.

4.1 BMI

As mentioned before, BMI is calculated by dividing the patient's weight (in kilograms) with the square of his/her height (in meters). Patients with BMI above 25 kg/m^2 are defined as overweight; above 30 kg/m^2 are obese. These are, again, divided into three subcategories: type I obesity ranging from 30 to 35 kg/m^2, type II or severe obesity ranging from 35 to 40 kg/m^2 and type III or morbid obesity with BMI levels above 40 kg/m^2.

Several studies have tried to substantiate the idea that obesity predisposes a person for the development of acute pancreatitis. Suazo-Barájona et al. in 1998 found a significant difference in the occurrence of severe acute pancreatitis between patients with BMI≥25 kg/m^2 (overweight and obese), and those with BMI<25 kg/m^2 (lean). The differentiation of the overweight and the obese into separate groups is performed only graphically. The graph shows a tendency of patients with higher BMI to develop severe acute pancreatitis more often. (Suazo-Barájona et al, 1998) Johnson et al. modified the APACHE II score by adding BMI into the scoring system. A value of 1 or 2 is added to the "classic" APACHE score depending on the value of BMI. (Johnson et al, 2004) The study, along with a study from Papachristou et al two years later, showed a positive correlation between the BMI and the disease' severity, though in the second study the APACHE-O score did not perform better than the original APACHE II score. (Papachristou et al, 2006) In 2006, a meta-analysis was performed by Martinez et al in order to determine the effect of BMI on the occurrence of local complications, systemic complications and mortality. The meta-analysis included 739 patients and clearly showed an increased incidence of local and systemic complications, as well as increased mortality. However, with respect to mortality, the odds ratio (OR) for the obese patients was 2.1, but with a 95% confidence interval (CI) ranging from 1.0 to 4.8 (figure 1). This implies an increased mortality risk in obese patients suffering acute pancreatitis, but it should be taken into careful consideration. (Martinez et al, 2006) In the period after 2006, several studies negating the effect of BMI on disease severity have been published. (Mentula et al, 2007; Stimac et al, 2007) The last meta-analysis published in 2011 (Wang et al, 2011) included 8 studies with 939 patients. The meta-analysis showed that the incidence rates of severe acute pancreatitis, local complications and mortality were all increased in overweight patients (OR 2.48, 2.58 and 3.81, respectively). The last meta-analysis did not show correlation between BMI and systemic complications, though.

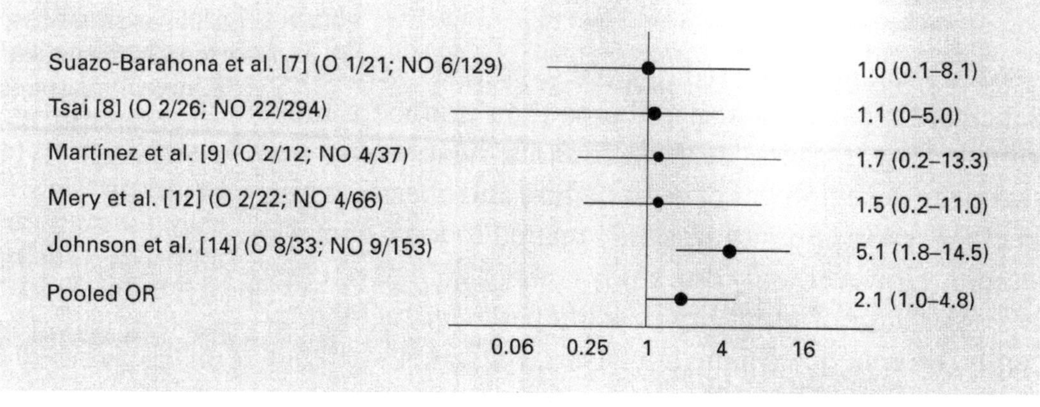

Fig. 1. The results of the meta-analysis performed by Martinez et al. (Martinez et al, 2006) The influence of obesity on the mortality in patients suffering acute pancreatitis is shown in the forest plot with a calculated pooled odds ratio (OR). O = Obese; NO = Nonobese

4.2 Waist diameter and waist-hip ratio

Waist diameter or circumference is the measurement of the shortest abdominal distance, halfway between the lower rib margin and the iliac crest. Men with a waist diameter <94 cm, 94-101.9 cm and ≥102 cm are defined as lean, overweight and obese. Similarly, in women the values are <80 cm, 80-87.9 cm and ≥88 cm, respectively.

Waist-to-hip or waist-hip ratio is calculated by dividing the waist diameter with the hip diameter. The hip diameter is acquired by measuring the abdominal diameter at the level of the hips. Again, the distribution is <0.90, 0.90-0.99 and ≥1.00 for lean, overweight and obese men. In women, the cut-off values are 0.80 and 0.85 (<0.80, 0.80-0.84 and ≥0.85).

The mentioned ranges are reference ranges defined for the European population. Differences exist among different populations. The American societies define the ranges somewhat higher, while the Asian societies tend to lower the ranges, mirroring the normal distribution of waist diameter and waist-hip ratio in the respective populations.

The idea of analyzing waist diameter and waist-hip ratio as a predictive factor in acute pancreatitis has emerged as early as in the 90's, but only several studies have been performed thus far. In 1999, Martinez et al. showed that waist diameter was greater in patients with severe acute pancreatitis than in patients with the mild form. (Martínez et al, 1999) A second study in which Torgerson et al. tried to determine the impact of obesity on the occurrence of gallstones, gallbladder disease and pancreatitis was limited by the small number of patients suffering acute pancreatitis. (Torgerson et al, 2003) The latest study published in 2010 by Duarte-Rojo et al. showed that waist diameter, waist-hip ratio and waist-thigh ratio all correlated well with the severity of acute pancreatitis. The study also showed that waist diameter correlated best with the subcutaneous abdominal fat, while the waist-hip ratio showed a similar correlation with intra-abdominal fat. (Duarte-Rojo et al, 2010)

Fluid sequestration in the retroperitoneal compartment affects both the BMI and the abdominal obesity measures. With fluid retention, the measures become inaccurate in assessing obesity as they tend to overestimate the amount of body fat, and become more accurate in predicting disease severity (the more the fluid is sequestered the more severe the course of the disease). That is perhaps the reason why some studies have shown a good correlation between obesity measures and disease severity, while others did not. In the case of fluid retention, abdominal measures should theoretically have a greater prognostic significance than BMI; one should note that this does not imply obesity as well. (Beger & Rau, 2007)

Whether BMI or abdominal measures are the best disease severity predictors still remains to be seen. Studies comparing the two are needed.

5. Treatment differences

Current approach to acute pancreatitis management depends mostly on the course the disease will follow. Specific therapy for acute pancreatitis does not exist, as medications which could impede the development of the disease or change its course have not been found yet. Therefore, the only therapy is symptomatic and depends on the patient's status.

In mild edematous pancreatitis, fluid resuscitation and oral food intake prohibition will enhance the patient's recovery. Even the lack of therapy would yield a similar result, as in this case the disease is self-limited. For this type of pancreatitis there are no differences in the management of obese and non-obese patients.

Severe necrotizing pancreatitis is the therapeutic nightmare for every gastroenterologist and intensivist. In the acute phase of the disease (within 7 days from onset), the main problem is organ failure. Obese patients tend to have more local and systemic complications, and respiratory failure is among the more common ones. Therefore, in the management of obese patients, aggressive fluid resuscitation with a special concern for respiratory function is of utmost importance. Since obesity carries the risk of type II diabetes, and glucose intolerance is rather often found in the acute phase of acute pancreatitis, insulin is usually added to glucose or Ringer solutions in order to maintain glucose levels under 10 mmol/L (180 mg/dL). (Di Carlo et al, 1981; Pisters & Ranson, 1992)

The main problem in the subacute phase of acute pancreatitis is the elevated risk of infection. Insulin resistance can impede the normal function of the immune system and lead to serious infections. (Turina et al, 2005) Therefore, antibiotic prophylaxis should be given in order to prevent this setting from taking place.

Since the predilection of obese patients for local and systemic complications is still under revision, the measures are opinion-based and not substantiated with evidence from RCTs. However, common sense dictates us to monitor such patients more closely in order to try to prevent the worst from happening.

6. Nutritional support

As obesity is (usually) a nutritional disorder, nutritional support in acute pancreatitis is separated from other therapeutic interventions. (Ionnanidis et al, 2008)

Due to the lack of specific therapy, the modern mainstay of therapy of acute pancreatitis is "pancreatic rest". (Cassim & Allardyce, 1974) This means that the pancreas should be stimulated as little as possible in order to enable it to contain the inflammation and give it time to heal itself. Again, the treatment approach for patients with mild pancreatitis differs from those suffering severe pancreatitis.

In mild pancreatitis food is withheld for several days, after which the patient is given oral food, first in the form of water and tea, followed by the so-called "pancreatic" diet (food rich in carbohydrates and scarce in fats). If the patient cannot tolerate oral intake, enteral or even parenteral feeding should be administered. Obese patients are treated the same way.

In severe pancreatitis, the approach is more invasive. Patients are fed enterally through a naso-jejunal tube. If they cannot tolerate enteral feeding, or enteral feeding is inadequate, parenteral feeding is added. Obese patients should be fed according to ideal weight and not the actual one. The target energy requirements include 25-35 kcal/kg of ideal body weight, with 1.2-1.5 g of nitrogen per kg of ideal body weight. (Choban & Dickerson, 2005; Elamin, 2005) One should note that this means that obese patients are 'permissively underfed'. In their case, weight reduction can have beneficial effects on insulin resistance and the overall status of the patient. (Martindale et al, 2009)

Plasma glucose levels should be monitored at least twice a day, more intensively in case of offset values. High glucose values (above 10.0 mmol/L) should be corrected with subcutaneous administration of insulin.

7. Treatment

The treatment of acute pancreatitis in obese patients is summarized in table 1.

Mild pancreatitis	
food restriction	(depending on clinical severity)
fluid resuscitation	(depending on laboratory values)
Severe pancreatitis	
enteral nutrition, parenteral if needed	(amount calculated according to ideal weight)
aggressive fluid resuscitation	(up to 4-6 L daily, depending on the state of the cardiovascular system)
insulin	according to plasma glucose levels
oxygen therapy	depending on oxygen saturation
antibiotic prophylaxis	(carbapenems, ciprofloxacin, metronidazole)

Table 1. Therapeutic approach in obese patients with acute pancreatitis

8. Conclusion

In the end, we will talk about the future and what it holds for obese patients suffering from acute pancreatitis.
Scientists and clinical practitioners are presently searching for new and better ways to help patients suffering from acute pancreatitis and are exploring ways to overcome and combat the disease.
In the field of diagnostics, most researches are battling with the issue of identifying prognostic factors for severe acute pancreatitis. The goal is to find a diagnostic tool that could predict and determine the course of the disease at admission. This is especially important for obese patients, as they tend to have a more complicated disease.
In the field of therapy, most researches are concentrated on finding a medication that could alter the course of the disease. A number of substances have been investigated in order to achieve this, but to no avail. Specific therapy would reduce the number of complications and mortality to ppm levels.
Finally, scientists are trying to find the best possible methods and interventions to treat acute pancreatitis complications. Again, it is an issue of utmost importance for the obese, as interventions are more difficult in these patients and carry out a greater risk of procedural complications and mortality.
Although the mentioned investigations are related to acute pancreatitis, there are a number of options available for implementing effective interventions for treating obesity. Will these obesity treatment procedures have positive effects on and will they become a part of acute pancreatitis treatment procedures, only time will show!

9. References

Bastard JP, Maachi M, Lagathu C, Kim MJ, Caron M, Vidal H, Capeau J, Feve B. Recent advances in the relationship between obesity, inflammation, and insulin resistance. *Eur Cytokine Netw.* 2006 Mar; 17(1): 4-12.

Beger HG & Rau BM. Severe acute pancreatitis: Clinical course and management. *World J Gastroenterol.* 2007 Oct 14; 13(38): 5043-51. Review.

Blomgren KB, Sundström A, Steineck G & Wiholm BE. Obesity and treatment of diabetes with glyburide may both be risk factors for acute pancreatitis. *Diabetes Care.* 2002 Feb; 25(2): 298-302.

Browning LM, Mugridge O, Dixon AK, Aitken SW, Prentice AM & Jebb SA. Measuring abdominal adipose tissue: comparison of simpler methods with MRI. *Obes Facts.* 2011; 4(1): 9-15.

Cassim MM & Allardyce DB. Pancreatic secretion in response to jejunal feeding of elemental diet. *Ann Surg.* 1974 Aug; 180(2): 228-31.

Choban PS & Dickerson RN. Morbid obesity and nutrition support: is bigger different? *Nutr Clin Pract.* 2005 Aug;20(4):480-7. Review.

Clement K & Langin D. Regulation of inflammation-related genes in human adipose tissue. *J Intern Med.* 2007 Oct; 262(4): 422-30. Review.

Di Carlo V, Nespoli A, Chiesa R, Staudacher C, Cristallo M, Bevilacqua G & Staudacher V. Hemodynamic and metabolic impairment in acute pancreatitis. *World J Surg.* 1981 May; 5(3): 329-39.

Duarte-Rojo A, Sosa-Lozano LA, Saúl A, Herrera-Cáceres JO, Hernández-Cárdenas C, Vázquez-Lamadrid J & Robles-Díaz G. Methods for measuring abdominal obesity in the prediction of severe acute pancreatitis, and their correlation with abdominal fat areas assessed by computed tomography. *Aliment Pharmacol Ther.* 2010 Jul; 32(2): 244-53.

Elamin EM. Nutritional care of the obese intensive care unit patient. *Curr Opin Crit Care.* 2005 Aug;11(4):300-3. Review.

Fantuzzi G & Faggioni R. Leptin in the regulation of immunity, inflammation, and hematopoiesis. *J Leukoc Biol.* 2000 Oct; 68(4): 437-46.

Frossard JL, Lescuyer P & Pastor CM. Experimental evidence of obesity as a risk factor for severe acute pancreatitis. *World J Gastroenterol.* 2009 Nov 14; 15(42): 5260-5.

Fuentes L, Roszer T & Ricote M. Inflammatory mediators and insulin resistance in obesity: role of nuclear receptor signaling in macrophages. *Mediators Inflamm.* 2010; 2010:219583. Epub 2010 May 20.

Goldacre MJ, Roberts SE. Hospital admission for acute pancreatitis in an English population, 1963-98: database study of incidence and mortality. *BMJ.* 2004 Jun 19; 328(7454): 1466-9.

Huang H, Park PH, McMullen MR & Nagy LE. Mechanisms for the anti-inflammatory effects of adiponectin in macrophages. *J Gastroenterol Hepatol.* 2008 Mar; 23 Suppl 1: S50-3. Review.

Ioannidis O, Lavrentieva A, Botsios D. Nutrition support in acute pancreatitis. *JOP.* 2008 Jul 10; 9(4): 375-90. Review.

Johnson CD, Toh SK & Campbell MJ. Combination of APACHE-II score and an obesity score (APACHE-O) for the prediction of severe acute pancreatitis. *Pancreatology.* 2004; 4(1): 1-6. Epub 2004 Feb 24.

Kamel EG, McNeill G & Van Wijk MC. Usefulness of anthropometry and DXA in predicting intra-abdominal fat in obese men and women. *Obes Res.* 2000 Jan; 8(1): 36-42.

Loffreda S, Yang SQ, Lin HZ, Karp CL, Brengman ML, Wang DJ, Klein AS, Bulkley GB, Bao C, Noble PW, Lane MD & Diehl AM. Leptin regulates proinflammatory immune responses. *FASEB J*. 1998 Jan; 12(1): 57-65.

Lord GM, Matarese G, Howard JK, Baker RJ, Bloom SR & Lechler RI. Leptin modulates the T-cell immune response and reverses starvation-induced immunosuppression. *Nature*. 1998 Aug 27; 394(6696): 897-901.

Lowenfels AB, Sullivan T, Fiorianti J & Maisonneuve P. The epidemiology and impact of pancreatic diseases in the United States. *Curr Gastroenterol Rep*. 2005 May; 7(2): 90-5.

Lowenfels AB, Maisonneuve P & Sullivan T. The changing character of acute pancreatitis: epidemiology, etiology, and prognosis. *Curr Gastroenterol Rep*. 2009 Apr; 11(2): 97-103.

Martindale RG, McClave SA, Vanek VW, McCarthy M, Roberts P, Taylor B, Ochoa JB, Napolitano L, Cresci G; American College of Critical Care Medicine; A.S.P.E.N. Board of Directors. Guidelines for the provision and assessment of nutrition support therapy in the adult critically ill patient: Society of Critical Care Medicine and American Society for Parenteral and Enteral Nutrition: Executive Summary. *Crit Care Med*. 2009 May; 37(5): 1757-61. Review.

Martínez J, Sánchez-Payá J, Palazón JM, Aparicio JR, Picó A & Pérez-Mateo M. Obesity: a prognostic factor of severity in acute pancreatitis. *Pancreas*. 1999 Jul; 19(1): 15-20.

Martínez J, Johnson CD, Sánchez-Payá J, de Madaria E, Robles-Díaz G & Pérez-Mateo M. Obesity is a definitive risk factor of severity and mortality in acute pancreatitis: an updated meta-analysis. *Pancreatology* 2006; 6: 206-9.

Masaki T, Chiba S, Tatsukawa H, Yasuda T, Noguchi H, Seike M & Yoshimatsu H. Adiponectin protects LPS-induced liver injury through modulation of TNF-alpha in KK-Ay obese mice. *Hepatology*. 2004 Jul; 40(1): 177-84.

Matyjek R, Herzig KH, Kato S & Zabielski R. Exogenous leptin inhibits the secretion of pancreatic juice via a duodenal CCK1-vagal-dependent mechanism in anaesthetized rats. *Regul Pept*. 2003 Jun 15; 114(1): 15-20.

Mentula P, Kylänpää ML, Kemppainen E, Repo H & Puolakkainen P. Early inflammatory response in acute pancreatitis is little affected by body mass index. *Scand J Gastroenterol* 2007 Nov; 42(11): 1362-8.

Ouchi N, Kihara S, Arita Y, Maeda K, Kuriyama H, Okamoto Y, Hotta K, Nishida M, Takahashi M, Nakamura T, Yamashita S, Funahashi T & Matsuzawa Y. Novel modulator for endothelial adhesion molecules: adipocyte-derived plasma protein adiponectin. *Circulation*. 1999 Dec 21-28; 100(25): 2473-6.

Ouchi N, Kihara S, Arita Y, Nishida M, Matsuyama A, Okamoto Y, Ishigami M, Kuriyama H, Kishida K, Nishizawa H, Hotta K, Muraguchi M, Ohmoto Y, Yamashita S, Funahashi T & Matsuzawa Y. Adipocyte-derived plasma protein, adiponectin, suppresses lipid accumulation and class A scavenger receptor expression in human monocyte-derived macrophages. *Circulation*. 2001 Feb 27; 103(8): 1057-63.

Ouchi N, Kihara S, Arita Y, Okamoto Y, Maeda K, Kuriyama H, Hotta K, Nishida M, Takahashi M, Muraguchi M, Ohmoto Y, Nakamura T, Yamashita S, Funahashi T & Matsuzawa Y. Adiponectin, an adipocyte-derived plasma protein, inhibits endothelial NF-kappaB signaling through a cAMP-dependent pathway. *Circulation.* 2000 Sep 12; 102(11): 1296-301.

Papachristou GI, Papachristou DJ, Avula H, Slivka A & Whitcomb DC. Obesity increases the severity of acute pancreatitis: performance of APACHE-O score and correlation with the inflammatory response. *Pancreatology.* 2006; 6(4): 279-85. Epub 2006 Apr 19.

Pisters PW & Ranson JH. Nutritional support for acute pancreatitis. *Surg Gynecol Obstet.* 1992 Sep; 175(3): 275-84. Review.

Santosa S, Demonty I, Lichtenstein AH, Cianflone K & Jones PJ. An investigation of hormone and lipid associations after weight loss in women. *J Am Coll Nutr.* 2007 Jun; 26(3): 250-8.

Satoh K, Shimosegawa T, Masamune A, Hirota M, Kikuta K, Kihara Y, Kuriyama S, Tsuji I, Satoh A, Hamada S & Research Committee of Intractable Diseases of the Pancreas. Nationwide epidemiological survey of acute pancreatitis in Japan. *Pancreas* 2011 May; 40(4): 503-7.

Spanier BW, Dijkgraaf MG & Bruno MJ. Epidemiology, aetiology and outcome of acute and chronic pancreatitis: An update. *Best Pract Res Clin Gastroenterol.* 2008; 22(1): 45-63.

Steppan CM, Bailey ST, Bhat S, Brown EJ, Banerjee RR, Wright CM, Patel HR, Ahima RS & Lazar MA. The hormone resistin links obesity to diabetes. *Nature.* 2001 Jan 18; 409(6818): 307-12.

Štimac D, Krznarić Zrnić I, Radić M & Žuvić-Butorac M. Outcome of the biliary acute pancreatitis is not associated with body mass index. *Pancreas* 2007 Jan; 34(1): 165-6.

Suazo-Baráhona J, Carmona-Sánchez R, Robles-Díaz G, Milke-García P, Vargas-Vorácková F, Uscanga-Domínguez L & Peláez-Luna M. Obesity: a risk factor for severe acute biliary and alcoholic pancreatitis. *Am J Gastroenterol.* 1998 Aug; 93(8): 1324-8.

Torgerson JS, Lindroos AK, Näslund I & Peltonen M. Gallstones, gallbladder disease, and pancreatitis: cross-sectional and 2-year data from the Swedish Obese Subjects (SOS) and SOS reference studies. *Am J Gastroenterol.* 2003 May; 98(5): 1032-41.

Trayhurn P, Wood IS. Adipokines: inflammation and the pleiotropic role of white adipose tissue. *Br J Nutr.* 2004 Sep; 92(3): 347-55. Review.

Turina M, Fry DE & Polk HC Jr. Acute hyperglycemia and the innate immune system: clinical, cellular, and molecular aspects. *Crit Care Med.* 2005 Jul; 33(7): 1624-33. Review.

Wang SQ, Li SJ, Feng QX, Feng XY, Xu L & Zhao QC. Overweight Is an Additional Prognostic Factor in Acute Pancreatitis: A Meta-Analysis. *Pancreatology.* 2011 May 17; 11(2): 92-98.

Wolf AM, Wolf D, Rumpold H, Enrich B & Tilg H. Adiponectin induces the anti-inflammatory cytokines IL-10 and IL-1RA in human leukocytes. *Biochem Biophys Res Commun.* 2004 Oct 15; 323(2): 630-5.

World Health Organization. Obesity: preventing and managing the global epidemic. Report of a WHO Consultation. Geneva, Switzerland: World Health Organization, 2000. (WHO technical report series 894).

Yamauchi T, Kamon J, Minokoshi Y, Ito Y, Waki H, Uchida S, Yamashita S, Noda M, Kita S, Ueki K, Eto K, Akanuma Y, Froguel P, Foufelle F, Ferre P, Carling D, Kimura S,

Nagai R, Kahn BB & Kadowaki T. Adiponectin stimulates glucose utilization and fatty-acid oxidation by activating AMP-activated protein kinase. *Nat Med.* 2002 Nov; 8(11): 1288-95. Epub 2002 Oct 7.

Zyromski NJ, Mathur A, Pitt HA, Lu D, Gripe JT, Walker JJ, Yancey K, Wade TE & Swartz-Basile DA. A murine model of obesity implicates the adipokine milieu in the pathogenesis of severe acute pancreatitis. *Am J Physiol Gastrointest Liver Physiol.* 2008 Sep; 295(3): G552-8. Epub 2008 Jun 26.

4

Acute Pancreatitis During Pregnancy

Tea Štimac and Davor Štimac[1]
Department of Gynecology & Obstetrics
[1]Division of Gastroenterology, Department of Internal Medicine
University Hospital Rijeka
Croatia

1. Introduction

Acute pancreatitis is rare and serious complication during pregnancy, estimated to occur in 1/1000 to 1/12000 pregnancies (Ramin et al., 1995). Discrepancy in incidence is because of the rarity of disease and because studies span different decades and countries. Acute pancreatitis appears to be more prevalent with advanced gestational stage, occurring more commonly in the second and the third trimester (Hernandez et al., 2007; Ramin et al., 2001). Ramin and al. noted that 19% of acute pancreatitis occurs in the first, 26% in the second, 53% in the third and 2% in the postpartum period, while others reported most of cases, 56%, in the second trimester (Hernandez et al., 2007; Ramin et al., 1995).

The most frequent etiology of acute pancreatitis in pregnancy is biliary caused by gallstones or sludge (Wang et al., 2009). Other causes are hyperlipidemia and alcohol abuse. Rarely it could be, also, caused by hyperparathyroidism, connective tissue diseases, abdominal surgery, infections (viral, bacterial or parasitic), blunt abdominal injuries or could be iatrogenic caused by medications (diuretics, antibiotics, antihypertensive drugs) (Wang et al., 2009; Ramin et al., 1995).

In pregnancy gallstones and sludge induce most of the cases of acute pancreatitis, they cause duct obstruction with pancreatic hyperstimulation that increases pancreatic duct pressure, trypsin reflux and activation of trypsin in the pancreatic acinar cells. This leads to enzyme activation within pancreas and causes autodigestion of the gland, followed by local inflammation. Pregnancy does not primarily predispose the pregnant woman to pancreatitis, but it does increase the risk of cholelithiasis and biliary sludge formation (Ramin et al., 1995). Theoretical reasons for the association of pregnancy and biliary tract diseases include increased bile acid pool size, decreased enterohepatic circulation, decreased percentage of chenodeoxycholic acid, and increased percentage of cholic acid and cholesterol secretion and bile stasis (Scott, 1992). Moreover, the steroid hormones of pregnancy decrease gallbladder motility (Ramin et al., 1995). Progesterone is a smooth muscle cell inhibitor that provokes gallbladder volume increase and slows emptying (Ramin et al., 1995). Estrogens increase cholesterol secretion and minimally alter gallbladder function (Ramin et al., 1995). Also in the third trimester when the acute pancreatitis is most frequent, the uterus is enlarged and intrabdominal pressure on the biliary ducts is increased (Berk et al., 1971).

2. Clinical features

Acute pancreatitis presents essentially in the same way during pregnancy as in the non-pregnant state. However, it is difficult to diagnose acute pancreatitis by history and physical examination because of similarity to many acute abdominal illnesses.

2.1 Symptomatology

Acute pancreatitis in pregnancy is mainly related to gallbladder disorders and correlates with cholelithiasis and biliary sludge (muddy sediment, precursor to gallstone formation) as the most likely predisposing causes (Ramin et al., 1995). The symptoms of gallbladder disease can be present or can precede the clinical presentation of acute pancreatitis. The symptoms include abdominal pain (colicky or stabbing) which may radiate to the right flank, scapula and shoulder. Onset of pain is rapid, with maximal intensity in 10 to 20 minutes. Pain is steady and moderate to severe. Band-like radiation of the pain to the back occurs in half of patients. Other symptoms of gallbladder disease include anorexia, nausea, vomiting, dyspepsia, low-grade fever, tachycardia and fatty food intolerance (Ramin et al., 1995).

2.2 Physical examination

Physical findings vary with the severity of illness, in moderate to severe pancreatitis the patient appears acutely ill and is found lying in the "fetal position" with flexed knees, hips and trunk. Abdominal tenderness is often found; in diffuse peritonitis muscle rigidity can be present. Bowel sounds, secondary to paralytic ileus, are usually hypoactive or absent. In severe pancreatitis the general physical examination may reveal abnormal vital signs if there are third-space fluid losses and systemic toxicity. Due to hypovolemia tachycardia up to 150/min and low blood pressure could be found. Also, because of severe retroperitoneal inflammatory process temperature may increase. Dyspnea, tachypnea and shallow respirations resulting with hypoxemia may be present. Altered maternal acid-base status can adversely affect fetal acid-base status. Acute fetal hypoxia activates some compensatory mechanisms for redistribution of blood that enable fetus to achieve a constancy of oxygen consumption in the fetal cerebral circulation and in fetal myocardium. Redistribution of blood to vital organs enable fetus to survive for moderately long period of limited oxygen supply, but during more severe or sustained hypoxemia, these responses were no longer maintained and decompensation with fetal tissue damage and even fetal death may occur (Crisan et al., 2009; Date et al., 2008).
Some physical findings point to a specific cause of acute pancreatitis: jaundice in biliary origin, spider angiomas in alcoholic or xanthomas and lipemia retinalis in hyperlipidemic pancreatitis.

3. Diagnosis

Acute pancreatitis in pregnancy is diagnosed by symptoms already described, by laboratory investigations and imaging methods.

3.1 Laboratory diagnosis

Laboratory investigations are the same as in non-pregnant and relies on at least a three-fold elevation of serum amylase and lipase levels in the blood. The total serum amylase level rises within 6 to 12 hours of onset of the disease, usually remain elevated for three to five days. However, there are several conditions (i.e. pathologic processes in salivary glands, fallopian tubes, bowel obstruction, cholecystitis, hepatic trauma, perforative dudoenal ulcer, hyperamylasemia on familial basis...) that may result in elevation of serum amylase. Serum lipase is elevated on the first day of ilness and remains elevated longer than the serum amylse. Specificity of serum lipase is greater than amylase, lipase level is normal in salivary gland disorder, tumors, gynecologic conditions and familial macroamylasemia. Calculation of an amylase to creatinine clearence ratio may be helpful in pregnancy, ratio greater than 5% suggests acute pancreatitis (Augustin&Majerovic, 2007).

3.2 Imaging methods

Imaging in pregnancy remains a controversial issue with concern of the effect of radiation on the developing fetus. Abdominal ultrasound (US) is the ideal imaging technique for detection of dilated pancreatic ducts and pseudocysts and focal accumulations larger than 2 to 3 cm. US has no radiation risk to the fetus, but is limited by operator skill, patient obesity and bowell dilatation. Computed tomography (CT) should be avoided, especially during the first trimester, because of radiation exposure to the fetus, but has to be performed when benefits out-weighed the risk. When a common bile duct stone is suspected, endoscopic ultrasound (EUS) has a high positive predictive value nearing 100%, even for small stones ≤ 2mm or sludge (Pitchumoni & Yegneswaran, 2009). EUS is considering to be the best imaging study to evaluate common bile duct, but requires expensive equipment, intravenous sedation and technical expertise. It is superior to magnetic resonance cholangiopancreatography (MRCP), an imaging method providing multi - planar large field of view images of the bilopancreatico-ductal system. There are some concerns about the safety of MRCP in the first trimester of pregnancy because radiofrequency pulses result in energy deposition and could potentially result in tissue heating (Leyendecker et al., 2004). MR procedures are indicated in pregnancy if other non-ionizing forms of diagnostic imaging studies are inadequate, or if the examination provides information that would otherwise require exposure to ionizing radiation. Endoscopic retrograde cholangiopancreatography (ERCP) as a diagnostic tool lost its value because of the risk of radiation and the availability of safer procedures (i.e. EUS or MRCP). ERCP should be used only as a therapeutic option in selected cases with confirmed bile duct stones. In cases of severe acute biliary pancreatitis (SABP) with or without cholangitis, early ERCP, preferably within 24 hours, is recommended (Banks&Freeman, 2006). Decompression of the common bile duct and removal of gallstones with subsequent papillotomy could prevent complications and reduce mortality in SABP. Before proceeding to therapeutic ERCP, a less-invasive diagnostic method such as MRCP or EUS should be performed. In pregnancy it is necessary to minimise radiation exposure during ERCP, the procedure should be carried out only by a very experienced endoscopic and radiologic team and the fetus should be shielded all the time (Chong & Jalihal, 2010; O'Mahony, 2007). With the advent of ERCP and MRCP, the need for IOC (intraopeartive cholangiogram) is minimal, although there have been no reports investigating the safety of IOC during pregnancy (Date et al., 2008). Laparoscopic US scan appears to be alternative to retained common bile duct stones (Date et al., 2008).

4. Treatment

4.1 Conventional treatment measures

The initial management of acute pancreatitis during pregnancy is similar to management in non-pregnant patients. Treatment consists of fluid restoration, oxygen, analgetics, antiemetics and monitoring of vital signs. Important additional measures during pregnancy include fetal monitoring, attention to the choice of medications and positioning of the mother to avoid inferior vena cava constriction.

Mild pancreatitis treated conservatively usually resolves within 7 days. Ten percent of patients have severe course, and they are best managed in an intensive care unit. The third space fluid sequestration is the most serious hemodynamic disorder leading to hypovolemia and organ hypoperfusion resulting in multiple organ failure. In volume-depleted patients the essential treatment modality is initial infusion of 500 to 1000 mL of fluid per hour (Gardner et al., 2008). Monitoring of hydration, cardiovascular, renal and respiratory functions is important for early detection of volume overload and electrolyte disturbances (Forsmark & Baillie, 2007).

Many pharmacological agents (somatostatin, octreotide, n-acetyl-cystein, gabexate mesylate, lexipafant and probiotics) have been investigated in acute pancreatitis, but because most of them have failed to show a positive effect they should be avoided in pregnancy.

Cessation of oral feeding has been thought to suppress the exocrine function of pancreas, and to prevent further pancreatic autodigestion. Bowel rest is associated with increased infectious complications, and total parenteral nutrition (TPN) and enteral nutrition (EN) have an important role in the management of acute pancreatitis. Keeping the patients "*nil by mouth*" with the use of TPN has been for years a traditional treatment of acute pancreatitis, but carries a significant risk of infections and metabolic distress. EN is physiological, helps the gut flora maintain the gut mucosal immunity, reduced translocation of bacteria, while simulataneously avoiding all the risks of TPN.

Mild cases of acute pancreatitis do not need nutritional support, as the clinical course is usually uncomplicated and a low-fat diet can be started within 3 to 5 days.

Treatment of severe necrotising pancreatitis should include enteral feeding by nasojejunal tube and if needed, should be supplemented by parenteral nutrition (Meier et al., 2006).

Prophylactic use of antibiotics is very controversial and the choice of antibiotic in pregnancy is difficult. There are concerns with regarding to the antibiotic being tranplacentally transferred to the fetus with a risk of teratogenicity. Antibiotics have no role in the treatment of mild acute pancreatitis. The use of prophylactic antibiotics in severe acute pancreatitis remains controversial. The available evidence demonstrates that antibiotic prophylaxis might have a protective effect against non-pancreatic infections, but failed to show a benefit on reduction of mortality, infected necrosis and need for surgical intervention (Bai Y et al., 2010; Jafri, 2009). Due to the lack of evidence on beneficial effect of antibiotics, an even more conservative approach is recommended in pregnancy.

4.2 Surgical treatment

Surgical treatment of pancreatitis has two aspects, which include operative intervention for the disease itself and surgical management of associated biliary tract disease once acute inflammation subsides (Ramin et al., 1995).

Since, first study published in 1963 (Greene et al., 1963), the dilemma, whether or not to treat pregnant patients with gall-stones conservatively, still exists. Risk of conservative treatment include risk to the fetus due to recurrent episodes, complications of gallstones, risk of malnutrition caused by lack of oral intake. Conversely, surgical treatment carries risk to the fetus from surgery and anaesthesia and risk specific to laparoscopic surgery. Laparoscopic cholecystectomy (once considered contraindicated during pregnancy) (Gadacz & Talamini,

1991), is today, probably, the best treatment for the patients failed to respond to conservative management or because of recurrent episodes (Cosenza et al., 1999; SAGES Guidelines, 2011). Benefits of laparoscopy during pregnancy appear similar to those non-pregnant patients including less postoperative pain, less postoperative ileus, significantly reduced hospitalization, decreased narcotic use and quick return to a regular diet and faster recovery. Other advantages of laparoscopy include less manipulation of the uterus and detection of other pathology that may be present and because of early mobility reduced risk of postoperative deep vein thrombosis (Date et al., 2008). Cholecystectomy is considered safe at all stages of pregnancy, and may be performed in any trimester of pregnancy without any increased risk to the mother or fetus (Cosenza et al., 1999; SAGES Guidelines, 2011). Historical recommendations to delay surgery until the second trimester or gestational age limit of 26 to 28 weeks of pregnancy have been refuted. Laparoscopy in pregnancy was conected with the fear of damage to the gravid uterus upon Veress or troacar insertion, technical difficulty in performing the surgery with the presence of an enlarged, gravid uterus and the concern of fetal acidemia due to decreased uterine blood flow because of increased intraabdominal pressure from insufflation and possible fetal carbon dioxide absorption (Wang et al, 2009). Also, maternal venous return secondary to increased intraperitoneal pressure from CO_2 insufflation could be present. The use of a uterine manipulator is contraindicated in pregnancy. At the begining of 2011, The Society of American Gastrointestinal and Endoscopic Surgeons (SAGES) updated its guidelines for laparoscopy during pregnancy (SAGES Guidelines, 2011). Recent reports suggest that the risk of fetal wasting and teratogenicity from gastrointestinal operation during pregnancy is minimal (Barone et al., 1999). However, some precautions should be followed: the use of an open technique for the insertion of the umbilical port, avoiding high intraperitoneal pressures, using of left lateral position to minimize aortocaval compression, avoiding rapid changes in the position of the patient and using electrocautery cautiously and away from uterus (Date et al., 2008).

Early cholecystectomy should be performed in patients with mild acute biliary pancreatitis while patients with SABP should undergo this procedure within 4 and 6 weeks, respectively, after hospital discharge (Forsmark & Baillie, 2007).

While sterile necrosis is treated conservatively, infected necrosis requires the use of antibiotics and surgical necrosectomy. Patients with infected necrosis should be treated surgically within 3 to 4 weeks after the onset of symptoms. Minimal invasive surgical techniques are new in the management of acute pancreatitis with only a few relatively small series reported to date (Van Santvoort et al., 2007).

A diagnostic and therapeutic alghorytm for acute pancreatitis in pregnancy is proposed in Diagramm 1 (Stimac & Stimac, *in press*)

5. Outcome

Prognosis for women with mild disease who respond to conservative management is excellent for mother and fetus. However, for more severe form of disease, mother mortality and fetal morbidity and mortality rates increase. In 1973 Wilkinson reviewed 98 cases of acute pancreatitis during pregnancy, 30 patients died (Wilkinson, 1973). Also, fetal death was noted in 60% of cases. Recently, the percentage of fatal outcomes of acute pancreatitis has been less than 5% (Talukdar & Vege, 2009) and is similar in pregnancy (Hernandez et al, 2007). In the past decades high perinatal mortality rate, up to 50% (Wilkinson, 1973) secondary to acute pancreatitis resulted from neonatal deaths after preterm delivery, but improvements in neonatal intensive and supportive care play important role in premature babies' survival. The mechanisms of demise include, also, placental abruption and profound metabolic disturbance, including acidosis. This highlights the importance of regular fetal monitoring and consideration of delivery if the maternal disease is deteriorating.

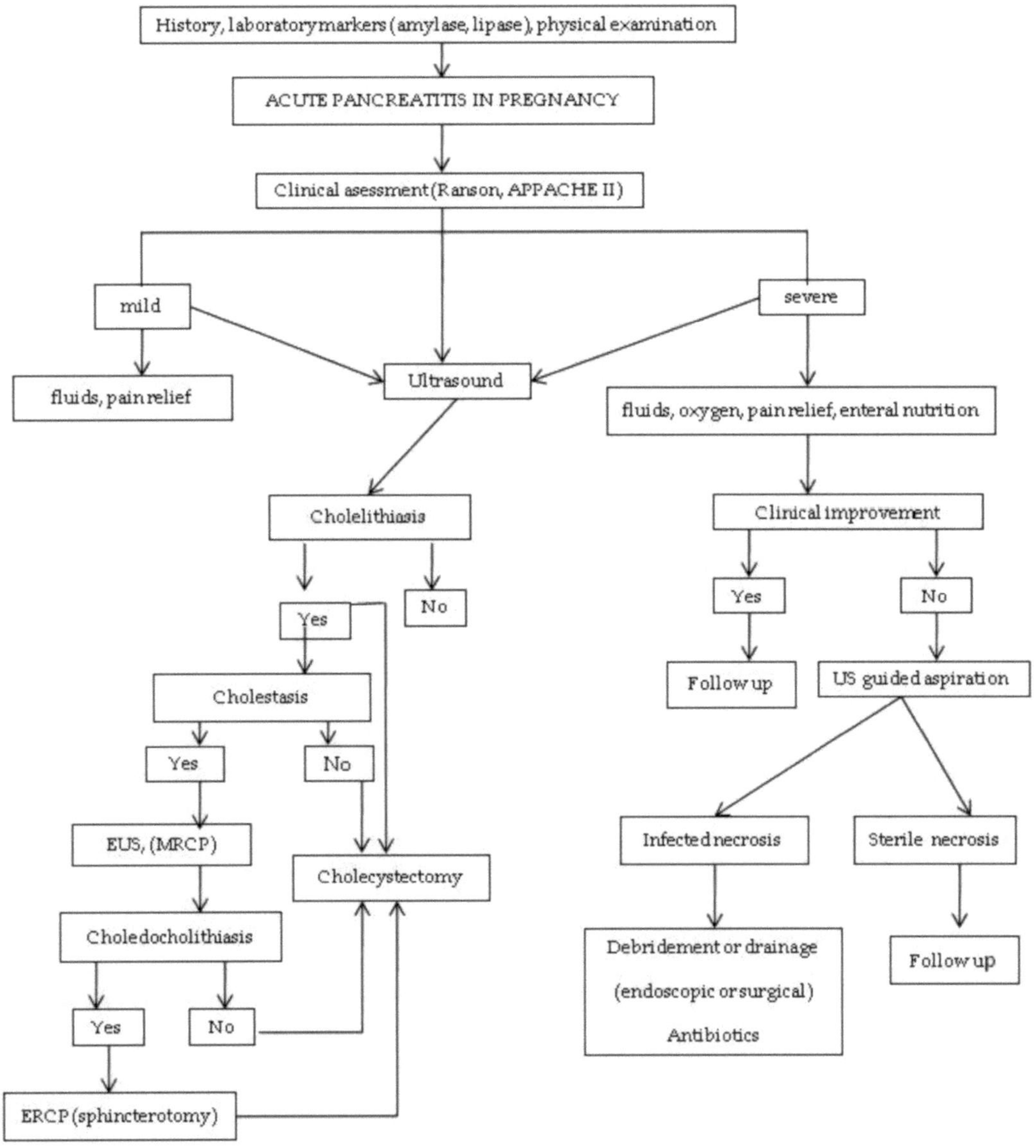

Diagramm 1. Diagnostic and therapeutic alghorithm - acute pancreatitis in pregnancy

6. Conclusions

Acute pancreatitisis is a rare entity in pregnancy, mainly caused by gallbladder disorders, in which symptoms of cholelithiasis and biliary sludge in many cases precede the symptoms and clinical picture of acute pancreatitis. Diagnosis is based on clinical presentation, laboratory investigations and imaging methods performed with precaution because of potential radiation risk to the fetus.

General management of mild AP in pregnancy is conservative and supportive, while severe AP deserves hospitalisation in intensive care unit and endoscopic or surgical interventions. The most common in pregnancy - biliary pancreatitis, can be resolved with urgent ERCP sphincterotomy and laparoscopic cholecystectomy preferably in second trimester, when technical conditions are optimal and risk for fetus and pregnant woman minimized. Although treatment of acute pancreatitis during pregnancy is similar to general approach in acute pancreatitis patients, a multidisciplinary team consisting of gastroenterologist, gastro-intestinal surgeon, radiologist and obstetrician should be included in the treatment and follow up of these patients.

7. References

Augustin, G. & Majerovic, M. (2007). Non-obstetrical acute abdomen during pregnancy. *Eur J Obstet Gynecol Reprod Biol* Vol.131, No.1, (Mar 2007), pp. 4-12

Bai, Y.; Gao, J.; Zou, DW. & Li, ZS. (2010). Antibiotics prophylaxis in acute necrotizing pancreatitis: an update. *Am J Gastroenterol* Vol. 103, No. 1, (Mar 2010), pp. 705-7

Banks, PA. & Freeman ML. (2006). Practice guidelines in acute pancreatitis. *Am J Gastroenterol* Vol. 101, No. 10, (Oct 2006), pp. 2379-400

Barone, JE.; Bears, S.; Chen, S.; Tsai, J. & Russell, JC. (1999). Outcome study of cholecystectomy during pregnancy. *Am J Surg* Vol. 177, No. 3 (Mar 1999), pp. 232-6

Berk, JE.; Smith, BH. & Krawi, MM (1971). Pregnancy pancreatitis. *Am J Gastroenterol* Vol. *56, No.* 2 (Sep 1971), pp.216-26

Chong, VH. & Jalihal, A. (2010). Endoscopic management of biliary disorders during pregnancy. *Hepatobiliary Pancreat Dis Int* Vol. 9, No. 2 (Apr 2010), pp. 180-5

Cosenza, CA.; Saffari, B.; Jabbour, N.; Stain, SC.; Garry, D.; Parekh, D. & Selby, RR. (1999). Surgical management of biliary gallstone disease during pregnancy. *Am J Surg* Vol. 178, No. 6 (Dec 1999), pp. 545-8

Crisan, LS.; Steidl, ET. & Rivera-Alsina, ME. (2008). Acute hyperlipidemic pancreatitis in pregnancy. *Am J Obstet Gynecol* Vol. 198, No. 5 (May 2008), pp.e57-9

Date, RS.; Kaushal, M. & Ramesh, A.(2008). A review of the management of gallstone disease and its complications in pregnancy. *Am J Surg* 2008; Vol. 196, No. 4 (Oct 2008), pp. 599-608

Forsmark, CE. & Baillie, J. (2007). AGA Institute technical review on acute pancreatitis. *Gastroenterology* Vol. 132, No. 5 (May 2007), pp. 2022-44

Gadacz, TR. & Talamini, MA. (1991). Traditional versus laparoscopic cholecystectomy. *Am J Surg* Vol. 161, No. 3 (Mar 1991), pp. 336-8

Gardner, TB., Vege, SS., Pearson, RK. & Chari, ST. (2008). Fluid resuscitation in acute pancreatitis. *Clin Gastroel Hepatol* Vol. 6, No. 10 (Oct 2008), pp. 1070-6

Guidelines for diagnosis, treatment, and use of laparoscopy for surgical problems during pregnancy: this statement was reviewed and approved by the Board of Governors of the Society of American Gastrointestinal and Endoscopic Surgeons (SAGES). (2008). *Surg Endosc* Vol. 22, No. 4 (Apr 2008), pp. 849-61

Hernandez, A., Petrov, MS., Brooks, DC., Banks, PA., Ashley, SW. & Tavakkolizadeh, A. (2007). Acute pancreatitis in pregnancy: a 10-year single center experience. *J Gastrointest Surg* Vol. 11, No. 12 (Dec 2007), pp.1623-7

Jafri, NS., Mahid SS, Idstein SR., Hornung, CA. & Galandiuk S. (2009). Antibiotic prophylaxis is not protective in severe acute pancreatitis: a systematic review and meta-analysis. *Am J Surg* Vol. 197, No. 6 (Jun 2009), pp. 806-13

Leyendecker, JR., Gorengaut, V. & Brown, JJ. (2004). MR imaging of maternal diseases of the abdomen and pelvis during pregnancy and the immediate postpartum period. *Radiographics* Vol. 24, No. 5 (Sep-Oct 2004), pp. 1301-16

Meier, R., Ockenga, J., Pertkiewicz, M., Pap, A., Milinic, N. & Macfie, J. (2006). ESPEN guidelines on enteral nutrition: pancreas. *Clin Nutr* Vol. 25, No. 2 (Apr 2006), pp. 275-84

O'Mahony, S. (2007). Endoscopy in pregnancy. *Best Pract Res Clin Gastroenterol* Vol. 21, No. 5 (May 2007), pp. 893-9

Pitchumoni, CS. & Yegneswaran, B. (2009). Acute pancreatitis in pregnancy. *World J Gastroenterol* Vol. 15, No. 45 (Dec 2009), pp. 5641-6

Ramin, KD., Ramin, SM., Richey, SD. & Cunningham, FG. (1995). Acute pancreatitis in pregnancy. *Am J Obstet Gynecol* Vol. 173, No. 1 (Jul 1995), pp. 187-91

Ramin, KD. & Ramsey, PS. (2001). Disease of the gallbladder and pancreas in pregnancy. *Obstet Gynecol Clin North Am* Vol. 28, No. 3 (Sep 2001), pp. 571-80

Stimac D. & Stimac T (in press). Acute pancreatitis in pregnancy. *EJGH (in press)*

Talukdar, R. & Vege, SS. (2009). Recent developments in acute pancreatitis. *Clin Gastroenterol Hepatol* Vol. 7, No. 11 Suppl. (Nov 2009), S3-S9

Van Santvoort, HC., Besselink, MG., Horvath, KD., Sinanan, MN., Bollen, TL., Van Ramshorst, B. & Gooszen, HG. (2007). Videoscopic assisted retroperitoneal debridement in infected necrotizing pancreatitis. *HPB* Vol. 9, No. 2 (Feb 2007), pp. 156-9

Wang, GJ., Gao, CF., Wei, D., Wang, C. & Ding, SQ. (2009). Acute pancreatitis: Etiology and common pathogenesis. *World J Gastroenterol* Vol. 15, No. 12 (Mar 2009), pp. 1427-30

Wilkinson, EJ. (1973). Acute pancreatitis in pregnancy: a review of 98 cases and a report of 8 new cases. *Obstet Gynecol Surv* Vol. 28, No. 5 (May 1973), pp. 281-303

5

Pancreatitis in Children

Alfredo Larrosa-Haro[1],
Carmen A. Sánchez-Ramírez[2] and Mariana Gómez-Nájera[3]
[1]*Instituto de Nutrición Humana, Centro Universitario de Ciencias de la Salud, Departamento de Clínicas de la Reproducción Humana, Crecimiento y Desarrollo Infantil, Universidad de Guadalajara. Guadalajara Jalisco,*
[2]*Universidad de Colima, Facultad de Medicina, Colonia Las Víboras, Colima, Col*
[3]*División de Pediatría, Hospital de Gineco-Pediatría # 48, Centro Médico del Bajío, Avenida México e Insurgentes, Colonia Los Paraísos, León Guanajuato*
México

1. Introduction

Decades ago acute pancreatitis was thought to be an unusual disease in children; therefore the diagnosis was delayed or even misdiagnosed. Recent published information regarding its incidence, etiological factors and clinical characteristics suggest two important issues: its prevalence and incidence seem to increase in the last decade and the concept of a benign entity has been challenged by the high proportion of cases with necrotic-hemorrhagic lesions demonstrated by image studies and the relatively frequent occurrence of relapses (1,2). It is not clear if these published data mean an actual increasing incidence or reflect the fact that pediatricians are testing more frequently for this disease. An increase in the number of cases of pancreatitis in children has been demonstrated by authors in the USA (2-8), Australia (9), Poland (10), México (11-13), and Taiwan (14).

2. Definition

The National Library of Medicine defines pancreatitis as an inflammatory disorder of the pancreas (http://www.ncbi.nlm.nih.gov). In order to diagnose pancreatitis at least two of the following criteria are required: 1) an increase in serum amylase >3 normal (>330 U/L) or in serum lipase >3 normal (>900 U/L); 2) clinical signs and symptoms consistent with the diagnosis (abdominal pain, vomiting, ileus and other signs like fever and jaundice); and 3) evidence of edema or hemorrhage and necrosis of the pancreas by ultrasonography and/or computed tomography (CT) (15). According to its evolution, pancreatitis may be classified as acute when it lasts days or a few weeks and is a reversible process. The term recurrent is used when more than one episode of acute pancreatitis occurs. Chronic pancreatitis implies the presence of pancreatic morphologic changes and losses of the exocrine and endocrine function that are not reversible.

3. Pathophysiology and etiology

Pancreatitis results from injury and inflammation of the pancreas that may be extended to peri-pancreatic tissues and remote organs. The process requires an initiating event that

triggers the acinar cells and activates the intracellular trypsinogen and other digestive enzymes. The resultant acinar cell damage produces pancreatic edema and a local inflammatory response associated with the release of inflammatory mediators (6,15-17).
In most cases of pancreatitis more than one etiological factor may be indentified; from this point of view pancreatitis is better defined as a complex multifactorial disease (Figure 1).

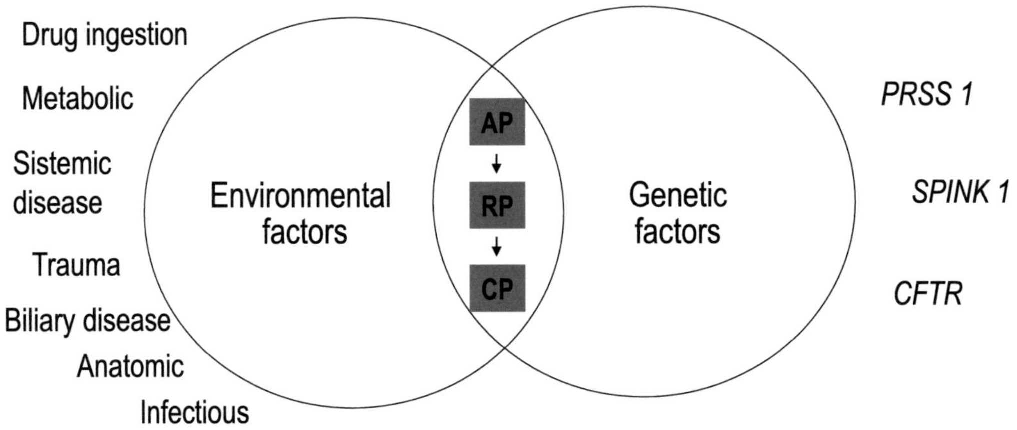

Fig. 1. Etiologic factors associated to pancreatitis. AP: acute pancreatitis; RP: recurrent pancreatitis; CP: chronic pancreatitis.

Studies performed in adults have described that the prevalence of the etiological factors have changed with time: the frequency of alcoholic induced chronic pancreatitis has decreased, biliary tract disease accounts for a higher percentage and etiologies as autoimmune and particularly hereditary/genetic pancreatitis are reported with increasing frequency (17-19).
In children, the spectrum of factors associated to pancreatitis is very broad. The etiological factors identified in some pediatric series are described in Table 1; the most common are biliary tract disease (cholelitiasis, lithogenic bile, choledocal cyst, sphincter of Oddi dysfunction), abdominal trauma, drug ingestion and viral infections. The family history of pancreatitis is an important etiological factor that has to be asked, since hereditary pancreatitis may be defined as two patients with history of pancreatitis within one generation or more than two patients in more than one generation (20). In 7.2 to 37.6% of children with acute pancreatitis, no etiological factors are identified and these cases are classified as idiopathic (3-5,9,10,14,21-25).
Another issue regarding etiology is the genetics of pancreatic disease. Recent evidence suggests that a significant proportion of cases with idiopathic pancreatitis, particularly recurrent and chronic, may be associated to mutations. The first pancreatitis susceptibility gene discovered was *PRSS1* (protease, serine 1). Mutations in *PRSS1,* which encodes cationic trypsinogen, were discovered in families with hereditary pancreatitis (26-28) and the most common *PRSS1* mutation results in an Arg122 His substitution, which eliminates the key autolysis site that allows for rapid trypsin self-destruction in solutions with a low calcium concentration, such as inside the acinar cell (Whitcomb, 1996). This means that trypsin activation and prolonged survival inside the acinar cell leads to pancreatitis due to a

premature trypsinogen activation and persistent trypsin activity as being key initiators of pancreatic injury, because all of the zymogens are activated by trypsin and thereby increase susceptibility to acute and chronic pancreatitis (29).

Author	Year	n	Biliary	Anatomic	Family history	Trauma	Drug ingestion	Metabolic	Infectious	Sistemic disease	Genetic	Idiopathic
Mao-Meng Tiao	2002	61	11.4		-	45.9	6.6		1.6	14.7	-	19.7
López	2002	274	10	-	-	19	5	-	-	53	-	17
Pezilli	2002	50	28	-	6	10	2	2	12	6	-	34
De Banto	2002	202	6.4	2.5	6.9	14.4	10.4	3.5	2.5	6.4	2.5	37.6
Werlin	2003	180	12.2	3.3	-	13.9	12.2	6.1	7.2	13.9	2.8	7.2
Choi	2003	56	29	2	-	11	30	-		9	-	12
Alvarez	2003	31	16.1	3.2	-	6.5	9.7	3.2	19.3	6.5	-	35.5
Sobczynska-Tomaszewska	2006	92	10.9	15.2	27.2	5.4	-	8.7	2.2	4.3	33.7	29.3
Nydegger	2007	279	5.4	-	-	36.3	3.2	5.8	2.2	22.2	-	25.1
Kandula	2008	87	5.7	-	-	8.0	8	-	21.8	34.5	-	21
Sánchez-Ramírez	2011	92	25	4.3	14.1	20	18.5	17.4	3.3	12	9.8	36.8

Table 1. Etiologic factors in 11 series of children with pancreatitis. Results are presented as percentages.

If trypsinogen becomes prematurely activated, a small fraction is directly inhibited by a pancreatic secretory trypsin inhibitor (PSTI), which is also known as serine protease inhibitor Kazal-type 1 (SPINK1). The importance of this specific trypsin inhibitor is that patients with mutated *SPINK1* develop recurrent acute and chronic pancreatitis.(30-32).

Another gene associated to the development of pancreatitis is the cystic fibrosis transmembrane conductance regulator (CFTR), which is a regulated anion channel that is located at the luminal surface of the duct cell and the key molecule in the pancreatic duct responsible for fluid secretion. The loss of bicarbonate secretion in the duct caused by *CFTR* mutations confers a less alkaline pancreatic juice that does not inhibits activated trypsin by interfering with the transition between trypsinogen and trypsin (33-35) and the ability to flush active enzymes out of the duct may be lost. The CFTR also protects the pancreas by quickly sweeping zymogens out of the pancreas. In 1998, two groups (34,35) demonstrated that *CFTR* mutations were also common in idiopathic and alcoholic chronic pancreatitis, which indicates that some of the 1,250 known *CFTR* gene sequence variants cause pancreatitis, particularly ΔF508 in which a three-base pair deletion causes loss of phenylalanine 508 and represents about 70% of CFTR mutations worldwide (36). The detection of mutations in the genes associated to pancreatitis is important since it has been demonstrated by other authors that the interaction of environmental and genetic factors (i.e. N34S + alcohol or PRSS1 + smoking) further increased the probability of a disease (20).

The majority of the cases with mutations in genes associated to pancreatitis get ill in childhood. However, in a significant number of cases the definite signs of chronic pancreatitis may be found only after a long follow-up period. Keim describes that approximately 80% of patients with SPINK1 mutations showed at least one of the definite signs of chronic pancreatitis after a follow-up time of 15 to 20 years. In 50% of the patients with a PRSS1 mutation, chronic pancreatitis may be diagnosed after 25 years of follow up. In addition, it has been demonstrated a geographical variation regarding etiology, particularly genetic variants.

The genetic variants (20) performed in pediatric population are very few compared to the studies performed in adult population. The mutations associated to pancreatitis that have been identified in some pediatric series are described in Table 2. There is a trend of a higher proportion of mutations in patients with RP and CP than in AP, although most of the studies included only patients with RP and CP and not cases with AP (10,31,37,38).

In a pediatric series of 92 children with AP and RP attended at the Hospital of Pediatría (Guadalajara, México), we identified mutations (R122H and N34S) in a group of AP exclusively; this represented a 13-fold increased risk of having AP compared with the general population in which we did not identified these mutations. The *SPINK1* N34S mutation was identified in 3/58 cases with AP, none in the group of RP nor in general population and it was found that the cases bearing the *SPINK1* N34S G allele exhibited a 10-fold increased risk of developing AP compared with the general population, suggesting that the *SPINK1* N34S mutation represents an etiological risk factor for the development of AP in our pediatric patients (25).

It is important to highlight that genetic testing in children with pancreatitis is not only useful for diagnosis but also as a predictive factor as it helps to identify individuals at risk for a more severe course of the disease.

4. Clinical, laboratory and image data

A summary of studies that report the frequency of the symptoms and signs in children with pancreatitis is presented in Table 3. The most common symptoms were abdominal pain followed by vomiting; in our series, ileus reached almost one-half of the cases studied (1,39,40). Abdominal pain is less commonly observed in children younger than 2 years, since it may be manifested by irritability (24,41).

In pediatric series with pancreatitis an elevation of serum amylase has been reported in 83.6 to 85.5% of the cases and of serum lipase in 82 to 90% (1,5,14). Although it has a relatively low sensitivity and specificity (75 to 92% and 20 to 60%, respectively), serum amylase remains as the test most frequently used to confirm pancreatitis. Serum amylase begins to increase 2 to 12 hours after the pancreatic insult and peaks at 12 to 72 hours after the onset of symptoms. Sensitivity and specificity of serum lipase is 86-100% and 50-99% respectively. By increasing the cutoff level to greater than three times the upper normal limit, sensitivity may increase to 100% and specificity to 99%. Lipase level remains elevated for a longer period of time in the plasma than amylase; increase occurs within 4 to 8 hours after symptom onset, peaks at 24 hours and decreases over 8 to 14 days. By using serum amylase and lipase determinations together, clinical sensitivity for the diagnosis of pancreatitis increases to 94% (15).

Imaging studies are a crucial tool to perform the diagnosis of pancreatitis. Ultrasound (US) is the primary imaging modality. However, the pancreas size is age-dependent and its echogenicity is variable; its reliability to identify pancreatitis seems to be higher in children. The US sensitivity in adults is 62-67% for acute and 50-80% for chronic pancreatitis, respectively (42). To our knowledge, in children there are no studies assessing the accuracy of US in the diagnosis of pancreatitis. The computed tomography (CT) provides additional information about potential etiologies besides the presence of necrosis and other complications (6); however, it involves radiation exposure and has poor sensitivity in detecting ductal abnormalities (6,43). The CT with IV contrast is useful to identify necrotic-hemorrhagic areas, fluid collections and peri-pancreatic inflammation; as pancreatic necrosis occurs 24 to 48 hour after the symptom onset it is recommended to perform the CT 48 to 72 hours after pain or vomiting appeared. In two pediatric series, CT identified abnormalities more frequently than US (1, 14).

Study	Year	Patients (n)	Clinical signs and symptoms (%)				
			Abdominal pain	Vomiting	Ileus	Fever	Jaundice
Mao-Meng Tiao, *et al.*	2002	61	95	37.7	-	29.5	|3.2
Pezzilli *et al.*	2002	50	96	-	-	-	-
Alvarez, *et al.*	2003	31	90	38	-	9.6	-
Werlin, *et al.*	2003	214	67.8	44.9	-	-	-
Sánchez-Ramírez, *et al.*	2007	55	94.5	85.5	47.3	27.3	9.1

Table 2. Mutations associated to acute (AP), recurrent (AR) or chronic (CP) pancreatitis in 624 children from different countries. Results are presented in percentages.

Author (year)	Country	n	SPINK (%)		PRSS1 (%)	
			AP	RP or CP	AP	RP or CP
Witt (2000)	Germany and Austria	96	-	19.6	-	6.2
Witt (2001)	Germany and Austria	164	-	20.7	-	4.2
Sobczynska-Tomaszewska (2006)	Poland	92	-	8.7	-	9.2
Werlin (2003)	USA	180	0.6	1.2	-	1.1
Sanchez-Ramírez (2011)	México	92	5.2	-	1.7	-

Table 3. Clinical characteristics in 411 children with pancreatitis from five pediatric series. Values of clinical signs and symptoms are presented as percentages.

The magnetic resonance cholangio-pancreaticography is non-invasive and do not expose the patients to radiation. It may provide a comprehensive morphological description of the biliary and pancreatic duct, making the endoscopic retrograde cholangio-pancreaticography (ERCP) unnecessary for diagnostic purposes (43).

5. Disease spectrum

Acute pancreatitis should be thought as an event and chronic pancreatitis as a process (16). Recurrent pancreatitis could be considered as a transition state until definite signs of chronic pancreatitis are detectable (20).The disease spectrum of pancreatitis is variable, ranging from mild edematous to severe fulminant pancreatitis, with potentially devastating complications.

DeBanto *et al.* (4) proposed a scoring system to predict the severity of pancreatitis in children. This scoring may permit to estimate the probability of having or not a severe disease; children who have a score of ≥3 on admission should be sent to a "step down" unit for close monitoring; if they reached the 48-h point with a score of ≤2, they would be transferred to a regular ward bed.
This scoring system has eight parameters, four to be scored on admission and four by 48h. The criteria for admission to an intensive care unit from the emergency room are: age <7 yr, weight <23 kg, white blood cell count >18,500 and lactic dehydrogenase >2,000. The 48h criteria are calcium <8.3 mg/dL, albumin <2.6 g/dL, fluid-sequestration >75 ml/kg/48 h and a rise in blood urea nitrogen >5 mg/dL.

6. Treatment

Once the diagnosis of acute pancreatitis has been confirmed, the approach during the acute phase is initially directed to maintain the homeostasis by means of an IV fluid, electrolyte and glucose infusion according to the patients needs for age, hydration status and electrolyte balance. An adequate hemodynamic condition will prevent ischemia and pancreatic necrosis. The cases with abdominal CT suggestive of severe hemorrhagic pancreatitis should be admitted to an intensive care unit; the DeBanto's score system on admission and at 48 hours may help the clinician to decide the admission to intensive care. A nasogastric tube with drainage by gravity will help to decompress the bowel and may improve the abdominal pain as well as the vomiting; in patients with ileus the nasogastric drainage will have intestinal or even fecal aspect (42,44,45).
Antibiotics are not recommended in all cases of children with acute pancreatitis. They should be used in the presence of biliary obstruction, pancreatic abscesses or in selected cases of necrotic-hemorrhagic pancreatitis. However, these recommendations have been outlined from adult series with pancreatitis; these criteria have been used somehow in children although systematic pediatric data are lacking (42,44,45). Management of abdominal pain is crucial as this symptom may be associated to an adverse outcome; narcotics are not recommended due to its potential effect on Oddi's sphincter (45).
Surgery may be indicated at least three weeks after the acute episode in patients with severe pancreatitis associated to extra-pancreatic fluid collections, abscesses and large pseudocysts (14,42). The surgical approach should be considered in particular cases.
The core goals of treatment are to support the involution of the pancreatic inflammation and to prevent the activation of the pancreatic enzymes. A logical way to achieve this goal is to avoid the physiologic stimulus of pancreatic secretion, namely the presence of macronutrients in the stomach and in the proximal duodenum (46). In children, this approach implies parenteral or enteral nutritional support.
Children with acute pancreatitis are at risk of acute malnutrition due to two conditions: a) an increase in energy and nutrient requirements related to their catabolic disease; and b) iatrogenic or spontaneous oral food restriction (47). The nutritional risk is inversely proportional to age as growth speed and energy/nutrient requirements are higher in younger children; this is a physiologic condition between catabolic states in children *versus* adults.
Fasting in adults with mild acute pancreatitis is not recommended and oral feedings may be initiated when pain stops. No benefit of enteral or parenteral nutrition has been

demonstrated in these patients (48). Parenteral or enteral nutrition have been widely used for more than two decades in adult patients when fasting must be prolonged beyond one week because the pancreatic inflammation persists or in the presence of hemorrhagic pancreatitis. Although these two modalities of nutritional intervention have shown their efficacy, evidence related to the advantages of enteral nutrition has gradually accumulated. The rationale for using enteral nutrition is that nutrient infusion ahead the duodenum diminishes or avoids the secretion of cholecystokinin, secretin and pancreozymin and consequently maintains a low pancreatic exocrine activity. However, there is controversy regarding the infusion site in the GI tract. Some authors have demonstrated that nasogastric infusion is a secure and well tolerated alternative although their data relate more to non-severe pancreatitis (49-53). There are no published data regarding enteral nutrition with a nasogastric infusion in pediatric patients with pancreatitis.

The *European Society for Clinical Nutrition and Metabolism* recommends initiating oral_ after abdominal pain has disappeared, when amylase and lipase concentration are almost normal, gastric emptying is normal and complications were solved out (48,53). A non-randomized study in adults with acute pancreatitis identified that 21% of patients presented a pain relapse and 12 day delay between onset of symptoms and oral refeeding. In a retrospective study in children with acute pancreatitis, 15.4% and 10.3% had recurrence of pain and amylasemia when oral feedings were started before the days 7th and 10th respectively (52,54,55).

An elemental diet or formulas with oligopeptides seem the best options to achieve a maximum suppression of the pancreatic enzyme secretion (48,53); however, a recent meta-analysis states that polymeric diets have similar efficacy in the nutritional support of adults with acute pancreatitis. In the last two decades a number of children with mild or severe pancreatitis have been managed with naso-jejunal enteral nutrition using an elemental diet with low recurrence and complication rates (54-57).

Adults with pancreatitis have increased energy and protein requirements; this has been estimated between 30 to 50% above normal daily requirements (Meier 2006). In children with pancreatitis this increased needs have been assumed for parenteral or enteral nutrition during the disease. In a series of children with pancreatitis managed with home enteral nutrition and energy intake of about 80% of the daily energy requirements an actual loss of weight was observed along the 14th to the 21th day of the intrevention (55). In a recent open clinical trial in 17 children with acute pancreatitis managed with enteral nutrition, an enteral energy supply of ~130% of daily energy requirements led to a stable weight along the trial and to a significant increase in serum albumin (57) .

Enteral nutrition prevents the systemic inflammatory response, luminal stasis, bacterial overgrowth and bacterial translocation (58). Besides maintaining the "pancreatic rest", enteral nutrition reduces the length and costs of hospitalization and the frequency of sepsis (59,60). In prospective studies it has been demonstrated that the early onset of enteral nutrition -within 48 hours after admission- actually prevents the severity of the pancreatic damage, maintains enteral function and improve oral tolerance.

The proposal of nutritional intervention in children with acute pancreatitis is supported in several facts: a) prevents acute malnutrition; b) provides nutrients for tissue healing; and c) modulates the systemic inflammatory response and thus prevents multiple organic failure (59). Published data related to nutritional support in children with acute pancreatitis are scanty. In the experience of the authors of this chapter in dealing with children with acute pancreatitis for about two decades, some facts may be underlined: a) children with mild or edematous pancreatitis managed NPO and IV saline/glucose solutions do present acute malnutrition with a loss of more than 1 standard deviation of weigh for height or triceps skinfold (13,39,54); b) fasting for less than 7 days has an increased risk of recurrence of abdominal pain, raise in amylase levels >3x and recurrence of US abnormalities in around 20% of cases (13,54); c) sepsis is almost inexistent in children managed with enteral nutrition; d) it is feasible to handle home enteral nutrition even with families with parents with mid educational level (55); e) decrease in amylase levels and symptomatic improvement are similar in children managed with total parenteral nutrition *versus* enteral nutrition (55); d) acute malnutrition may be prevented with the infusion of ~ 130% of the daily recommended intake of energy and macronutrients (56,57).

The suggested nutritional intervention protocol for children with acute pancreatitis is presented in Table 4. The enteral infusion may be initiated once the ileum is resolved (the nasogastric drainage is clear, peristalsis is normal and the patient is passing gas and stools), even in the presence of abdominal pain. The enteral tube must be located in the jejunum and the infusion should be continuous for 24 hours if the patient remains hospitalized or discontinued for six hours (from 24 PM to 6 AM) if the patient is managed at home. The energy target is ~130% of daily recommended intake of energy for age and sex and the recommended formula is an elemental diet; the authors do not have experience with the management of semi-elemental or polymeric formulas. The large amount of fluids required to reach this goal are tolerated quite well (56-57).

Enteral tube	Naso-jejunal feeding tube (2-way, radio-opaque tube) Infusion site placed ahead the angle of Treitz (verify tube placement with abdomen X-ray) Tube marked with permanent ink at the nostril fixation level
Enteral formula	Elemental formula (free amino-acids, glucose polymers and essential fatty acids). 80g of formula = carbohydrate 63g, protein 12.6g and fat 0.81g.
Enteral infusion	24-hour continuous infusion in hospitalized patients, 18-hour infusion in home enteral nutrition. Initial infusion: 100% of DRI of energy for age and sex; increase 15% daily to a target of ~ 130%
Re-feeding	Oral refeeding; edematous pancreatitis 7 days and severe pancreatitis 14 days after de symptom onset (in absence of abdominal pain and serum amylase and lipase not higher than 2x) Re-feeding diet: Diet high in carbohydrate and moderate in fat and protein starting with 70% of energy DRI and increasing 10% daily to reach 100% DRI.

DRI: Daily recommended intake

Table 4. Enteral nutrition recommendations in children with acute pancreatitis.

7. References

[1] Sánchez- Ramírez CA, Larrosa-Haro A, Flores-Martínez S, Sánchez-Corona J, Villa-Gómez A, Macías-Rosales R. Acute and recurrent pancreatitis in children: etiological factors. Acta Paediatr. 2007;96:534–537.

[2] Bai HX, Lowe ME, Husain SZ. What have we learned about acute pancreatitis in children? J Pediatr Gastroenterol Nutr. 2011;52:262-270.

[3] Lopez M. The changing incidence of acute pancreatitis in children: a single-institution perspective. J Pediatr. 2002;140:622–624.

[4] DeBanto J, Goday P, Pedroso M, Iftikhar R, Fazel A, Nayyar S, *et al.* Acute pancreatitis in children. Am J Gastroenterol. 2002;97:1726–1731.

[5] Werlin S, Kugathasan S, Cowan B. Pancreatitis in children. J Pediatr Gastroenterol Nutr. 2003;37:592–595.

[6] Lowe M, Greer J. Pancreatitis in children and adolescents. Curr Gastroenterol Rep. 2008;10:128-135.

[7] Park A, Latif SU, Shah AU, Tian J, Werlin S, Hsiao A, *et al.* Changing referral trends of acute pancreatitis in children: A 12-year singe-center analysis. J Pediatr Gastroenterol Nutr. 2009;49:316-322.

[8] Morinville V, Barmada M, Lowe M. Increasing incidence of acute pancreatitis at an American pediatric tertiary care center: is greater awareness among physicians responsible? Pancreas. 2010;39:5-8.

[9] Nydegger A, Heine R, Ranuh R, Gegati-Levy R, Crameri J, Oliver M. Changing incidence of acute pancreatitis: 10-year experience at the Royal Children´s Hospital, Melbourne. J Gastroenterol Hepatol. 2007;22:1313-1316.

[10] Sobczynska-Tomaszewska A, Bak Daniel, Oralewska B, Oracz G, Norek A, Czerska K, et al. Analysis of CFTR, SPINK1, PRSS1 and AAT mutations in children with acute or chronic pancreatitis. J Pediatr Gastroenterol Nutr. 2006;43:299–306.

[11] Larrosa A, Sánchez C, Villa A, Macías R, Martínez E. Increasing incidence of acute pancreatitis as an emergent syndrome. J Pediatr Gastroenterol Nutr. 2006;43:E31.

[12] Larrosa-Haro A, Macías-Rosales R, Hurtado-López E, Cámara-López ME, Rodríguez-Anguiano K, Luna-Pech A. Desnutrición secundaria en el Servicio de Gastroenterología y Nutrición de un hospital pediátrico de referencia. Rev Gastroenterol Mex. 2006;71:157.

[13] Larrosa-Haro A, Sánchez-Ramírez CA, Villa-Gómez A, Macías-Rosales R, Martínez-Puente E. Pancreatitis aguda y recurrente: Incremento en la incidencia. Pancreatitis como un síndrome emergente. Rev Gastroenterol Mex. 2006;71:157.

[14] Mao-Meng Tiao, Jiin-Haur Chuang, Sheung-Fat Ko, Hsin-Wei Kuo, Chi-Di Liang, Chao-Long Chen. Pancreatitis in children: clinical analysis of 61 cases in Southern Taiwan. Chang Gung Med J. 2002;25:162-168.

[15] Pietzak M. Thomas D. Pancreatitis in childhood. Pediatr. Rev. 2000;21:406-412.

[16] Whitcomb D. Mechanisms of disease: advances in understanding the mechanisms leading to chronic pancreatitis. Nat Clin Pract Gastroenterol Hepatol. 2004;1:46–52.

[17] Lucidi V, Alghisi F, Dall'Oglio L, D'Apice MR, Monti L, De Angelis P, *et al.* The etiology of acute recurrent pancreatitis in children: a challenge for pediatricians. Pancreas. 2011;40:517-521.

[18] Bai Y, LiuY, Jiang H, Ji M, Lv Nonghua, Huang K, *et al.* Severe acute pancreatitis in China. Pancreas. 2007;35:232-237.

[19] Joergensen M, Brusgaard K, Gylling Cru¨ger D, Gerdes A, Schaffalitzky de Muckadell. Incidence, prevalence, etiology, and prognosis of first-time chronic pancreatitis in young patients: A Nationwide Cohort Study. Dig Dis Sci. 2010;55:2988–2998.
[20] Keim V. Role of genetic disorders in acute recurrent pancreatitis. World J Gastroenterol. 2008 Feb 21;14(7):1011-5.
[21] Pezzilli R, Morselli, Labate A, Castellano E, Barbera C, Corrao S, *et al.* Acute pancreatitis in children. An Italian multicenter study. Digest Liver Dis. 2002;34:343-348.
[22] Choi B, Lim Y, Yoon C, Kim E, Park Y, Kim K. Acute pancreatitis associated with biliary disease in children. J Gastroenterol Hepatol. 2003;18:915-21.
[23] Alvarez-Catalayud G, Bermejo F, Morales L, Claver E, Huber B, Abunaji J, *et al.* Pancreatitis aguda en la infancia. Rev Esp Enferm Dig. 2003;95:40-44.
[24] Kandula L, Lowe M. Etiology and outcome of acute pancreatitis in infants and toddlers. J Pediatr. 2008;152:106–110.
[25] Sánchez-Ramírez CA, Flores-Martínez S, García-Zapién A, Montero-Cruz S, Larrosa-Haro A, Sánchez-Corona J. Screening of R122H and N29I Mutations in the PRSS1 Gene and N34S Mutation in the SPINK1 Gene in Mexican Pediatric Patients with Acute and Recurrent Pancreatitis. Pancreas. 2012 (in press).
[26] Whitcomb D, Gorry M, Preston R, Furey W, Sossenheimer M, Ulrich C, *et al.* Hereditary pancreatitis is caused by a mutation in the cationic trypsinogen gene. Nat Genet.1996;14:141-145.
[27] Whitcomb D. Genetic predispositions to acute and chronic pancreatitis. Med Clin North Am. 2000;84:531-547.
[28] Howes N, Lerch M, Greenhalf W, Stocken D, Ellis I, Simon P, *et al.* Clinical and genetic characteristics of hereditary pancreatitis in Europe. Clin Gastroenterol Hepatol. 2004;2:252-261.
[29] Teich N, Ockenga J, Hoffmeister A, Manns M, Mössner J, Keim V. Chronic pancreatitis associated with an activation peptide mutation that facilitates trypsin activation. Gastroenterology. 2000;119:461-465.
[30] Witt H, Luck W, Hennies H, Classen M, Kage A, Lass U, et al. Mutations in the gene encoding the serine protease inhibitor, Kazal type 1 are associated with chronic pancreatitis. *Nat Genet.* 2000;25:213–216.
[31] Witt H. Gene mutations in children with chronic pancreatitis. Pancreatology. 2001;1:432–438.
[32] Pfützer R, Barmada M, Brunskill A, Finch R, Hart P, Neoptolemos J, *et al.* SPINK1/PSTI polymorphisms act as disease modifiers in familial and idiopathic chronic pancreatitis. Gastroenterology. 2000;119: 615-623.
[33] Bennett W, Huber R. Structural and functional aspects of domain motions in proteins. CRC Crit Rev Biochem. 1984;15:291-384.
[34] Sharer N, Schwarz M, Malone G, Howarth A, Painter J, Super M, *et al.* Mutations of the cystic fibrosis gene in patients with chronic pancreatitis. N Eng J Med.1998; 339: 645-652.
[35] Cohn J, Friedman K, Noone P, Knowles M, Silverman L, Jowell P. Relation between mutations of the cystic fibrosis gene and idiopathic pancreatitis. N Engl J Med.1998;339:653-658.
[36] Choudari C, Glen A, Stuart S. Pancreatitis and cystic fibrosis gene mutations. Gastroenterology Clinics. 1999;3:543-549.

[37] Drenth J, Morsche R, Jansen J. Mutations in serine protease inhibitor Kazal type I are strongly associated with chronic pancreatitis. Gut 2002;50:687-692.

[38] Kaneko K, Nagasaki Y, Furukawa T, Mizutamari H, Sato A, Masamune A, *et al.* Analysis of the human pancreatic secretory trypsin inhibitor (PSTI) gene mutations in Japanese patients with chronic pancreatitis. J Hum Genet. 2001;46:293–297.

[39] García-Rodríguez E, Álvarez-López MC, Martínez-Puente EO, Larrosa-Haro A, Rodríguez-Alvarez TH, Coello-Ramírez P. Pancreatitis aguda en niños. Rev Gastroenteol Mex. 1995;60 (Supl):89.

[40] Villa-Gómez A, Larrosa-Haro A, Martínez-Puente EO, Bojórquez-Ramos MC, Castillo de León YA, Macías-Rosales R, Sánchez-Ramírez CA, García-Salazar O. Acute pancreatitis *versus* acute recurrent pancreatitis: Clinical and biochemical associated factors. J Pediatr Gastroenterol Nutr. 2004;39 (Suppl 1):S-366.

[41] Park A, Latif SU, Ahmad M, Bultron G, Orabi A, Bhandari V, *et al.* A comparison of presentation and management trends in acute pancreatitis between infants/toddlers and older children. J Pediatr Gastroenterol Nutr. 2010;51:167-70.

[42] Nydegger A, Couper RT, Oliver MR.Childhood pancreatitis.J Gastroenterol Hepatol. 2006 ;21:499-509.

[43] Darge K, Anupindi S. Pancreatitis and the role of US, MRCP and ERCP. Pediatr Radiol. 2009;Suppl 2:S153-S157.

[44] Bragg JD, Cox KR, Despins L, Hall LW, Bechtold ML. Improvements in care in acute pancreatitis by the adoption of an acute pancreatitis algorithm. JOP. 2010;11:183-185.

[45] Takeda K, Takada T, Kawarada Y, Hirata K, Mayumi T, Yoshida M, *et al.* JPN Guidelines for the management of acute pancreatitis: medical management of acute pancreatitis. J Hepatobiliary Pancreat Surg. 2006;13:42-47.

[46] McClave SA. Nutrition support in acute pancreatitis. Gastroenterol Clin North Am. 2007;36:65-74,vi.

[47] Curtis CS, Kudsk KA. Nutrition support in pancreatitis. Surg Clin North Am. 2007;87:1403-15, viii.

[48] Meier R, Ockenga J, Pertkiewicz M, Pap A, Milinic N, Macfie J (German Society for Nutritional Medicine), Löser C, Keim V; ESPEN (European Society for Parenteral and Enteral Nutrition). ESPEN Guidelines on Enteral Nutrition: Pancreas. Clin Nutr. 2006;25:275-284.

[49] Eatock FC, Chong P, Menezes N, Murray L, McKay CJ, Carter CR, *et al.* A randomized study of early nasogastric versus nasojejunal feeding in severe acute pancreatitis. Am J Gastroenterol. 2005;100:432-439.

[50] Petrov MS, Pylypchuk RD, Uchugina AF. A systematic review on the timing of artificial nutrition in acute pancreatitis. Br J Nutr. 2009;101:787-793.

[51] Kumar A, Singh N, Prakash S, Saraya A, Joshi YK. Early enteral nutrition in severe acute pancreatitis: a prospective randomized controlled trial comparing nasojejunal and nasogastric routes. J Clin Gastroenterol. 2006;40:431-434.

[52] Petrov MS, van Santvoort HC, Besselink MG, Cirkel GA, Brink MA, Gooszen HG. Oral refeeding after onset of acute pancreatitis: a review of literature. Am J Gastroenterol. 2007;102:2079-2084.

[53] Ioannidis O, Lavrentieva A, Botsios D. Nutrition support in acute pancreatitis. JOP. 2008 ;9:375-390.

[54] Martínez-Puente EO, Larrosa-Haro A, Rodríguez-Álvarez TH. Pancreatitis aguda en niños: Protocolo prospectivo de soporte nutricional en su casa con nutrición enteral y dieta elemental. Rev Gastroenterol Mex. 1996;61(Suppl):38.
[55] Martínez-Puente EO, Larrosa-Haro A. Home nutritional support with a duodenal infusion of an elemental diet in children with acute pancreatitis. J Pediatr Gastroenterol Nutr. 2000;31(Suppl 2):S152.
[56] Gómez-Nájera M, Larrosa-Haro A. Alimentación enteral con infusión yeyunal de dieta elemental en la prevención de desnutrición aguda en niños con pancreatitis aguda. Rev Gastroenterol Mex. 2009;74(Supl 2):90.
[57] Gómez-Nájera M, Larrosa-Haro A, Bojórquez-Ramos MC, Macías-Rosales R, Castillo de León Y, García Salazar O. Enteral Nutrition in Children with Acute Pancreatitis: Open Clinical Trial. Proceedings, Annual Meeting of the North American Society for Pediatric Gastroenterology, Hepatology and Nutrition. Orlando FL, Oct 2010.
[58] Petrov MS, Kukosh MV, Emelyanov NV. A randomized controlled trial of enteral versus parenteral feeding in patients with predicted severe acute pancreatitis shows a significant reduction in mortality and in infected pancreatic complications with total enteral nutrition. Dig Surg. 2006;23:336-344.
[59] O'Keefe SJ, Sharma S. Nutrition support in severe acute pancreatitis. Gastroenterol Clin North Am. 2007;36:297-312, vii.
[60] Qin HL, Su ZD, Hu LG, Ding ZX, Lin QT. Effect of parenteral and early intrajejunal nutrition on pancreatic digestive enzyme synthesis, storage and discharge in dog models of acute pancreatitis. World J Gastroenterol. 2007;13:1123-1128.

6

Pancreatitis in Cystic Fibrosis and CFTR-Related Disorder

Michael J. Coffey[1] and Chee Y. Ooi[1,2]
[1]*School of Women's and Children's Health, Faculty of Medicine, University of New South Wales,*
[2]*Department of Gastroenterology, Sydney Children's Hospital Randwick, Sydney, New South Wales, Australia*

1. Introduction

Named after the pathologic changes seen in the pancreas, cystic fibrosis (CF) is the most common lethal genetic disease in Caucasians, occuring in around 1 in 3000 live births. CF is uncommon among Asians (1 in 31,000 live births) and African Americans (1 in 15,000 live births) (Maitra & Kumar, 2005). It is caused by disease-causing mutations on both cystic fibrosis transmembrane conductance regulator (*CFTR*) alleles. Acute, recurrent-acute and chronic pancreatitis in association with *CFTR* mutations can develop in the setting of either CF disease or CFTR-related pancreatitis, which belong within the spectrum of disorders associated with CFTR dysfunction.

2. Cystic fibrosis (mucoviscidosis)

Cystic fibrosis was historically considered to be a multi-system disease which manifested clinically either at birth (with intestinal obstruction due to meconium ileus) or in infancy/early childhood (with failure to thrive due to pancreatic insufficiency and recurrent/chronic sino-pulmonary disease). Our understanding of this disease has changed in recent times, particularly after the discovery of the *CFTR* gene. Any one, or all of the manifestations of CF can occur at any point, from before birth through to childhood, adolescence and even in adulthood.

The *CFTR* gene responsible for CF is located on chromosome band 7q31.2, and encodes for a cyclic adenosine monophosphate (cAMP)-dependent chloride channel (Fig. 1). This particular chloride channel is located in the apical membrane of secretory and absorptive epithelium of the pancreas, intestine, liver, airway, vas deferens and sweat glands. The manifestations of CF generally arise from ductal and glandular obstruction due to an inability to hydrate macromolecules within the ductal lumen.

3. Pancreatic diseases associated with CF and CFTR-related diseases

Immunohistologic and pathologic studies have identified localisation of CFTR protein at the apical domain of the pancreatic ductal cells. Obstruction of proximal intralobular ducts by inspissated protein plugs (obstructive tubulopathy) has been shown as early as during the in-utero period in CF (Oppenheimer & Esterly, 1976). The susceptibility of the pancreas to intraductal obstruction resulting from CFTR dysfunction is thought to be due to the high macromolecule concentration of the secretions and the dependence on the CFTR chloride (and bicarbonate) channel for maintaing fluid balance. Progressive ductal obstruction and fibrosis of acinar tissue presents as pancreatic insufficiency either at birth or in early childhood (Waters et al. 1990). Complete pancreatic exocrine deficiency is the seen in 85% to 90% of patients with CF (Durno et al., 2002; Ooi et al., 2011a).

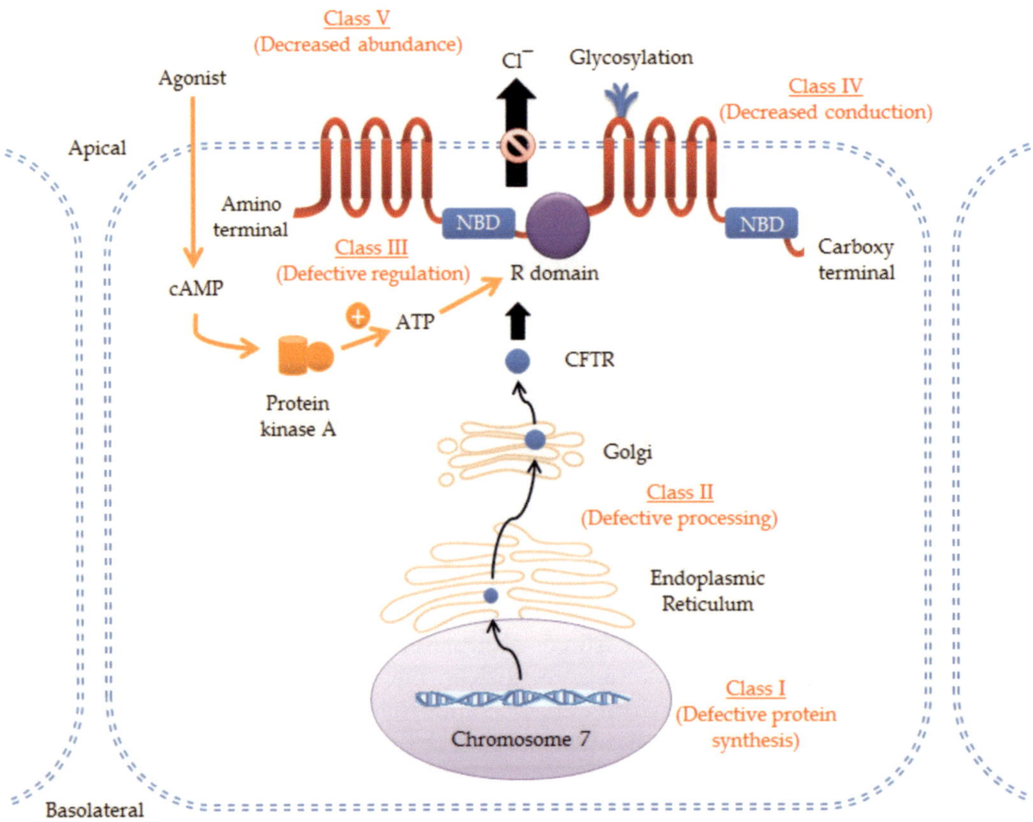

Fig. 1. Schema illustrating the processing, structure and function of the CFTR protein. The classes of genetic mutations (discussed later) and their effects on the CFTR processing/function are illustrated. The CFTR protein consists of two transmembrane domains, two nucleotide-binding domains (NBD), and a regulatory R domain. Normal functioning involves an agonist such as acetyl-chloine binding to epithleial cells, resulting in an increase in cAMP, which activates protein kinase A (PKA). PKA phosphorylates the CFTR protein at the R domain, thus resulting in opening of the chloride (Cl^-) channel. ATP, adenosine triphosphate; c-AMP, cyclic adenosine monophosphate; CFTR, cystic fibrosis transmembrane conductance regulator.

The majority of CF patients carrying functionally severe mutations on both alleles (Class I-III and VI) have a pancreatic insufficient (PI) phenotype (85% to 90%). A small proportion (2-3%) of patients carrying severe mutations on both alleles are pancreatic sufficient (PS) at diagnosis, but most experience gradual transition from PS to PI (Waters et al.,1990; Wilschanski & Durie, 2007). It is well established that PS-CF patients, who are often diagnosed at an older age, with more subtle disease manifestations, have mean sweat chloride values that are significantly lower than the current diagnostic reference criteria of 60 mmol/L (Farrell et al., 2008; Gilljam et al., 2004). Without sufficient enzyme activity (or enzyme replacement), PI patients suffer from malabsorption of proteins, fats and fat-soluble vitamins, and to a lesser extent, carbohydrates. Clinical manifestations of PI include: steatorrhoea, failure to thrive/poor weight gain, abdominal distension, a reduction in subcutaneous fat and muscle tissue, and fat-soluble vitamin deficiencies. In adolescents, absence of a pubertal growth spurt and delayed maturation may occur (Rosenstein, 2006).

With the increasing life expectancy of CF patients, it has become recognised that a significant proportion of PI-CF patients develop glucose intolerance, and up to 32% of patients over 25 years of age progress to insulin-requiring CF-related diabetes mellitus (Moran et al., 1999; Rosenstein, 2006). CF-related diabetes is characterised by an insidious onset and mild clinical course (e.g. gradual weight loss).

4. Pancreatitis in CF and CFTR-related disease: Pathogenesis

Pancreatitis is a well-known but uncommon manifestation in CF disease. This is not surprising as the majority of patients who carry functionally severe mutations on both alleles are PI. Since the presence of residual pancreatic acinar tissue is necessary for pancreatitis to occur, symptomatic pancreatitis does not (or rarely) occur in PI patients, but is not uncommon in PS-CF patients. Approximately 20% of PS-CF patients develop pancreatitis (Ooi et al., 2011a). Several studies have shown that individuals with idiopathic recurrent-acute or chronic pancreatitis have an increased incidence of mutations in the *CFTR* gene (Bishop et al., 2005; Cohn et al., 1998; Sharer et al.,1998). Bishop et al. (2005) showed that 43% and 11% of patients with idiopathic recurrent-acute or chronic pancreatitis carried at least one, and two *CFTR* mutations (and/or variants), respectively; the diagnostic criteria of CF could be fulfilled in 21% of these patients.

Whilst obstructive tubulopathy of the pancreas due to CFTR dysfunction is thought to be primary pathogenic factor, the exact mechanism of pancreatitis associated with *CFTR* mutations is still unknown. Based on murine models, CFTR dysfunction may also affect pancreatic acinar cells by impairing apical endocytosis through diminished ductal bicarbonate secretion and subsequently reduced alkalinization of the acinar lumen (Freedman et al., 2001). A recent study also suggests an important role of pH dysregulation in the development of pancreatitis. Co-release of protons (H^+) with proteins from secretory granules of acinar cells during pancreatic secretion was demonstrated (Behrendorff et al., 2010). Acidification of the pancreatic lumen led to a loss of tight junction integrity, which allowed the leakage of zymogens into the interstitial fluid. Abberant activation of calcium channels may also occur and result in the release and premature activation of zymogens, thus causing tissue damage and inflammation. The findings of this study fits with the development of pancreatitis in the setting of *CFTR* mutation(s) or CFTR dysfunction; reduced CFTR function impairs entry of bicarbonate into the ducts, and results in a more acidic and dehydrated pancreatic lumen. These studies support the complex interactions that exist between the ductular and acinar components of the pancreas in the development of pancreatitis.

Parodoxically, *CFTR* genotypes associated with otherwise mild phenotypic effects have a greater risk of causing pancreatitis, when compared with genotypes associated with moderate to severe disease phenotypes. Patients with enough functional *CFTR* to confer a phenotypically functional pancreas have an increased risk of pancreatitis, as sufficient pancreatic acinar tissue is required for obstructive ductal lesions to cause disease (Fig. 2).

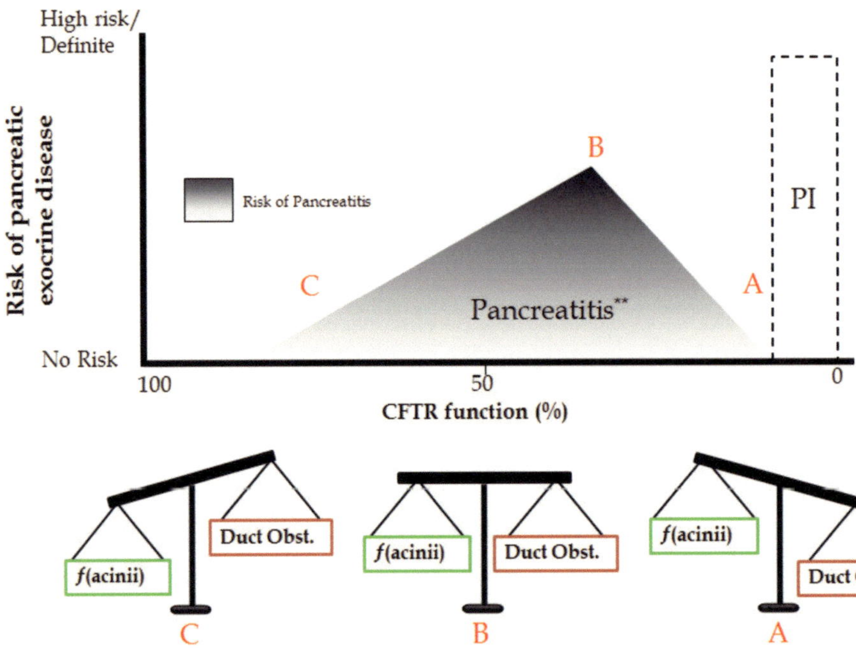

Fig. 2. Risk of pancreatitis in relation to severity of CFTR dysfunction. **The gradient within the pancreatitis curve reflects the relative risk of pancreatitis. A delicate balance between the degree of residual acinar tissue present and severity of ductal obstruction exists, and this balance correlates to the risk of pancreatitis. A. Patients with severe CFTR dysfunction have minimal/no risk of developing clinical pancreatitis despite severe ductal obstruction, as there is insufficient residual pancreatic acinar tissue. B. The risk of pancreatitis increases with decreasing CFTR dysfunction and is highest when there is adequately pathogenic ductal obstruction and sufficient residual acinar tissue present. C. With further increases in CFTR function, the degree of ductal obstruction is minimal, thus the risk of pancreatitis is low despite large amounts of pancreatic acinar tissue. The exception to this is when non-CFTR modifier factors play a role. CFTR, cystic fibrosis transmembrane conductance regulator; Duct Obst., degree of ductal obstruction; f(acinii), residual acinar function; PI, pancreatic insufficient.

5. *CFTR* mutations

Since the discovery of the *CFTR* gene in 1989, advances in molecular analysis techniques have identified > 1800 *CFTR* mutations (Dorfman, 2011). Mutation in this context simply refers to a molecular alteration in the DNA sequence of a gene, with no inference made concerning the effect of this alteration on gene expression, protein function and, therefore, clinical phenotype. For many of the *CFTR* mutations which have been identified, the effect of the mutation on gene expression or function of the protein product is unknown. This is especially true for missense mutations (a base pair substitution in the DNA sequence) which represent approximately 40% of the identified mutations. To explain the use and interpretation of *CFTR* mutation analysis in clinical practice, the European Cystic Fibrosis Society (ECFS) published a consensus paper in 2008 which categorised mutations into four groups based on their predicted clinical consequences: (*i*) CF-causing mutations, (*ii*) mutations associated with *CFTR*-related disease, (*iii*) mutations with no known clinical consequence, and (*iv*) mutations with unknown clinical relevance (Castellani et al., 2008). Mutations which are associated with both PS and PI phenotypes are listed in Table 1. Note the more conservative list of mutations which are included on the recommended panel of CF-causing mutations for population screening developed by the American College of Medical Genetics (Farrell et al., 2008). This list is not entirely exhaustive, as other mutations can be predicted to be CF-causing if the molecular alteration results in a change in amino acid sequence that: severely affects CFTR synthesis and/or function; introduces a premature termination signal; or alters invariant nucleotides of intron splice sites. However, the vast majority of known mutations do not fulfill the accepted criteria for CF-causing mutations (Castellani et al., 2008; Farrell et al., 2008).

In CF, disease-causing mutations are often identified on newborn screening panels. In recent times, several diseases that resemble CF at an organ-specific level (e.g. pancreatitis, bronchiectasis and obstructive azoospermia) have also been found to be strongly associated with mutations in the *CFTR* gene (Ooi et al., 2010b). The functional consequence(s) of many *CFTR* gene alterations is unknown and unable to be determined. This is due to the interplay of mild and severe mutations, as well as the variation in genotype-phenoytpe expression, which is affected by non-*CFTR* modifiers (genetic and/or environmental).

The complex and heterogenous presentation of CF disease and CFTR-related disorders is associated with a continuous spectrum of CFTR dysfunction. A clear relationship between the number and functional severity of *CFTR* gene alterations, with the range of CFTR-mediated ion channel abnormalities has been established (Bishop et al., 2005; Wilschanski, 2006). This observation has helped develop our understanding of the threshold of CFTR-mediated ion channel function that is required for disease pathogenesis and diagnosis.

A 5-class classification system for *CFTR* mutations was originally developed to categorize the molecular characteristics of different mutations (Fig. 3) (Tsui, 1992). On the basis of its molecular defect, mutations in Classes I-III could be predicted to have severe functional and phenotypic consequences. Conversely, Classes IV-V may confer residual CFTR function and thus, be predicted to be associated with milder phenotypic consequences. Remarkably, genotype-phenotype studies demonstrated an excellent correlation between Classes I-III with a PI phenotype, and Classes IV-V with a PS phenotype (Ahmed et al., 2003; Kristidis et al.,1992). A 6th mutation class has subsequently been proposed which is also associated with severe functional and phenotypic consequences. In general, patients homozygous or compound heterozygous for severe mutations (class I-III, and VI) will be PI. Alternatively, patients with at least one mild mutation (class IV or V), will often be PS, as the milder of the two mutations confers a dominant phenotypic effect. In very young infants, *CFTR* genotype may not be closely associated with pancreatic phenotype; particularly those identified by newborn screening. This is almost certainly due to the fact that some infants carrying severe mutations on both alleles have some residual exocrine pancreatic function at birth. However, almost all of the patients who are homozygous or compound heterozygous for severe mutations will develop PI within the first two years of life (Waters et al., 1990).

***CFTR* mutations and their associated clinical consequences**

Association	Mutations			Phenotype
CF-causing	F508del*	6542X*	G85E*	**Usually PI**
	R553X*	G551D*	711+1G>T*	
	R1162X*	W1282X*	1898+1G>A	
	R1158X	N1303K*	S549N	
	2184delA*	621+1G>T*	E822X	
	2184insA	1717-1G>A*	1078delT	
	3120+1G>A*	1898+1G>T*	2789+5G>A*	
	I507del*	R560T*	3659delC*	
	1677delTA			
	A455E*	711+3A>G	D1152H	**Usually PS**
	R334W*	3849+10kbC>T*	L206W	
	R347P*	R117H-T5*	TG13-T5	
CFTR-related disease	R117H-T7*	TG12-T5	TG11-T5	**Usually PS**
	D1152H	S997F	R74W-D1270N	
	TG13-T5	R297Q	R668C-G576A-	
	D565G	L997F	D443Y	
		G576A	M9521	
No clinical consequences	I148T	T854T	1521F	-
	R75Q	P1290P	F508C	
	875+40A/G	2752-15G/C	I506V	
	M470V	I807M	TG11-T5	
	E528E			
Unknown or uncertain clinical consequence	Mainly missense mutations with subclinical molecular consequences (e.g. M470V), which may co-segregate on the same chromosome and exert a more potent, cumulative phenotypic effect.			-

Table 1. List of *CFTR* mutations with their associated clinical consequence(s) and pancreatic exocrine phenotype(s). Adapted from Castellani et al., 2008. Underlined are the mutations associated with both PS and PI phenotypes. * The CFTR mutations included on the recommended panel of CF-causing mutations for population screening (Farrell et al., 2008). CF, cystic fibrosis; CFTR, cystic fibrosis transmembrane conductance regulator; PI, pancreatic insufficient; PS, pancreatic sufficient.

Although this class system is useful as a conceptual framework, it does have several limitations which include (Ooi et al., 2010b): (*i*) molecular changes of different mutations within the same class (especially classes IV and V), may have varying functional consequences, (*ii*) mutations may have overlapping molecular defects which may be assigned to more than one class, (*iii*) the molecular consequences of the majority of rare

CFTR mutations, particularly missense alterations are unknown or cannot be predicted, and (*iv*) inferred properties of many mutations remain to be confirmed by functional studies.

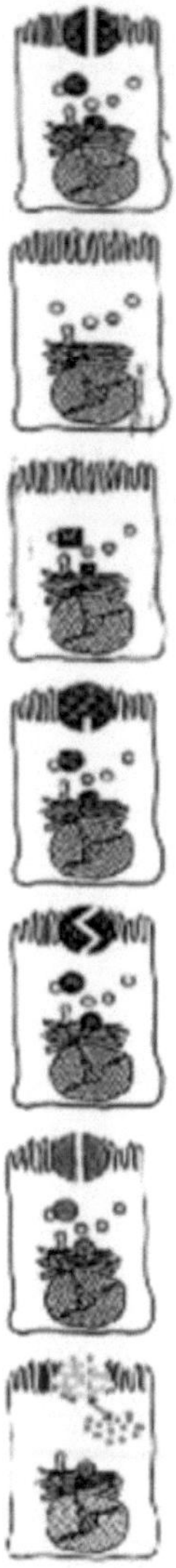

Normal — Normal CFTR protein function

I — **Defective protein synthesis**: Nonsense or frameshift mutations associated with a complete lack of CFTR protein at the apical membrane (e.g. G542X, 394delTT and 1717-1G>A)

II — **Abnormal protein folding, processing, and trafficking**: Misfolded functional CFTR protein is largely degraded intracellularly, so there is a complete lack of CFTR protein at the apical membrane (e.g. F508del and N1303K)

III — **Defective regulation:** Mutations prevent channel activation by inhibiting binding and hydrolysis of ATP at one of the two nucleotide-binding domains. Thus the CFTR protein on the apical surface is nonfunctional (e.g. G551D)

IV — **Decreased conductance:** Abnormal anion conductance results in impaired protein function (e.g. R117H and R347P)

V — **Reduced abundance:** Abnormal splicing, promoter mutations or inefficient trafficking results in a reduced number of normally functioning protein at the apical membrane (e.g. A455E and 3849+10kbC>T)

VI — **Decreased stability or altered regulation of separate ion channels:** Mutations which cause inherent lability of the CFTR protein or alter regulation of other ion channels

Fig. 3. Classes of *CFTR* mutations according to the functional consequences of the gene product with respect to chloride regulation. Severe mutations (classes I-III and VI) confer little or no functional CFTR at the apical membrane, whilst mild mutations (classes IV and V) confer some partial CFTR function. Adapted from Tsui, 1992; Wilschanski & Durie, 2007.CFTR, cystic fibrosis transmembrane conductance regulator.

A new surrogate measure for the severity of *CFTR* mutations, known as the Pancreatic Insufficiency Prevalence (PIP) score, was recently developed and validated (Dorfman et al., 2010; Ooi et al., 2011a). The PIP scoring system permitted a more refined classification of the functional severity of *CFTR* mutations, and in a far greater number of patients than previous methods of classification. The PIP score is based upon a direct assessment of the effect of each genotype on exocrine pancreatic phenotype; which had been objectively determined in a large population-based CF database. This classification system is based on several premises: (*i*) the well-established correlation between severity of *CFTR* mutations and exocrine pancreatic function, (*ii*) the dominant phenotypic effect conferred by the milder of the 2 *CFTR* mutations, and (*iii*) the availability of a comprehensive database containing large numbers of CF patients, with stringent determination of clinical diagnosis and exocrine pancreatic status. Ooi et al. (2011a) described how mutations can be classified as either mild (≤0.25) or moderate-severe (>0.25) on the basis of the PIP score (Table 2).

Pancreatic Insufficiency Prevalence (PIP) Scores for Common, Well-Defined *CFTR* Mutations

Mutation	Class	Total PI	Total PI + PS	PIP Score	Phenotype
R117H	IV-V	1	25	0.04	
3849+10kbC>T	IV-V	2	22	0.09	Mild
R334W	IV-V	1	10	0.10	
2789+5G>A	IV-V	6	16	0.38	
A455E	IV-V	18	37	0.49	
G85E	I-III,VI	16	22	0.73	
G551D	I-III,VI	59	67	0.88	
R1162X	I-III,VI	12	13	0.92	
N1303K	I-III,VI	45	48	0.94	
W1282X	I-III,VI	19	20	0.95	Moderate-
1717-1G>A	I-III,VI	20	21	0.95	severe
F508del	I-III,VI	1276	1324	0.96	
G542X	I-III,VI	74	75	0.99	
I507del	I-III,VI	11	11	1.00	
R553X	I-III,VI	24	24	1.00	
711+1G>T	I-III,VI	36	36	1.00	
621+1G>T	I-III,VI	96	96	1.00	

Table 2. PIP scores for common, well-defined *CFTR* mutations based on the prevalence of PI in a large and well-defined cohort of Canadian CF patients (n=2481) (Ooi et al., 2011a). The PIP score for a specific mutation is the ratio between the PI patients carrying the mutation (Total PI), and all PI and PS patients (Total PI + PS) carrying the same mutation when in a homozygous state or heterozygous combination with F508del, G551D or class I mutations (bona fide severe mutations). For example, a ratio of 1.00 indicates that all patients with 621+1G>T are PI. Similarly, a ratio of 0.1 demonstrates that 10% of subjects with R334W are PI. CFTR, cystic fibrosis transmembrane conductance regulator; PI, pancreatic insufficient; PIP, pancreatic insufficiency prevalence; PS, pancreatic sufficient.

Using the PIP score, a relationship between severity of *CFTR* genotypes with risk of pancreatitis was observed among PS-CF patients. Patients with genotypes associated with mild phenotypic (PIP score ≤ 0.25) effects have a greater risk of developing pancreatitis than patients with genotypes associated with moderate-severe phenotypes (PIP score > 0.25);

among the patients who developed pancreatitis, 70% had a mild genotype, while 30% carried a moderate-severe genotype (P = 0.004) (Ooi et al., 2011a). The genotype associated with mild PIP scores had a hazard ratio of 2.4 for pancreatitis (95% confidence interval, 1.3-4.5; P = 0.006). Furthermore, there was a gradation of risk of developing pancreatitis according to severity of each allele carried: highest risk seen in CF patients who carried 2 mild mutations (mild/mild) followed by those who carried 1 mild mutation (mild/moderate-severe), compared with those who carried functionally moderate-severe mutations on both alleles (Fig. 4). Thus, this is the first systematic study to date, demonstrating an association between higher risks of pancreatitis with different degrees of genotype mildness (based on the PIP score).

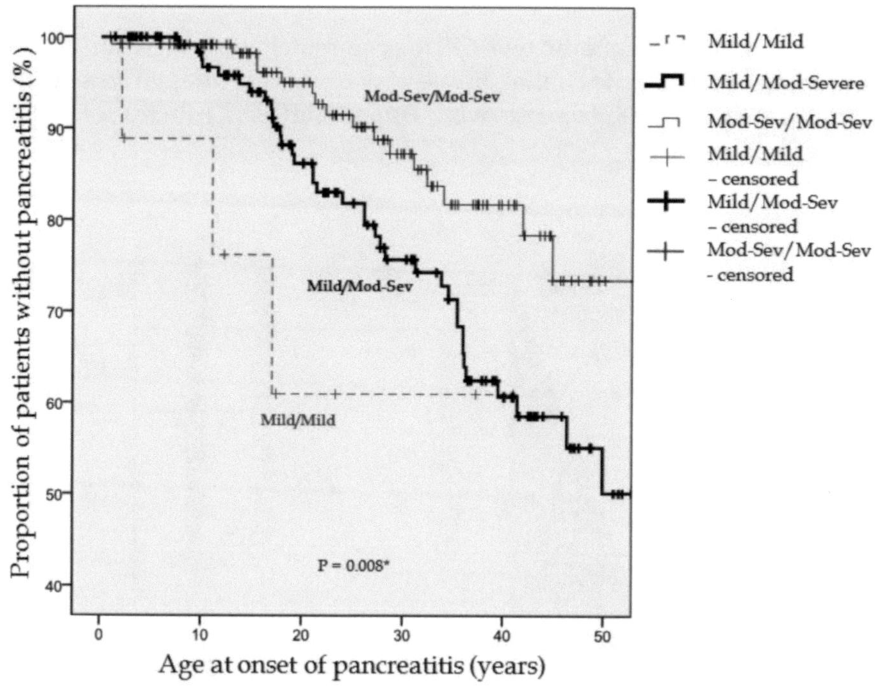

	0	10	20	30	40	50
Mild/Mild	9	7	3	2	1	0
Mild/Mod-Sev	138	115	84	58	34	10
Mod-Sev/Mod-Sev	130	111	82	54	28	7

Fig. 4. Survival curves (Kaplan-Meier estimate) comparing time to pancreatitis in patients grouped according to severity of both *CFTR* alleles (mild/mild *vs.* mild/moderate-severe *vs.* moderate-severe/moderate-severe). The survival table (below the curve) indicates the number of patients/"survivors" at risk of pancreatitis at 0, 10, 20, 30, 40 and 50 years respectively. Adapted from Ooi et al., 2011a. * Log-rank test CFTR, cystic fibrosis transmembrane conductance regulator; Mod-Sev, moderate-severe.

All classification systems are limited by the fact that the heterogenous CF disease spectrum is not just explained by *CFTR* genotype, but is also influenced by environmental and other genetic modifying factors. Genes such as cationic trypsinogen (*PRSS1*), anionic trypsinogen (*PRSS2*), pancreatic secretory trypsin inhibitor (*SPINK1*), and chymotrpsinogen C (*CTRC*) have been demonstrated to be involved in the regulation of trypsinogen autoactivation and also play a role in cases of idiopathic recurrent-acute and chronic pancreatitis (Ooi et al., 2010a). The interactions with environmental factors such as cigarette smoking, alcohol and diet are also highly complex, and are only beginning to unravel.

6. The spectrum of CFTR dysfunction

The notion of a spectrum of CFTR dysfunction is supported by the observation that CF may manifest at different ages, in different organs and with variable severity. Cystic fibrosis and CFTR-related disorders comprise of pancreatic exocrine insufficiency, pancreatitis, chronic sinopulmonary disease, intestinal diseases, hepatobiliary disease, and obstructive azoospermia in men.

Individuals who carry one or two *CFTR* gene mutation(s) show an overlapping clinical spectrum, ranging from no clinical disease at one extreme, through those with CFTR-related disorders, to those with CF disease (with/without sufficient pancreatic function) at the other extreme (Fig. 5).

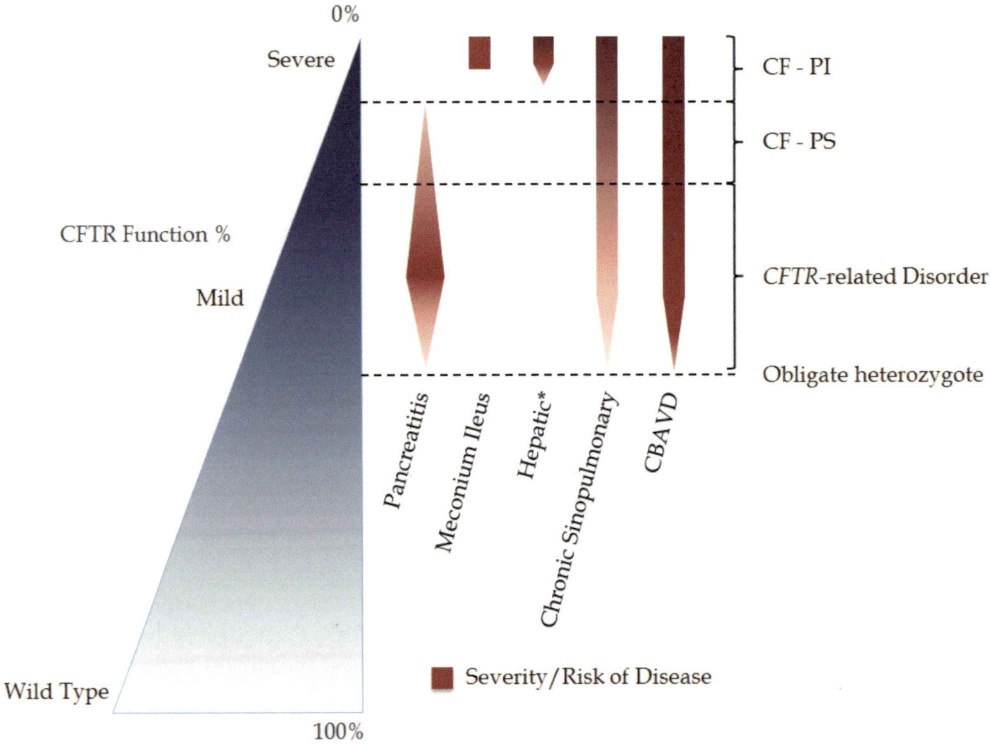

Fig. 5. Spectrum of disorders associated with the level of CFTR function and the respective severity/risk of disease. * Severe CF liver disease with cirrhosis ± portal hypertension. CBAVD, congenital absence of the vas deferens; CF, cystic fibrosis; CFTR, cystic fibrosis transmembrane conductance regulator; PI, pancreatic insufficient; PS, pancreatic sufficient.

There is considerable debate and difficulty on where to draw the diagnostic line between CF disease and CFTR-related disorder. Although they can be divided into two entities, they form part of a continuous spectrum of diseases associated with CFTR dysfunction. Similarly, ion channel measurements in the sweat gland (sweat test) and nasal epithelium (nasal potential difference test) show a continuum of values with overlap, and no clear delineating point between individuals without CF (healthy controls and obligate heterozygotes) and patients with CF (pancreatic sufficient and insufficient). Consequently our ability to establish or exclude CF disease has become increasingly problematic.
The subset of clinically heterogeneous patients who are diagnosed with CF in adolescence and adulthood, who do not resemble the typical clinical presentation in infancy or early childhood are discussed later in this chapter.

7. Pancreatitis in CF and CFTR-related disorder: Clinical presentation and diagnosis

The initial clinical presentation of acute, recurrent-acute and chronic pancreatitis due to CFTR dysfunction can be indistinguishable from idiopathic pancreatitis. The clinical features and diagnostic criteria for pancreatitis are covered by companion chapter(s) in this textbook.
The most recent United States Cystic Fibrosis Foundation (USCFF) consensus report (Farrell et al., 2008), agreed that a diagnosis of CF can be made in individuals who present with a characteristic clinical phenotype or a history of CF in a sibling, *in the presence of* an abnormal sweat chloride value ≥ 60 mmol/L and/or two CF-causing mutations. It is important to note that a diagnosis of CF cannot be made based on the identification of *CFTR* mutations on both alleles alone, especially when one or both are not designated as disease-causing mutations.
Due to the vast array of phenotypes associated with *CFTR* mutations, the diagnosis of patients with CF disease has become increasingly difficult, and the demarcation line between those with CF and those not classified as having CF by current diagnostic criteria has blurred. To deal with the spectrum of disease, the USCFF consensus report stated that the classification of this disease should be limited to two terms (Farrell et al., 2008): (*i*) CF disease, to describe patients who fulfil the currently accepted diagnostic criteria, and (*ii*) "CFTR-related disorder," to describe individuals with a CF phenotype in at least one affected organ *plus* evidence of CFTR dysfunction, but insufficient to fulfil the diagnostic criteria for CF disease (e.g. borderline sweat test and/or 1 - 2 non-CF causing mutation(s)). Using this terminology, patients with recurrent-acute or chronic pancreatitis due to CFTR dysfunction , may receive a diagnosis of CF pancreatitis or CFTR-related pancreatitis.
Individuals with a CFTR-related disorder are recognised to be *at risk for developing CF disease* (Farrell et al., 2008). Therefore, a diagnosis of CFTR-related pancreatitis may precede a diagnosis of CF, as it may be the initial manifestation of CFTR dysfunction, or it may be associated with other CFTR-related disorders at the time of presentation (e.g. infertile males with pancreatitis) or later on. Consequently, if repeat sweat chloride values remain in the intermediate range (40-59 mmol/L), further assessment has been recommended at a CF care center to clarify the diagnosis. Further assessment may include: clinical assessment, expanded genetic testing, exocrine pancreatic function testing, and respiratory tract culture for CF-associated pathogens. Depending on the clinical presentation, assessment may also include ancillary tests, such as pulmonary function testing and urogenital evaluation in males (genital examination, rectal ultrasound, and sperm analysis). It is important to

emphasise that treatment should be dependent on the disease presentation, and not on presence or absence of a diagnostic label.

7.1 Sweat chloride testing

The sweat chloride test has been in clinical use for over 50 years, and it still remains the principal test for the confirmation of the diagnosis of CF in the genomic era (Gibson & Cooke, 1959). Although the test is now commonly available in most diagnostic laboratories, appropriate performance of the sweat test in accordance to recommended standards is crucial for accurate diagnosis. The sweat test involves transdermal administration of pilocarpine by iontophoresis to stimulate sweat gland secretion, followed by collection and quantitation of sweat onto gauze or filter paper, or into a Macroduct coil. The reference ranges for sweat chloride concentration which we use today, were defined using studies of CF patients presenting with classical symptoms of CF at an early age (most were PI); there were no "truly healthy" controls, and the technical aspects of the sweat test methodologies would not meet currently accepted guidelines (Farrell et al., 2008; Shwachman & Mahmoodian, 1967). Furthermore, there has also been no study to accurately determine the reference ranges for sweat chloride values in infants and young children less than 5 years of age (Farrell et al., 2008). Several studies have also reported patients being diagnosed with CF (PS and PI), who have sweat chloride values < 60mmol/L (Desmarquest et al., 2000; Highsmith et al., 1994; Stewart et al., 1995). This is especially true among the well described CF disease-causing mutations associated with normal or intermediate sweat chloride values (e.g. 3849+10kbC>T).

Sweat chloride values are traditionally interpreted categorically. Due to the aforementioned limitations, it is not surprising that the reference values for the various sweat chloride categories are not universally agreed upon. According to the USCFF consensus guideline, sweat chloride values can be categorised as the following among individuals > 6 months old: normal ≤ 39 mmol/L, intermediate 40-59 mmol/L, or abnormal ≥ 60 mmol/L; the intermediate range is extended to 30-59 mmol/L in infants up to 6 months old (Farrell et al., 2008). This differs from the reference ranges recommended by the ECFS: normal ≤ 29 mmol/L, intermediate 30-60 mmol/L, and abnormal > 60 mmol/L, for all ages (De Boeck et al., 2006).

There is preliminary data to suggest that the individual sweat chloride value, taken into account with the clinical context, is of more value to the clinician than categorical interpretation (Ooi et al., 2011b). This study evaluated the diagnostic performance of sweat testing in the general population and in patients with idiopathic pancreatitis who were referred to a gastroenterology (GI)-CF clinic. This study raised an important point that sweat test parameters and results are dependent on the patient population and disease incidence in each population. When comparing the general population to symptomatic pancreatitis patients in a GI-CF clinic: the pre-test probability for CF is 1 in 3608 vs. 10%; the carrier rate is 4% vs. 50%; and the PI:PS CF ratio is 8:1 vs. all patients with pancreatitis being PS (Bishop et al., 2005; Castellani et al., 2010; Dupuis et al., 2005; Durno et al., 2002). It has also been reported that a diagnosis of CF can be made in 10% of idiopathic pancreatitis patients (referred to a GI-CF clinic), based on sweat testing and/or genotyping, however the diagnosis may be equivocal in up to 20% of patients (Bishop et al., 2005; Ooi et al., 2010a). As expected, there were vast differences in the diagnostic performance of sweat chloride testing in the two populations (Table 3).

An important observation from this study is the dramatic increase in the positive predictive value (PPV) of sweat chloride values ≥ 55 mmol/L in the general population, and the not clinically insignificant high PPV in those who present with symptomatic pancreatitis and have sweat chloride values ≥ 40mmol/L (Fig. 6). These results demonstrate how the individual sweat chloride result (whilst also taking in to account the clinical context of the patient), may be more valuable to the clinician than using the traditional categorical interpretation.

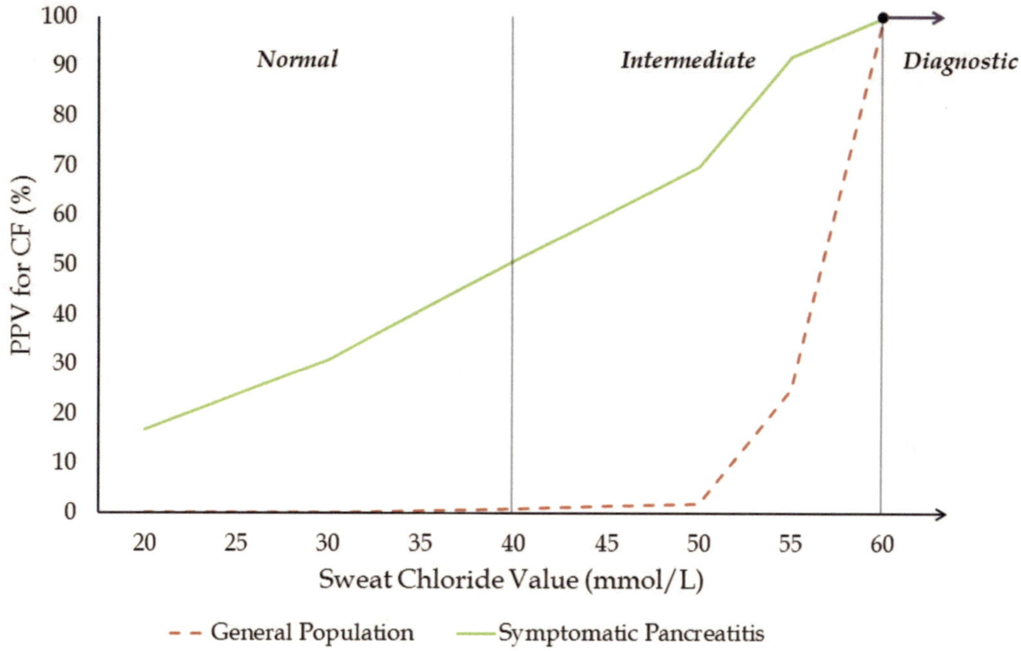

Fig. 6. PPV of sweat chloride testing in the general population and patients with idiopathic pancreatitis referred to a GI-CF clinic (Ooi et al., 2011b).CF, cystic fibrosis; CFTR, cystic fibrosis transmembrane conductance regulator; PPV, positive predictive value.

Sw Cl (mmol/L)	General Population				GI-CF Clinic			
	Sens	Spec	PPV	NPV	Sens	Spec	PPV	NPV
20	100	54	0.1	100	98	48	17	100
30	99	83	0.2	100	94	77	31	99
40	98	97	0.9	100	81	91	51	98
50	97	99	2	100	77	96	70	97
55	97	100	25	100	73	99	92	97
60	96	100	100	100	64	100	100	96

Table 3. Diagnostic performance parameters for various sweat chloride values in a general population and patients at a GI-CF clinic. (Ooi et al., 2011b). CF, cystic fibrosis; GI, gastroenterology; NPV, negative predictive value; PPV, positive predictive value; Sens, sensitivity; Spec, specificity; Sw Cl, sweat chloride.

7.2 Genotyping

Despite the considerable optimism that genotyping would supersede the traditional sweat test, there remains considerable misunderstanding of the role of *CFTR* genotyping as a diagnostic aid in CF. In patients with a suspected, but unproven diagnosis of CF, mutation testing (including complete sequencing of the *CFTR* gene) appears to be the least helpful diagnostic tool and may be potentially misleading. In fact, carefully performed sweat chloride testing has been reported to be more sensitive and specific than complete sequencing in patients presenting with a single organ manifestation of CF including pancreatitis (Bishop et al., 2005; Gilljam et al., 2004; Wilschanski, 2006). In a cohort of 46 CF patients diagnosed in adulthood, only 15 (33%) fulfilled the diagnostic criteria of CF based on genotyping alone; all except one of the 15 (6.7%) had an abnormal sweat test > 60 mmol/L. Sweat testing alone diagnosed CF in 30 (65%) subjects and when sweat testing was combined with genotyping, the diagnostic sensitivity only improved slightly to 67% (n=31) (Gilljam et al., 2004).

If a clinician decides to assess a patient's genotype, it is important to consider that most patients presenting in adolescence and adulthood and/or those who present with single-organ disease, frequently carry one or more rare *CFTR* mutations which are often not included in screening panels. However, extensive genotyping or complete sequencing of the *CFTR* gene has major limitations also. The majority of mutations have unknown functional consequences, while some are considered to be benign polymorphisms with no pathogenic potential. Furthermore, some mutations are known to form complex alleles i.e. > 1 mutation occurs only on one allele and hence, may be mis-interpreted as the presence of mutations on both alleles. With all these variables, there is a potential risk of informing a patient with pancreatitis that they have *CFTR* mutations, and implying they have CF. Misinterpretation of genotyping results carries enormous psychosocial and medical implications, as well as affecting potential insurability. In a study reporting the outcomes from a commercially available extensive *CFTR* mutation test, 84% of patients identified with 2 *CFTR* mutations were incorrectly labeled as having CF (Keiles & Kammesheidt, 2006; Ooi et al., 2010a).

7.3 Transepithelial nasal potential difference testing

The transepithelial nasal potential difference (NPD) test is an electrophysiological test that assesses CFTR activity by measuring transepithelial potential difference of the nasal epithelium. This test is based on the characteristic bioelectric properties of amiloride-dependent sodium (Na^+) absorption (via ENaC) and CFTR-mediated Cl^- diffusion (Schuler et al., 2004). NPD has been used in CF research for decades but due to a lack of validated reference values and standardisation, it has only been cautiously applied in clinical practice as an adjunctive test to assist in clarifying the diagnosis of CF, especially for individuals with intermediate sweat chloride values (Farrell et al., 2008).

NPD is measured between a fluid-filled exploring bridge positioned on the nasal respiratory mucosa, and a reference bridge inserted into the subcutaneous space. Both bridges are linked by Ag/AgCl electrodes (or saturated calomel half-cells) to a high-impedence voltmeter. An otoscope is used to help place the tip of the exploring catheter on the respiratory mucosa inferior to the concha nasalis inferior. A basal potential difference is established once consistent baseline NPD measurements are obtained. Different solutions/drugs can be administered via the exploring catheter, and the changes in transepithelial potential difference as a response to superfusion can be measured. The findings of a high potential difference during baseline measurements, followed by an absent or very low voltage response to zero-chloride plus isoproterenol perfusion, are indicative of CF (Knowles et al., 1995).

Patients who have equivocal sweat chloride results and/or CFTR mutation analysis may also have equivocal NPD measurements, and a consensus of what constitutes a borderline result is lacking (Ooi et al., 2010b). In addition, the procedure is complex to perform, labour intensive, and operator dependent. Although NPD testing has been reported in infants and young children, the accurate performance of this test requires undivided cooperation from the subject. False positives can occur with incorrect placement of the measuring catheter, minor perturbations of nasal epithelium, allergies, respiratory infections, and smoking (Cantin et al., 2006).

7.4 Intestinal ion channel measurement

Intestinal ion channel measurement (ICM) is an ex vivo test performed in an Ussing chamber using a freshly obtained rectal biopsy and measuring its electrical response to a series of secretagogues. Intestinal epithelia of CF subjects have been evaluated by two different laboratory methods (circulating vs. continuously perfused) (De Jonge et al., 2004; Mall et al., 2004). The common finding of both approaches demonstrates absent or diminished chloride secretion after stimulation with agonists that act via intracellular cAMP. Intestinal ICM has been reported to be useful in clarifying the diagnosis of CF in cases of uncertainty, but again the absence of standardisation and well-established reference values limits its use in clinical practice (Farrell et al., 2008).

7.5 Imaging in CF and CFTR-related pancreatitis

The typical changes of the pancreas on imaging in patients with CF are neither specific nor diagnostic for CF and CFTR-related pancreatitis. In CF, fatty replacement of the pancreatic parenchyma, with or without glandular atrophy (56-93%) is the most common finding at imaging in adult patients, and the mean age of fatty replacement is 17 years (Robertson et al., 2006; Shanbhogue et al., 2009). Other radiological findings include pancreatic calcifications (7%); cyst formation (pancreatic cystosis); and abnormalities of the pancreatic duct, including strictures, beading, dilatation, and obstruction (Shanbhogue et al., 2009). The pancreatic duct can be poorly demonstrated with ultrasonography (US) in CF patients with pancreatic atrophy and fatty replacement, and is best demonstrated with magnetic resonance cholangiopancreatography (MRCP) or endoscopic retrograde cholangiopancreatography (ERCP) (Robertson et al., 2006). Imaging has no role in monitoring of exocrine pancreatic function but has a yet to-be-defined role in surveillance for pancreatic adenocarcinoma.

8. Management of pancreatitis in CF and CFTR-related disorder

The management of pancreatitis associated with CF or *CFTR* mutations per se, is currently no different to other forms of pancreatitis (covered in companion chapters). Affected patients however should be referred to a CF clinic or gastroenterologist with interests/expertise in CF for a thorough evaluation. The main considerations in these patients are a progression from PS to PI, and the risk of developing CF disease and/or disease in other CF-affected organs (e.g. bronchiectasis) (Gilljam et al., 2004; Ooi et al.,

2011a). In addition, there are increasing concerns of an increased risk of pancreatic adenocarcinoma among those with CF and CFTR-related pancreatitis.

8.1 Pancreatic function testing

The exocrine pancreas has a large reserve capacity and requires between 90% and 99% of enzyme secretory capacity to be lost before a subject develops clinical manifestations of PI. It is recommended that patients with PS-CF and CFTR-related pancreatitis have their pancreatic exocrine function assessed. Individuals who have sufficient pancreatic function at presentation need to be assessed periodically, or when new symptoms suggestive of PI develop, as some may progress to PI (Gilljam et al., 2004; Ooi et al., 2011a). Progression of PI is dependent on the following factors: (1) the carriage of moderate-severe mutations on both alleles, and (2) the development of symptomatic pancreatitis. PS-CF patients with mild genotypes (i.e. those otherwise expected to remain PS) who develop pancreatitis are at an increased risk of progressing from PS to PI (odds ratio = 5.5) (Ooi et al., 2011a).

Exocrine pancreatic function can be measured through non-invasive and invasive methods. Currently, non-invasive pancreatic function tests are commonly utilised for defining the exocrine pancreatic phenotype. The 72-hour faecal fat balance test, expressed as the coefficient of fat absorption (CFA), is considered the gold standard as far as non-invasive tests are concerned (Ooi et al., 2010b). However, the test is inconvenient and not well tolerated by patients or laboratory staff. Faecal elastase-1 is an alternative indirect stool marker for pancreatic function, as elastase (an endogenous pancreatic secretion enzyme) is resistant to gastrointestinal degradation. Using a cut-off of 200 µg/g stool, the sensitivity for mild, moderate, severe and all patients with PI, was reported to be 63%, 100%, 100% and 93% respectively, whilst the specificity was 93% (Loser et al., 1996). Because of its ease of use, faecal elastase-1 is recommended for evaluating pancreatic function at diagnosis and for follow-up monitoring. Currently, a value of < 100 µg/g in individuals over the age of 2 to 3 years is considered indicative of PI. Values from 100 µg/g to 200 µg/g are associated with significant loss of pancreatic function, although not necessarily of sufficient severity to confer PI, and warrant the need for pancreatic enzyme supplementation (Farrell et al., 2008). In addition, there are differences in the diagnostic performance parameters (sensitivity and specificity) between monoclonal and polyclonal assays for faecal elastase; the monoclonal assay is superior due to less cross-reactivity and can be used whilst patients are on pancreatic enzyme therapy (Pezzilli et al., 2005). False positivity can occur due to malabsorption from an intestinal cause, particularly if there is stool dilution from severe diarrhoea (Beharry et al., 2002). Other indirect methods for assessing pancreatic function include the measurement of faecal concentrations of the pancreatic enzymes, trypsin and chymotrypsin. However, both faecal trypsin and chymotrypsin are prone to intestinal degradation and faecal chymotrypsin cross-reacts with exogenously administered enzyme therapy.

Serum trypsinogen has been used for newborn screening for more than two decades, and has been shown to help define pancreatic functional status in CF patients older than 7 years of age (Durie et al., 1986). This test has the added benefit of being able to predict the progression of pancreatic status from PS to PI (Couper et al., 1995). Serum trypsinogen is also capable of identifying the presence of pancreatic disease and dysfunction (loss of pancreatic reserve or pancreatitis) in individuals with a CFTR-related disorder (Ooi et al., 2010b).

Alternatively, the invasive direct pancreatic stimulation test allows assessment of both pancreatic acinar (enzyme) and ductular (electrolyte and fluid) status. There is currently no standardized methodology for direct pancreatic stimulation testing and various techniques are used throughout the world. Measurements and diagnosis of exocrine pancreatic status based on pancreatic stimulation testing warrants careful interpretation and can be misleading if not performed accurately. The quantitative pancreatic stimulation test that uses perfusion markers with multiple sampling periods is sensitive, highly specific, and capable of evaluating the entire range of pancreatic function (Groman et al., 2004). This technique is regarded as the true gold standard in direct pancreatic stimulation testing. Nevertheless, this test is time consuming, technically complex to perform and not routinely available. Consequently, alternative and simpler direct pancreatic stimulation techniques (non-quantitative), are used at many clinical centers. These generally utilise a single-lumen duodenal tube or endoscope to aspirate duodenal pancreatic secretions, either as a spot sample and/or over a timed sampling period (Choi et al., 2001; Monaghan et al., 2004; Rohlfs et al., 2002; Suaud et al., 2007). Despite their popularity, non-quantitative techniques have a high false positive rate for misdiagnosing PI and have not been proven superior over non-invasive indirect pancreatic function tests. In fact, Schibli et al. (2006) demonstrated that these techniques carry the greatest risk of misclassifying a PS patient as PI, especially among PS patients with a secretory capacity between the threshold of PI and the lower limit of normal (Grody et al., 2001; Schibli et al., 2006).

8.2 Referral to a CF care centre

As mentioned previously, CF and CFTR-related disease may manifest with variable severity, in single or multiple organs, and at different ages. For the clinician at hand dealing with a patient with pancreatitis associated with borderline or abnormal sweat test results and/or *CFTR* mutations, a more detailed assessment of other affected organ systems may be necessary. The phenotypic features of CF which should be kept in mind are summarised in Table 4. Furthermore, other organs affected by CFTR dysfunction may not be clinically evident at the time of diagnosis, thus overall assessment and routine follow-up is crucial. Referral should be made to a multidisciplinary CF care centre that can provide comprehensive diagnostic testing, determination of involvement of all affected organs (e.g. pulmonary disease), timely intervention, disease-specific counseling (e.g. fertility and smoking cessation for pancreatitis and lung disease), genetic counseling, and monitoring. Beyond the well-established phenotypic features of CF, cystic-fibrosis-related diabetes (CFRD) should also be tested for and monitored, particularly among those confirmed as having CF and who progress to PI.

8.3 Prognosis

Data from the Canadian CF registry shows that the median survival age in patients with CF has risen from 29.1 years in 1988 to 46.6 years in 2008 (Canadian Cystic Fibrosis Foundation, 2008). Similar improvements have occurred in other countries, but differences in survival persist (Fogarty, 2000). End-stage lung disease is the primary cause of morbidity and mortality in CF, but discussions on the respiratory aspects of CF are beyond the scope of this chapter. For patients with CFTR-related pancreatitis, the long-term outcomes are unknown.
A recent study reported an association between *CFTR* mutations and a higher risk of pancreatic adenocarcinoma (OR 1.82; 95% CI, 1.14-2.94; P = 0.011) (McWilliams et al., 2010). Carriers of *CFTR* mutations were seen to be diagnosed at a younger age than non-carriers, with the effect exclusively seen in ever-smokers (median 60 years vs. 65 years; P = 0.028).

Phenotypic Features of CF	
Gastrointestinal Abnormalities	*i.* Pancreatic: PI, recurrent-acute pancreatitis, chronic pancreatitis *ii.* Intestinal: meconium ileus, distal intestinal obstruction syndrome, rectal prolapse *iii.* Hepatic: prolonged neonatal jaundice, chronic hepatic disease (focal biliary cirrhosis or multilobular cirrhosis) *iv.* Nutritional: failure to thrive, hypoproteinemia and oedema, fat-soluble vitamin deficiency syndromes
Male Genital Tract Disease	*i.* Obstructive azoospermia due to congenital absence of the vas deferens
Chronic Sinopulmonary Disease	*i.* Persistent colonisation/infection with typical CF pathogens (Staphylococcus aureus, nontypeable Haemophilus influenza, mucoid and nonmucoid Pseudomonas aeruginosa, Stenotrophomonas maltophilia, and Burkholderia cepacia) *ii.* Chronic cough and sputum production *iii.* Persistent chest radiographic findings (e.g bronchiectasis, atelectasis, infiltrates, and hyperinflation) *iv.* Airway obstruction, with wheezing and air-trapping *v.* Nasal polyps *vi.* Digital clubbing

Table 4. Phenotypic features of CF. (Adapted from Farrell et al., 2008). CF, cystic fibrosis; PI, pancreatic insufficiency.

9. Areas for future research

Greater understanding of the true prevalence of CFTR-related disorders, including CFTR-related pancreatitis is much needed, and long-term studies in these patients are lacking.

Despite CF being a monogenic disease, the development of pancreatitis in CF and CFTR-related disorder is dependent on complex interactions with non-CFTR genetic, environmental and anatomic factors. Future research is needed to investigate the complex interaction between *CFTR*, other known (e.g. *PRSS1* and *SPINK1* mutations) and unknown genetic factors, and their interplay with environmental factors. Future studies are needed to determine the risk and protective modifier factors (genetic and environmental) that lead to the different single organ phenotypes in CFTR-related disorders (i.e. "why do individuals with the same combinations of *CFTR* mutations present heterogeneously?"). This in turn may also lead to additional therapeutic potentials.

One such therapeutic potential in the pipeline are small molecule therapies, known as CFTR correctors and potentiators. These therapies may have a role in not only patients with CF, but also those with CFTR-related pancreatitis; in view of our recent increased understanding of the relationship between CFTR dysfunction and risk of pancreatitis (Ooi et al., 2011a). A recent study of a CFTR mutation-specific potentiator reported improvement in CFTR function (measured using NPD and sweat chloride testing) and lung function in affected CF patients with a G551D mutation (Accurso et al., 2010).

With increased longevity of patients with CF, the relatively infrequent condition of pancreatic adenocarcinoma is anticipated to become more clinically relevant. In view of its associated high mortality rates, future studies into optimal screening regimens and modalities in patients with genetic causes of chronic pancreatitis are needed.

10. Conclusion

There has been a vast expansion in our understanding of the wide range of phenotypes associated with CFTR dysfunction since the discovery of the *CFTR* gene. Pancreatitis is one such phenotype, which is almost exclusively seen in patients who are PS. In addition, a relationship between the severity of *CFTR* genotypes and the risk of pancreatitis has been established. Paradoxically, genotypes associated with otherwise mild phenotypic effects have the greater risk for causing pancreatitis; compared with genotypes associated with moderate to severe disease phenotypes.

Idiopathic acute, recurrent-acute and chronic pancreatitis may be the initial manifestation of CF and CFTR-related disorder. However, diagnosing CF or CFTR-related disorder can be challenging. Sweat chloride testing is the principal diagnostic test and effectively diagnoses CF patients with the severe PI phenotype but it may have a limited ability to conclusively establish or exclude a diagnosis of CF disease. Careful interpretation of sweat chloride values and repeated testing may be necessary. *CFTR* genotyping for investigation of idiopathic pancreatitis has a limited diagnostic yield, may be misleading and may have uncertain "real life" consequence(s). Referral to a tertiary CF centre for further assessment is recommended, and periodical reassessment may be necessary to detect, monitor and intervene in treatable co-morbidities, even if the diagnostic criteria for CF cannot be fulfilled. Development of symptomatic pancreatitis is a strong risk factor for progressive decline in exocrine pancreatic function in patients with cystic fibrosis and possibly also in CFTR-related pancreatitis; thus, it is important to monitor for the development of exocrine pancreatic insufficiency over time.

11. References

Accurso, F.J.; Rowe, S.M.; Clancy, J.P.; Boyle, M.P.; Dunitz, J.M.; Durie, P.R.; et al. (2010). Effect of VX-770 in persons with cystic fibrosis and the G551D-CFTR mutation. *New England Journal of Medicine*, Vol.363, No.21, (November 2010), pp. 1991-2003, ISSN 0028-4793

Ahmed, N.; Corey, M.; Forstner, G.; Zielenski, J.; Tsui, L.; Ellis, L.; et al. (2003). Molecular consequences of cystic fibrosis transmembrane regulator (CFTR) gene mutations in the exocrine pancreas. *Gut*, Vol.52, No.8, (August 2003), pp. 1159-1164, ISSN 0017-5749

Beharry, S.; Ellis, L.; Corey, M.; Marcon, M. & Durie, P. (2002). How useful is fecal pancreatic elastase 1 as a marker of exocrine pancreatic disease?. *Journal of Pediatrics*, Vol.141, No.1, (July 2002), pp. 84-90, ISSN 0022-3476

Behrendorff, N.; Floetenmeyer, M.; Schwiening, C. & Thorn, P. (2010). Protons released during pancreatic acinar cell secretion acidify the lumen and contribute to pancreatitis in mice. *Gastroenterology*, Vol.139, (November 2010), pp. 1711-1720, ISSN 0016-5085

Bishop, M.D.; Freedman, S.D.; Zielenski, J.; Ahmed, N.; Dupuis, A.; Martin, S.; et al. (2005). The cystic fibrosis transmembrane conductance regulator gene and ion channel function in patients with idiopathic pancreatitis. *Human Genetics*, Vol.118, No.3-4, (December 2005), pp. 372-381, ISSN 0340-6717

Canadian Cystic Fibrosis Foundation (Ed.). (2008). Canadian Cystic Fibrosis Patient Data Registry Report 2008, In: *Cystic Fibrosis Canada*, 08.06.2011, Available from: http://www.cysticfibrosis.ca/assets/files/pdf/CPDR_ReportE.pdf

Cantin, A.M.; Hanrahan, J.W.; Bilodeau, G.; Ellis, L.; Dupuis, A.; Liao, J.; et al. (2006). Cystic fibrosis transmembrane conductance regulator function is suppressed in cigarette smokers. *American Journal of Respiratory and Critical Care Medicine*, Vol.173, No.10, (May 2006), pp. 1139-1144, ISSN 1073-449X

Castellani, C.; Macek, M.Jr.; Cassiman, J.J.; Duff, A.; Massie, J.; ten Kate, L.P.; et al. (2010). Benchmarks for cystic fibrosis carrier screening: a European consensus document. *Journal of Cystic Fibrosis*, Vol.9, No.3, (May 2010), pp. 165-178, ISSN 1569-1993

Castellani, C.; Cuppens, H.; Macek, M.; Cassiman, J.J.; Kerem, E.; Durie, P.; et al. (2008). Consensus on the use and interpretation of cystic fibrosis mutation analysis in clinical practice. *Journal of Cystic Fibrosis*, Vol.7, No.3, (May 2008), pp. 179-196, ISSN 1569-1993

Choi, J.Y.; Muallem, D.; Kiselyov, K.;Lee, M.G.; Thomas, P.J. & Muallem, S. (2001). Abberant CFTR-dependent HCO3- transport in muations associated with cystic fibrosis. *Nature*, Vol.410, No.6824, (March 2001), pp. 94-97, ISSN 0028-0836

Cohn, J.A.; Friedman, K.J.; Noone, P.G.; Knowles, M.R.; Silverman, L.M. & Jowell, P.S. (1998). Relation between mutations of the cystic fibrosis gene and idiopathic pancreatitis. *New England Journal of Medicine*, Vol.339, No.10, (September 1998), pp. 653-658, ISSN 0028-4793

Couper, R.T.; Corey, M.; Durie, P.R.; Forstner, G.G. & Moore, D.J. (1995). Longitudinal evaluation of serum trypsinogen measurement in pancreatic-insufficient and pancreatic-sufficient patients with cystic fibrosis. *Journal of Pediatrics*, Vol.127, No.3, (September 1995), pp. 408-413, ISSN 0022-3476

De Boeck, K.; Wilschanski, M.; Castellani, C.; Taylor, C.; Cuppens, H.; Dodge, J. & Sinaasappel, M. (2006). Cystic Fibrosis: terminology and diagnostic algorithms. [Review]. *Thorax*, Vol.61, No.7, (July 2006), pp. 627-635, ISSN 0040-6376

De Jonge, H.R.; Ballmann, M.; Veeze, H.; Bronsveld, I.; Stanke, F.; Tummler, B. & Sinaasappel, M. (2004). Ex vivo CF diagnosis by intestinal current measurements (ICM) in small aperture, circulating Ussing chambers. *Journal of Cystic Fibrosis*, Vol.3 Supplement 2, (August 2004), pp. 159-163, ISSN 1569-1993

Desmarquest, P.; Feldman, D.; Tamalat, A.; Boule, M.; Fauroux, B.; Tournier, G. & Clement, A. (2000). Genotype analysis and phenotypic manifestations of children with intermediate sweat chloride test results. *Chest*, Vol.118, No.6, (December 2000), pp. 1591-1597, ISSN 0012-3692

Dorfman, R. (April 2011). Cystic Fibrosis Mutation Database, 08.06.2011, Available from: http://www.genet.sickkids.on.ca/cftr

Dorfman, R.; Nalpathamakalam, T.; Taylor, C.; Gonska, T.; Keenan, K.; Yuan, X.W.; et al. (2010). Do common in silico tools predict the clinical consequences of amino-acid substitutions in the CFTR gene?. *Clinical Genetics*, Vol.77, No.5, (May 2010), pp. 464-473, ISSN 0009-9163

Dupuis, A.; Hamilton, D.; Cole, D.E. & Corey, M. (2005). Cystic fibrosis birth rates in Canada: a decreasing trend since the onset of genetic testing. *Journal of Pediatrics*, Vol.147, No.3, (September 2005), pp. 312-315, ISSN 0022-3476

Durie, P.R.; Forstner, G.G.; Gaskin, K.J.; Moore, D.J.; Cleghorn, G.J.; Wong, S.S. & Corey, M.L. (1986). Age-related alterations of immunoreactive pancreatic cationic trypsinogen in sera from cystic fibrosis patients with and without pancreatic insufficiency. *Pediatric Research*, Vol.20, No.3, (March 1986), pp. 209-213, ISSN 0031-3998

Durno, C.; Corey, M.; Zielenski, J.; Tullis, E.; Tsui, L. & Durie, P. (2002). Genotype and phenotype correlations in patients with cystic fibrosis and pancreatitis. *Gastroenterology*, Vol.123, No.6, (December 2002), pp. 1857-1864, ISSN 0016-5085

Farrell, P.M.; Rosenstein, B.J.; White, T.B.; Accurso, F.J.; Castellani, C.; Cutting, G.R.; et al. (2008). Guidelines for diagnosis of cystic fibrosis in newborns through older adults: Cystic Fibrosis Foundation consensus report. *The Journal of Pediatrics*, Vol.153, No.2, (August 2008), pp. S4-S14, ISSN 0022-3476

Fogarty, A. (2000). International comparison of median age at death from cystic fibrosis. *Chest*, Vol.117, No.6, (June, 2000), pp. 1656-1660, ISSN 0012-3692

Freedman, S.D.; Kern, H.F. & Scheele, G.A. (2001). Pancreatic acinar cell dysfunction in CFTR(-/-) mice is associated with impairments in luminal pH and endocytosis. *Gastroenterology*, Vol.121, No.4, (October 2001), pp. 950-957, ISSN 0016-5085

Gibson, L.E. & Cooke, R.E. (1959). A test for concentration of electrolytes in sweat in cystic fibrosis of the pancreas utilizing pilocarpine by iontophoresis. *Pediatrics*, Vol.23, No.3, (March 1959), pp. 545-549, ISSN 0031-4005

Gilljam, M.; Ellis, L.; Corey, M.; Zielenski, L.; Durie, P. & Tullis, D.E. (2004). Clinical manifestations of cystic fibrosis among patients diagnosed in adulthood. *Chest*, Vol.126, No.4, (October 2004), pp. 1215-1224, ISSN 0012-3692

Grody, W.W.; Cutting, G.R.; Klinger, K.W.; Richards, C.S.; Watson, M.S.; Desnick, R.J. & Subcommittee on Cystic Fibrosis Screening, Accreditation of Genetic Services Committee, ACMG. American College of Medical Genetics. (2001). Laboratory standards and guidelines for population-based cystic fibrosis carrier screening. *Genetics in Medicine*, Vol.3, No.2, (March-April 2001), pp. 149-54, ISSN 1098-3600

Groman, J.D.; Hefferon, T.W.; Casals, T.; Bassas, L.; Estivill, X.; Des Georges, M.; et al. (2004). Variation in a repeat sequence determines whether a common variant of the cystic fibrosis transmembrane conductance regulator gene is pathogenic or benign. *American Journal of Human Genetics*, Vol.74, No.1, (January 2004), pp. 176-179, ISSN 0002-9297

Highsmith, W.E.; Burch, L.H.; Zhou, Z.; Olsen, J.C.; Boat, T.E.; Spock, A.; et al. (1994). A novel mutation in the cystic fibrosis gene in patients with pulmonary disease but normal sweat chloride concentrations. *New England Journal of Medicine*, Vol.331, No.15, (October 1994), pp. 974-980, ISSN 0028-4793

Keiles, S. & Kammesheidt, A. (2006). Identification of CFTR PRSS1 and SPINK1 mutations in 381 patients with pancreatitis. *Pancreas*, Vol.33, No.3, (October 2006), pp. 221-227, ISSN 0885-3177

Knowles, M.R.; Paradiso, A.M. & Boucher, R.C. (1995). In vivo nasal potential difference – techniques and protocols for assessing efficacy of gene transfer in cystic fibrosis. *Human Gene Therapy*, Vol.6, No.4, (April 1995), pp. 445-455, ISSN 1043-0342

Kristidis, P.; Bozon, D.; Corey, M.; Markiewicz, D.; Rommens, J.; Tsui, L.C. & Durie, P. (1992). *American Journal of Human Genetics*, Vol.50, No.6, (June 1992), pp. 1178-1184, ISSN 0002-9297

Loser, C.; Mollgaard, A. & Folsch, U.R. (1996). Faecal elastase 1: a novel, highly sensitive, and specific tubeless pancreatic function test. *Gut*, Vol.39, No.4, (October 1996), pp. 580-586, ISSN 0017-5749

Maitra, A. & Kumar, V. (2005). Diseases of Infancy and Childhood, In: *Robbins and Cotran Pathologic Basis of Disease* (7th ed.), Kumar, V.; Abbas, A. & Fausto, N. (Eds.), 469-508, Elsevier Saunders, ISBN 978-0-7216-0187-8, Phildelphia, USA

Mall, M.; Hirtz, S.; Gonska, T. & Kunzelmann, K. (2004). Assessment of CFTR function in rectal biopsies for the diagnosis of cystic fibrosis. *Journal of Cystic Fibrosis*, Vol.3 Supplement 2, (August 2004), pp. 165-169, ISSN 1569-1993

McWilliams, R.R.; Petersen, G.M.; Rabe, K.G.; Holtegaard, L.M.; Lynch, P.J.; Bishop, M.D. & Highsmith, W.E.Jr. (2010). Cystic fibrosis transmembrane conductance regulator (CFTR) gene mutations and risk for pancreatic adenocarcinoma. *Cancer*, Vol.116, No.1, (January 2010), pp. 203-209, ISSN 0008-543X

Monaghan, K.G.; Highsmith, W.E.; Amos, J.; Pratt, V.M.; Roa, B.; Friez, M.; et al. (2004). Genotype-phenotype correlation and frequency of the 3199del6 cystic fibrosis mutation among I148T carriers: Results from a collaborative study. *Genetics in Medicine*, Vol.6, No.5, (September-October 2004), pp. 421-425, ISSN 1098-3600

Moran, A.; Hardin, D.; Rodman, D.; Allen, H.; Beall, R.; Borowitz, D.; et al. (1999). Diagnosis, screening and management of CF related diabetes mellitus: a consensus conference report. *Diabetes Research & Clinical Practice*, Vol.45, No.5, (August 1999), pp. 61-73, ISSN 0168-8227

Ooi, C.Y.; Dorfman, R.; Cipolli, M.; Gonska, T.; Castellani, C.; Keenan, K.; et al. (2011). Type of CFTR mutation determines risk of pancreatitis in patients with cystic fibrosis. *Gastroenterology*, Vol.140, No.1, (January 2011), pp. 153-161, ISSN 0016-5085

Ooi, C.Y.; Dupuis, A.; Keenan, K.; Tullis, E. & Durie, P.R. (2011). Role of sweat testing in patients with idiopathic pancreatitis. *Gastroenterology*, Vol.140, No.5, Supplement 1, (May 2011), pp. S-854-S-855, ISSN 0016-5085

Ooi, C.Y.; Gonska, T.; Durie, P.R. & Freedman, S.D. (2010). Genetic Testing in Pancreatitis. *Gastroenterology*, Vol.138, No.7, (June 2010), pp 2202-2206, ISSN 0016-5085

Ooi, C.Y.; Tullis, E. & Durie, P. (2010). Diagnostic Approach to CFTR-related Disorders, In: *Cystic Fibrosis. Lung Biology in Health and Disease Series*, Allen, J.; Rubenstein, R. & Panitch, H. (Eds.), 103-122, Informa Healthcare, ISBN 978-1-4398-0182-6, New York, USA

Oppenheimer, E.H. & Esterly, J.R. (1976). Pathology of cystic fibrosis: review of the literature and comparison with 146 autopsied cases. *Perspectives in Pediatric Pathology*, Vol.2, (n.d. 1976), pp. 241-278, ISSN 0091-2921

Pezzilli, R.; Morselli-Labate, A.M.; Palladoro, F.; Campana, D.; Piscitelli, L.; Tomassetti, P. & Corinaldesi, R. (2005). The ELISA fecal elastase-1 polyclonal assay reacts with different antigens than those of the monoclonal assay. *Pancreas*, Vol.31, No.2, (August 2005), pp. 200-201, ISSN 0885-3177

Robertson, M.B.; Choe, K.A. & Joseph, P.M. (2006). Review of the abdominal manifestations of cystic fibrosis in the adult patient. *Radiographics*, Vol.26, No.3, (May-June 2006), pp. 679-690, ISSN 0271-5333

Rohlfs, E.M.; Zhou, Z.; Sugarman, E.A.; Heim, R.A.; Pace, R.G.; Knowles, M.R.; et al. (2002). The I148T CFTR allele occurs on multiple haplotypes: a complex allele is associated with cystic fibrosis. *Genetics in Medicine*, Vol.4, No.5, (September-October 2002), pp. 319-323, ISSN 1098-3600

Rosenstein, B.J. (2006). Cystic Fibrosis, In: *Oski's Pediatrics* (4th ed.), McMillan, J.A.; Feigin, R.D.; DeAngelis, C. & Jones, M.D. (Eds.), 1426-1438, Lippincott Williams & Wilkins, ISBN 0-7817-3894-6, Philadelphia, USA

Schibli, S.; Corey, M.; Gaskin, K.J.; Ellis, L. & Durie, P.R. (2006). Towards the ideal quantitative pancreatic function test: analysis of test variable that influence validity. *Clinical Gastroenterology and Hepatology*, Vol.4, No.1, (January 2006), pp. 90-97, ISSN 1542-3565

Schuler, D.; Sermet-Gaudelus, I.; Wilschanski, M.; Ballmann, M.; Dechaux, M.; Edelman, A.; et al. (2004). Basic protocol for transepithelial nasal potential difference measurements. [Review]. *Journal of Cystic Fibrosis*, Vol.3 Supplement 2, (August 2004), pp. 151-155, ISSN 1569-1993

Shanbhogue, A.K.; Fasih, N.; Surabhi, V.R.; Doherty, G.P.; Shanbhogue, D.K. & Sethi, S.K. (2009). A clinical and radiologic review of uncommon types and causes of pancreatitis. *Radiographics*, Vol.29, No.4, (July-August 2009), pp. 1003-1026, ISSN 0271-5333

Sharer, N.; Schwarz, M.; Malone, G.; Howarth, A.; Painter, J.; Super, M. & Braganza, J. (1998). Mutations of the cystic fibrosis gene in patients with chronic pancreatitis. *New England Journal of Medicine*, Vol.339, No.10, (September 1998), pp. 645-652, ISSN 0028-4793

Shwachman, H. & Mahmoodian, A. (1967). Pilocarpine ionophoresis sweat testing results of seven years' experience. *Bibliotheca Paediatrica*, Vol.86, (n.d. 1967), pp. 158-182, ISSN 0301-357X

Stewart, B.; Zabner, J.; Shuber, A.P.; Welsh, M.J. & McCray, P.B.J. (1995). Normal sweat chloride values do not exclude the diagnosis of cystic fibrosis. *American Journal of Respiratory and Critical Care Medicine*, Vol.151, No.3 Pt 1, (March 1995), pp. 899-903, ISSN 1073-449X

Suaud, L.; Yan, W. & Rubenstein, R.C. (2007). Abnormal regulatory interactions of I148T-CFTR and the epithelial Na+ channel in Xenopus oocytes. *American Journal of Physiology. Cell Physiology*, Vol.292, No.1, (January 2007), pp. C603-611, ISSN 0363-6143

Tsui, L. (1992). The spectrum of cystic fibrosis mutations. *Trends in Genetics*, Vol.8, No.11, (November 1992), pp. 392-398, ISSN 0168-9525

Waters, D.L.; Dorney, S.F.; Gaskin, K.J.; Gruca, M.A.; O'Halloran, M. & Wilcken, B. (1990). Pancreatic function in infants identified as having cystic fibrosis in a neonatal screening program. *New England Journal of Medicine*, Vol.322, No.5, (February 1990), pp. 303-308, ISSN 0028-4793

Wilschanski, M. & Durie, P.R. (2007). Patterns of GI disease in adulthood associated with mutations in the CFTR gene. *Gut*, Vol.56, No.8, (August 2007), pp. 1153-1163, ISSN 0017-5749

Wilschanski, M. (2006). Mutations in the cystic fibrosis transmembrane regulator gene and in vivo transepithelial potentials. *American Journal of Respiratory and Critical Care Medicine*, Vol.174, No.7, (October 2006), pp. 787-794, ISSN 1073-449X

7

Diabetes or Diabetes Drugs: A Cause for Acute Pancreatitis

Leann Olansky
Cleveland Clinic,
USA

1. Introduction

About a decade ago, a question was raised about glyburide, a widely used sulfonylurea, as a possible cause for acute pancreatitis (Blomgren). Since then, several systemic reviews reveal the incidence of acute pancreatitis in patients with type 2 diabetes 1.5 to 3-fold increase risk compared to non-diabetic subjects in each of 3 large health data bases (Noel, Garg, Girman). Five years after the concern was raised about glyburide and soon after the first of the incretin based, exenatide, had gained a significant market share, reports of pancreatitis again began to surface. This was followed by a similar concern when the first in class of the next new class of diabetes agents, the dipeptyl depeditidase-4 inhibitor (DPP-4 inhibitor), sitagliptin had achieved a significant market share. Exenatide is a glucagon like peptide one (GLP-1) agonist and DPP-4 inhibitors increase to action of endogenous GLP-1 by slowing the degradation of endogenous GLP-1, as well of other gut derived hormones, so a common etiology was implied. Examination of two different insurance data bases, again reveal no real increase over other agents used to treat type 2 diabetes. Review of the incidence of acute pancreatitis from the adverse event data from the clinical trials of the two GLP-1 agonists and the three DPP-4 inhibitors available currently on the US market reveals similar rates of acute pancreatitis with each agent and with the comparators during blinded clinical trials, providing more evidence that it is the disease state, not the agent causing the increase in incidence.

This chapter will cover the wide variety of drugs that have been associated with acute pancreatitis as well as the studies that substantiate increase in acute pancreatitis in type 2 diabetes. The rate of acute pancreatits in incretin based agents and other agents as mentioned above seems the same as the rate in the population of type 2 diabetic as a whole. The rates of acute pancreatitis from clinical trial data of the five agents available in the US and the comparators afford the best prospective data on this subject.

2. Background

In 2002 Blomgren reported the association of acute pancreatitis with obesity and glyburide therapy in type 2 diabetic subjects (Blomgren). The first of a new class of incretin-mimetic agents, exendatide (Byetta) was introduced for the treatment of diabetes in 2005 and by 2006 the first report of acute pancreatitis was made by Denker (Denker) and soon others began to immerge. In 2007, the first of the dipeptyl depeditidase-4 (DPP-4) inhibitors (Januvia) entered the US market and by 2009 there were 88 reports of acute pancreatitis in patients treated with this agent (FDA). These agents shared a common pathway in improving metabolic control in diabetes by increasing the occupancy of GLP-1 receptors. The incretin-mimetic agents are synthetic agonists for the gut hormone, glucagon like peptide 1 (GLP-1)receptors, and the DPP-4 inhibitors extend the action of endogenous incretin hormones including GLP-1 and also gastric inhibitory peptide (GIP) as well other gut derived hormones by delaying their degradation. Perhaps, the fact that the pathway involved with each of these new types of agents has the potential to affect the gastrointestinal tract, there was concern that this might be responsible for precipitating acute pancreatitis.

Acute pancreatitis in the general population appears to be increasing in Western countries with 70–80% attributed to alcohol or gallstones but at least 20% has no clear etiology. Diabetic comorbidities of hypertriglyceridemia and obesity may increase their risk for acute pancreatitis. New etiologies continue to be described as evidenced by the report by Frulloni and colleagues of an autoimmune pancreatitis identified by a novel antibody directed at an epitope homologous to a protein from *Helicobacter pylori* (Frulloni). Type 2 diabetes is associated with obesity and hyperlipidemia, each of which has been considered a risk factor for pancreatitis (Trivedi, Blomgren). It is estimated that 2-5% of cases of acute pancreatitis are drug-induced. Many drugs have been associated with acute pancreatitis, yet these include drugs from varied classes, with very different modes of action and metabolic degradation pathways without any uniform explanation. Only alcohol, which both stimulates exocrine pancreatic secretion and contraction of the outlet sphincter (of Oddi) can be explained. In a 2005 review, Trivedi reported that, of the top 100 prescribed drugs in the United States, 44 have been associated with acute pancreatitis (Trivedi). These include over-the-counter agents such as acetaminophen, common antibiotics such as trimethoprim/ sulfamethoxazole and erythromycin, commonly used agents such as furosamide, glucocortiods, statins, angiotensin conversion inhibitors as well as agents used to treat human immunodeficiency virus acquired immunodeficiency syndrome, and oncologic agents. No clear pathophysiologic basis connects the various agents.

3. Diabetes and acute pancreatitis

The association of diabetes and acute pancreatitis was noticed at least a century ago and reported by Korte (Korte). His data was included in a large review by Shumacker along with many of Shumacker's own observations (Shumacker). Korte' s observation preceded any pharmacologic agents for diabetes and at a time of Schumacker's reports, only insulin was available to treat diabetes. While the emphasis of Shumacker's paper appears to be acute pancreatitis causing diabetes, he does report some patients who were known to have diabetes prior to the episode of acute pancreatitis. Schumacker also noted cholelithiasis and/or cholecystitis in patients with acute pancreatitis. Gall bladder disease is known to be increased in diabetes as well as a cause for acute pancreatitis (Pagliarulo). K. Warren made a similar case for pancreatitis causing diabetes in five cases (Warren 1950). However, S. Warren reported acute pancreatitis in 12 patients 6 months to 13 years after the diagnosis of diabetes in a pathology text dealing with pathology of diabetes (Warren 1952). Root reported 5 cases of acute pncreatitis with diabetes, four of which were shown at autopsy to have fatty livers, which suggests type 2 diabetes with accompanying insulin resistance (Root). Bossak's report seemed to be the first to emphasize acute pancreatitis complicating diabetes mellitus rather than causing diabetes (Bossak,). She noted 3 cases of acute pancreatitis in hospitalized patients with previously diagnosed diabetes which prompted an examination of the records of 103 patients admitted to Mount Sinai Hospital, New York City between 1936 and 1954. She found 5 more cases of acute pancreatitis in patients with pre-existing diabetes. Again, these observations were made in an era prior to any anti-diabetic therapies other than insulin. As more recent reports of acute pancreatitis have been published in association with agents used to treat diabetes, the earlier association of acute pancreatitis in the diabetic patient has not been acknowledged. Since these early twentieth century reports have been primarily in the way of case reports of acute pancreatitis in subjects with diabetes on a particular agent used in the treatment of diabetes or its comorbidities. Drugs such as metformin, ACE inhibitors and statins have been reported. The only series is that by Blomgren suggesting glyburide could increase the risk of acute pancreatitis and the relationship of that agent and the other agents has been primarily circumstantial (Balani, Blomgren, Jeandidier, Singh). The most common etiologies of acute pancreatitis accounting for 70-80% of cases are alcohol and gallstones. Chapman reported in 1996 a higher prevalence of gallstone disease based on ultrasound examination or report of cholecystectomy in diabetics (32.7%) compared to controls (20.8%, $p<0.001$) (Chapman, 1996). The difference was even greater for females were prevalence was 41.8% for female diabetic compared to controls 23.1% ($p<0.001$).

Drug Class	Agents
Cardiovascular	
ACE Inhibitors	Captopril, Enalopril, Lisinopril, Ramipril
Angiotensin Receptor Blocker	Losartan
Centrally acting	Metyldopa
Loop diuretic	Furosemide
Thiazide diuretic	Chlorothiazide, hydrocholthiazide
HMG-CoA reductase inhibitors	Simvastatin, pravastatin, fluvastatin, atrovastatin, rosuvastatin
Fibrate	Benzafibrate
Antidiabetic	Metformin, glyburide, exenatide, sitagliptin

Table 1. Common Agents used in treating diabetic patients with reports of acute pancreatitis

The increased prevalence of gall bladder disease in subjects with diabetes has been addressed more recently in the medical literature than the association with acute pancreatitis. In 1990 Haffner reported an increased incidence of gallbladder disease in non-insulin dependent diabetes mellitus (NIDDM, now referred to as type 2 diabetes) patients compared to those without diabetes in San Antonio Heart Study (Haffner). The relative risk was 1.6, 95% CI 1.08-2.37. There was an even greater risk in Mexican-American women compared to non Hispanic white women where the relative risk was 2.21, 95% CI 1.50-3.28. The San Antonio Heart Study was a landmark study that early on identified the insulin resistance with an increased risk for cardiovascular disease. The increased risk for gallbladder disease as well as cardiovascular disease in this population known to have resistance to insulin suggests that insulin resistance might be the common thread. Jorgensen failed to find an increased prevalence of gall stones in diabetic subjects in a Danish population after adjusting for obesity in a population not known for insulin resistance (Jorgensen). Chapman, in contrast, found an increased risk for gallstones in female diabetic subjects in New Zealand but no statistically increase in male diabetics after controlling for other know risk factors of BMI, HDL cholesterol, and TG, common comorbidities associated with type 2 diabetes (Chapman, 1996). Chapman reported increased gallbladder volume in type 2 diabetic subjects even without stones not seen in type 1 diabetics (Chapman 1998). It has been suggested that this reflects stasis or poor gallbladder emptying that could predispose to stone formation. Ruhl examined 5,653 adults as part of the third Unites States National Health and Nutrition Examination Survey (NHANES 1988-1994) a cross section of the US population, using ultrasound examinations, fasting glucose and insulin levels in a population not known to have diabetes (Ruhl). After controlling for other known risks for gall bladder disease, she found that women with undiagnosed diabetes (fasting blood glucose above 126 mg/dl (>7 mmole/L)) were at an almost 2-fold risk for gall stones (1.91, 95% CI 1.29-2.83). This risk increased as the fasting serum insulin increased comparing the highest to lowest quintiles. She suggested that it was the insulin resistance rather than diabetes that accounted for the increase in gall bladder disease even though this relationship was not seen in those who only had impaired fasting glucose (fasting glucose 110-125 mg/dl (6.1-6.9 mmole/L)). Boland reported gallbladder disease severe enough to lead to hospitalization in the Atherosclerosis Risk in Communities (ARIC) study of 3.8 per thousand person years increasing with an increase in BMI (Boland 2002). She also noted association to hyperinsulinemia, low HDL, hypertriglyceridemia and hormone replacement in diabetic women. Noel examined a US insurance data base for comorbidities of type 2 diabetes, acute pancreatitis and gall bladder disease and found relative risk for gall bladder disease to be quite similar to the investigators above (Noel). Girman examined health records covering 2003- 2007 from the General Practice Research Database (GPRD) in the UK and found rates that were not dissimilar (Girman). It is not a great leap to infer that increased rates of acute pancreatitis relate to the greater risk for gall bladder disease, a known risk factor for acute pancreatitis as suggested by Pagliarulo (Pagliarulo).

Author	Population	RR	95% CI	P value
Haffner	San Antonio Heart Study (all)	1.6	1.08-2.37	
	Mexican American vs Non Hispanic Women	2.21	1.50-3.82	
Jorgensen	Denmark	NS		
Chapman	New Zealand Women DM vs Non DM	1.8		<.001
	Women Type 2 DM vs Non DM	2.10		<0.001
	Women Type 1 DM vs Non DM	1.57		<0.05
	Men Type 2 DM vs Non DM	1.83		<0.05
	Men Type 1 vs Non DM	0.86		ns
Ruhl	USA Women DM vs Non DM	1.91	1.29-2.83	
Noel	US Type 2 DM vs Non DM	1.91	1.81-1.99	
Girman	UK Type 2 DM vs Non DM Adjusted	1.49	1.31-1.70	

Table 2. Risk of gall bladder disease in diabetic subjects.

The examine more directly the relative risk for acute pancreatitis in subjects with type 2 diabetes three separate large health data bases, two in the USA and one in United Kingdom, have been examined. Noel reported a 2.83 fold risk of acute pancreatitis as well as 1.91 fold risk for biliary tract disease in type 2 diabetic members by examining a large US health care claims database covering more than 100,000 person-years over the period from 1999-2005, a period predating GLP-1 or DPP4 therapies (Noel). Garg and Girman each examined other large health databases, Garg a US database and Girman one from the UK (Garg, Girman). Garg reports a 2.1 (95 % CI: 1.7-2.5) fold increase in acute pancreatitis in type 2 patients. Girman examined data from the (GPRD) found that 0.2% of type 2 diabetic subjects experienced acute pancreatitis from 2003 to 2007. Girman reports a similar increased risk for acute pancreatitis in type 2 diabetes of 2.89 (95% CI: 2.56-3.27) but after correction for age, gender and obesity the relative risk was 1.49 (95% CI:1.31-1.70). Only Girman made adjustment for obesity.

It is likely that the increase in acute pancreatitis in type 2 diabetic subjects is secondary to the gallbladder dysfunction. The increase in gallbladder disease is attributed to the secretion of lithogenic bile in the setting of obesity, insulin resistance and dyslipidemia. Which of these is primary is not known but studies by Grundy of bile composition in Pima Indian women, a group known to have a high risk for both type 2 diabetes and gallbladder disease, demonstrated an increase secretion of cholesterol and a reduced secretion of bile salts compared to non-stone forming Caucasian women and compared to Pima Indian men (Grundy, Sampliner). Lithogenic bile develops in the setting of inadequate bile salts or phospholipids to maintain cholesterol in solution (Dowling). Stones or sludge form due to supersaturation with cholesterol. Patients can have symptoms of gallbladder dysfunction even when no stones are present, a situation known as acalculous gallbladder disease presumably from this sludge (Fink-Bennett). The relationship of gallbladder disease risk to lipid metabolism in highlighted by Boland's finding in the ARIC study that Apo E4/E4 genotype subjects had a reduced risk to be hospitalized for gallbladder disease compared to all the other genotypes (Boland 2006). Apo E regulate metabolism of triglyceride rich lipid particles. The enzyme CYP7A1 appears to be key to the regulation of cholesterol conversion to bile salts (Pandak). CYP7A1 is regulated by LXR *alpha*, the nuclear oxysterol receptor liver X receptor *alpha* (Goodwin) and that regulation is complex but it has been shown that LXR alpha null mice feed a high cholesterol diet accumulate cholesterol in the liver and eventually die of liver failure. The relationship to insulin resistance and type 2 diabetes has yet to be elucidated but this may be a model for non-alcoholic liver disease seen with increasing frequency in obese type 2 diabetic subjects with dyslipidemia.

4. Diabetes and incretin-based antidiabetic therapies

The association acute pancreatitis with diabetes and with exenatide and sitagliptin usage has been examined systematically by Dore as well as Garg (Dore, Garg). Dore examined similar large health data base covering 2005 to 2008 and was able to compare the risk of acute pancreatitis in over 27,000 exenatide users and matched metformin or glyburide users and found the relative risk for acute pancreatitis was 1.0 (95% CI: 0.6-1.7). He compared over 16,000 sitagliptin users with matched metformin or glyburide users and found the relative risk for acute pancreatitis to be 1.0 (95% CI 0.5-2.0). Garg examined another large US health claims database of 786,656 patients and found the incidence of acute pancreatitis to be 1.9 per 1000 patients years in non-diabetic control group compared to 5.6 per 1000 patient years in the diabetic control group. Exenatide users incidence for pancreatitis was 5.7 and for sitagliptin users 5.6 cases per 1000 patient years. This data is retrospective.

Is there any prospective data that is relevant to this subject? If we examine the adverse event reporting from the clinical trials that lead to approval of incretin based therapies, we see very similar incidence rates. These were fairly large trials with balanced patient demographics and fairly complete data collection as these event were undoubtedly Severe Adverse Events (SARs) requiring extensive follow-up reporting to the FDA. **Exenatide:** Examination of the clinical trial data deposited with the FDA shows that in the exenatide development program, six cases of acute pancreatitis were observed in about 3,489 subject-years of exposure (1.7 per 1,000 subject-years), compared with one case in about 336 subject-years with placebo (3.0 per 1,000 subject-years) and one case in about 497 subject-years (2.0 per 1,000 subject-years) with insulin (FDA.gov/Drugs/DrugSafey). **Liraglutide:** The second GLP-1 agonist to market, showed a similar risk of acute pancreatitis, with seven cases in 3,900 patients receiving liraglutide compared with one case in a patient taking comparator diabetes agents. Liraglutide incidence was similar to that seen in exenatide clinical trials but the control goup had fewer than expected, suggesting an ascertainment bias or that comparison groups might have been underreported. **Sitagliptin.** The pooled analysis of controlled clinical trials revealed incidence rates to be (0.8 events vs. 1.0 events per 1000 patient-years for comparators. **Saxagliptin** the second DPP-4 inhibitor to reach the US market. reported an incidence of acute pancreatitis of 0.2% in 3,422 patients receiving saxagliptin and 0.2% in 1,066 controls in mostly shorter termed trials. **Linagliptin**, the most recent addition to the US DPP-4 inhibitor agents showed 0.2% incidence of acute pancreatitis (1 case in 538 person years and 0 in 433 patient-years in the comparators). The risk of acute pancreatitis in each of these trials is similar to that found by Noel, Garg and Girman during periods predating most of these agents (Noel, Garg, Girman). Despite this reassuring data, the FDA requires warnings for each product and continues post-marketing surveillance for acute pancreatitis. As new antidiabetic agents enter the market and their use becomes common, we expect similar rates of acute pancreatitis to be reported, just as was reported in by Blomgren in 2002 for glyburide as it was reaching peak popularity (Blomgren).

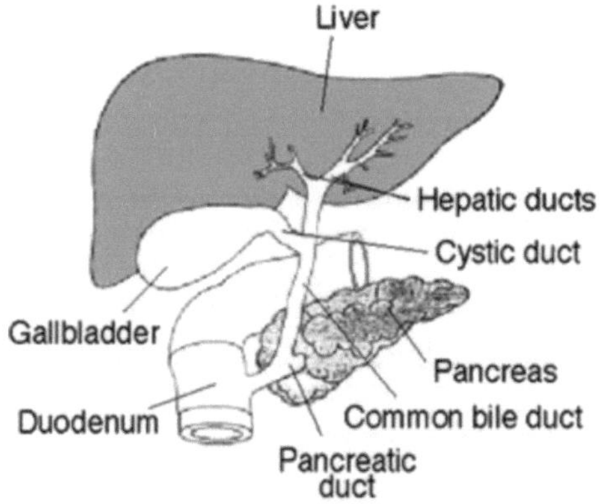

Fig. 1. Pathophysiology of gallbladder disease and acute Pancreatitis in type 2 diabetes. Liver produces lithogenic bile that forms stones or sludge. The occlusion of the common bile duct obstructs the pancreatic duct leading to acute pancreatitis.

5. Discussion

The medical literature over the past century reflects an increase in gallblader disease and acute pancreatitis in patients with diabetes, particularly those with type 2 diabetes. These patients are often obese, with dyslipidemia. The association of dyslipidemia with lithogenic bile may be the explanation for the increased incidence of gallbladder disease in type 2 diabetic subjects and this is the likely explanation for the increase in acute pancreatitis as illustrated in Figure 1. If any agent would be predicted to be associated with an increase in gallbladder disease and acute pancreatitis, it might be colesevelam, a bile sequesterant with glucose lowering action, due to the loss of bile salts but no reports of an increase in acute pancreatitis with this agent have immerged. It is unlikely that any one class of medications used to treat diabetes has significantly altered this risk. It would be helpful if the risk for acute pancreatitis associated with type 2 diabetes were more generally known so that as each new agent is not accused of causing the problem when it achieves a significant level or use.

6. References

Balani B, Grendel JH (2008). Drug-induced pancreatitis. *Drug Safety*. 31:p823-827.

Blomgren KB, Steineck G, Sundstrom A, Wiholm BE (2002). Obesity and treatment of diabetes with glyburide may both be risk factors for acute pancreatitis. *Diabetes Care*. 25: pp 298-302.

Boland LL, Folsom AR, Rosamond WD (2002). Hyperinsulinemia, dyslipidemia, and obesity as risk factors for hospitalized gallbladder disease: A prospective study. *Ann. Epidemiol.* 12: pp131-40.

Boland LL, Folsom AR, Boerwinle E (2006). Apolipolipoprotein E genotype and gallbladder disease risk in a large population-based cohort. *Ann Epidemiol* 10: pp 763-9.

Bossak ET Joelson RH. (1956). Acute pancreatitis complicating diabetes mellitus. *A.M.A. Archives Int Med.* 97: pp 201-207.

Chapman BA, Wilson IR, Frampton CM, Chisholm RJ, Stewart NR, Eagar GM, et al (1996) Prevalence of gallbladder disease in diabetes mellitus. *Digestive Dis and Sciences* 41: pp2222-2228.

Chapman BA, Chapman TM, Frampton CM, Chisholm RJ, Allan RB, Wilson IR, et al (1998) Gallbladder volume: comparison of diabetics and controls. *Digestive Dis and Sciences* 43: pp344-48.

Denker PS, Demarco PE. (2006) Exenatide (Exendin-4)-induced pancreatitis. *Diabetes Care* 29: p 471.

Dore DD, Seeger JD, Arnold Chan K. (2009) Use of a claims-based active drug safety surveillance system to assess the risk of acute pancreatitis with exenatide or sitagliptin compared to metformin or glyburide. *Curr Med Res Opin* 25: pp1019-27.

Dowling RH. (2000) Review: pathogenesis of gallstones. *Aliment Pharmacol Ther* 14 (suppl.2): pp 39-47.

http://www.FDA.gov/Drugs/DrugSafety (2011).

Fimognari FL, Corsonello A, Pastorell R, Antonelli-Incalzi R (2006) Metformin-induced pancreatitis. *Diabetes Care* 29:p 1183.

Fink-Bennett D, DeRidder P, Kolozsi WZ, Gordon R, Jaros R (1991) Cholecystokinin cholescinitigraphy: Detection of abnormal gallblader motor function in patients with chronic acalculous gallbladder disease. *J Nuc Med* 32: pp1695-99.

Frulloni L, Lunardi C, Simone R, Dolcino M, Scattolini C, Falconi M, et al. (2009) Identification of a novel antibody associated with autoimmune pancreatitis. *N Engl J Med* 361: pp 2135-42.

Garg R, Chen W, Pendergrass M (2010) Acute pancreatitis in Type 2 diabetes treated with exenatide or sitagliptin: a restrospective observational pharmacy claims analysis. *Diabetes Care* 33: pp 2349-2354.

Girman CJ, Kou TD, Cai B, Alexander CM, O' Neill EA, Williams-Herman DE, Katz L (2010) Patients with type 2 diabetes have higher risk for acute pancreatitis compared with those without diabetes. *Diabetes Obes and Metab* 12: pp 766-771.

Goodwin B, Watson MA, Kim H, Miao J, Kemper JK, Kliewer SA (2003) Differential regulation of rat and human CYP7A1 by the nuclear oxysterol receptor liver X receptor-*alpha*. *Molecular Endocrinol* 17: pp 386-94.

Grundy SM, Metzger AL, Adler RD (1972) Mechanisma of lithogenic bile formation in American Indian women with cholesterol gallstones. *J Clin Invest* 51: pp 3026-43.

Haffner SM, Diehl AK, Mitchell BD, Stern MP, Hazuda HP (1990) Increased prevalence of clinical gall bladder disease in subjects with non-insulin-dependent diabetes mellitus. *Am J Epidemiol* 132: pp327-335.

Jeandidier N, Klewansky M, Pinget M (1995) Captopril-induced acute pancreatitis. *Diabetes Care* 18:pp410-411.

Jorgensen T (1989) Gall stones in a Danish populationa. Relationship to weight, physical activity, smoking, coffee consumption, and diabetes mellitus. *Gut* 30: pp 528-534.

Korte W. (1911) Die chirurgische Behandlung der acuten pankreatitis. *Archiv klinische Chirurgia* 96: pp 557-615.

Mallick S (2004) Metformin indiced acute pancreatitis precipitiated by renal failure. *Postgraduate Med* 80: pp239-240.

Noel RA, Patterson RE, Braun DK, Bloomgren GL. (2009) Increased risk for acute pancreatitis and biliary disease observed in patients with type 2 diabetes. *Diabetes Care.* 32: pp 834-38.

Pagliarulo M, Fornari F, Fraquelli M, Zoli M, Giangregorio F, Grigolon A, Peracchi M, Conte D. (2004) Gallstone disease and related risk factors in a large cohort of diabetic patients. *Dig Liver Dis.* 36: pp 130-4.

Pandak WM, Schwarz C, Hyleemon PB, Mallonee D, Valerie K, Heuman DM, et al (2001) Effects of CYP7A1 overexpressionon cholesterol and bile salt homeostatis. *Am J Physiol Gastrointest Liver Physiol* 281: pp G878-89.

Root HF.(1937) Diabetic coma and acute pancreatitis with fatty livers. *JAMA* 108: pp 777-780.

Ruhl CE, Everhart JE (2000) Association of diabetes, serum insulin and c-peptide with gall bladder disease. *Hepatology* 31: pp 299-303.

Sampliner RE, Bennett PH, Comess LJ, Rose FA, Burch TA. (1970) Gallbladder disease in Pima Indians: Demonstration of high prevalence and early onset by cholecystography. *N Engl J Med* 283: pp 1358-64.

Shumacker HB. (1940) Acute pancreatitis and diabetes. *Annals Surgery* 112: pp 177-200

Singh S, Nautiyal A, Dolan JG (2004). Recurrent acute pancreatitis possibly induced by atrovastatin and rosuvastatin. Is statin induced pancreatitis a class effect? *J Pancreas* 5: pp 502-504.

Trivedi CD, Pitchumoni CS. (2005) Drug-induced pancreatitis: an update. *J Clin Gastroenterol.* 39: pp 709-16.

Warren KW, Fallis LS, Barron J. (1950) Acute pancreatitis and diabetes. *Annals Surgery* 132: pp 1103-1110.

Warren S, Le Compte (1952) *The Pathology of Diabetes Mellitus*, Philadelphia. Lea & Febiger, pp 68-69.

Part 2

Pathogenesis

8

Role of Peritoneal Macrophages on Local and Systemic Inflammatory Response in Acute Pancreatitis

Marcel Cerqueira Cesar Machado and Ana Maria Mendonça Coelho
University of São Paulo,
Brazil

1. Introduction

Severe acute pancreatitis is a serious disease with high morbidity and mortality.[1,2] Despite many experimental and clinical studies its pathophysiology is yet not completely understood. It is well accepted that activation of enzymes within the pancreatic tissue is the initial event in acute pancreatitis followed by a cascade of events that modify not only the local process but also affect distant organs and systems.[3] Indeed, previous studies have demonstrated that acute pancreatitis is associated with an increase in inflammatory mediators that induce the systemic inflammatory response syndrome (SIRS) and are associated with distant organ dysfunction being responsible for the morbidity and mortality related to disease.[4,5] Acute pancreatitis is characterized by release of proteolytic enzymes from the pancreas and activation of several signaling pathway in macrophages resulting in the releasing of TNF-α.[6,7]

2. Macrophages

Macrophages are released from bone marrow migrate to many tissues and undergo to final differentiation into specific type of resident macrophages. Macrophages are concentrated in lungs, spleen, liver (Kupffer cells), lymphnodes, and in the serosal membrane of pleural and peritoneal cavity. Activation of macrophages by different insults may result in the production of many substances that interfere in the immune response. Inflammation lymphocytes activation and secretion of various cytokines are some of the many function of macrophages.

The degree of macrophages activation seems to be an important factor determining the severity of acute pancreatitis.[8-10] In the pancreatic tissue, besides enzymatic activation, and acinar cells production of TNF-α, macrophages and monocytes are the main inflammatory cells involved in the pathogenesis of local and systemic inflammation. The production of proinflammatory substances by these cells results in amplification of the inflammation to distant organs as liver, lungs kidneys intestines and might result in multi organs failure.[11-13] Following pancreatic inflammation several organs like liver, spleen and lungs with a large population of macrophages function as important source of cytokines production further amplifying the inflammatory response.[14] In spite the production of cytokines macrophages also induce the activation of enzymes as inducible nitric oxide synthase (iNOS) or

cyclooxygenase 2 (COX-2) involved in the production of nitric oxide and arachdonic acid.[15] The severity of acute pancreatitis seems to be related to the levels of proinflammatory cytokines as IL-1, IL-6, IL-8, and TNF-α, PAF, and C-reactive protein.[3,16] Administration of agents that antagonize or diminish the production of TNF-α is associated with decreasing of the systemic effects of acute pancreatitis.[17,18]
In a previous study we have showed that treatment of rats with acute pancreatitis by administration of hypertonic saline solution reduces the production of inflammation markers (inducible nitric oxide synthase, cyclooxygenase 2, TNF-α, and IL-6) in pancreatic tissue. The volume of ascitic fluid and level of cytokines in ascitic fluid were also reduced, decreasing the systemic inflammatory response in experimental acute pancreatitis.[19] In this study pancreatic enzymes activation was not reduced in animals receiving hypertonic saline, therefore ascitic fluid volume and TNF-α reduction were probably caused by decrease of peritoneal macrophages proinflammatory response.[20,21] Administration of hypertonic saline solution reduces the production of cytokines by these cells and reduces the systemic inflammatory response in experimental acute pancreatitis.[19]

	Pancreatic TNF-α	Pancreatic IL-6	Pancreatic IL-10	Pancreatic IL-10/TNF- α ratio
Control (without AP)	12,6± 0,9	9,3 ±1,9	2,7 ± 0,27 *	0.22
AP Non-treated	45,0 ± 6,9 *	44,1 ± 5,6 *	14,6 ± 2,1	0,32
AP hypertonic saline-treated	23,1 ± 4,2 #	18,7 ± 1,2 #	16,4 ± 2,8	0,88*

Pancreatic levels of TNF- α, IL-6; and IL-10 were measured in homogenates of pancreas (pg/mg protein). Date are expressed of mean ± SEM *, #$p<0.05$

Table 1. Effect of hypertonic saline solution on pancreatic inflammation in acute pancreatitis (AP).

	COX-2	iNOS
Control (without AP)	100 ± 0	100± 0
AP Non-treated	329 ± 16 *	505 ± 105 *
AP hypertonic saline-treated	206 ± 38 #	213 ± 48#

Date are expressed of mean ± SEM *, #$p<0.05$

Table 2. Effect of hypertonic saline solution on the expression of COX-2 and iNOS (Western blot analysis) in the pancreas in acute pancreatitis (AP)

	Ascitic Fluid Volume (ml)	Ascitic Fluid TNF-α (pg/ml)
Control (without AP)	0	0
AP Non-treated	1.8 ± 0.3*	192 ± 23 *
AP hypertonic saline-treated	0.8 ± 0.2 #	64 ± 10#

Date are expressed of mean ± SEM *, #p<0.05

Table 3. Effect of hypertonic saline solution on peritoneal inflammation in acute pancreatitis (AP).

In the early stage of inflammatory response there is activation of macrophages (M1 macrophages) that release proinflammatory cytokines as TNF-α IL-1β and IL-6.[15] Besides M1 macrophages another population of macrophages was observed (M2a) called alternative related to wound healing. This population of macrophages is unable to produce NO and to present antigen to T cells. This population of macrophages up regulates mannose receptor expression and arginase II [22,23] and seems to act in the production of extracellular matrix. There is yet another population of macrophages (M2b) found in the later stages of inflammation which are related to the production of IL-10 and TGF beta with inhibition of the production of proinflammatory mediators.[24]

2.1 Peritoneal macrophages

Peritoneal macrophages in spite to be a small fraction of the total population seem to performing an important role in the defense against infection in the peritoneal cavity and in the severity of acute pancreatitis.

Previous study demonstrated that trypsin stimulates the production of cytokines from peritoneal macrophages in vitro and in vivo.[25] In acute pancreatitis there is activation and leakage of enzymes from the intracellular compartment to pancreatic interstitium, peripancreatic tissues and peritoneal cavity[26], therefore activating peritoneal macrophages and increasing the production of TNF-α[25] Peritoneal macrophages from animals with acute pancreatitis are more efficient in the production of TNF-α than controls when challenged with LPS.[27] Indeed some investigators in 1970s proposed that most of the mediators of inflammatory process in acute pancreatitis could be found in the peritoneal cavity and should be removed in order to attenuate the systemic inflammatory syndrome associated with acute pancreatitis.[28] Endotoxin can also increase the production of TNF-α by peritoneal macrophages that makes infected pancreatic necrosis extremely dangerous. Many investigators demonstrated that pancreatitis associated ascitic fluid has noxious effects on mitochondria[29], kidney and lungs besides an apoptosis-inducing-factor.[30] The key point in these studies is to understand the importance of peritoneal macrophages on the systemic inflammatory response in acute pancreatitis.[31,32] Peritoneal macrophages represent a small fraction of the total macrophage population however they are strategically located lining the serosal peritoneal membrane. Activated peritoneal macrophages have many activities such

as lymphocyte activation, tissue damage and microbiocidal activity through the production of several cytokines as TNF-α, IL-1, IL-8 TGF-β1, superoxide and nitric oxide.[30]
Overproduction of these substances however, may be dangerous inducing systemic inflammatory response. Reducing the production or removal of these substances may have beneficial effects on the inflammatory response in acute pancreatitis. Indeed, previous study has shown the beneficial effect of peritoneal lavage in acute pancreatitis. [28]
Recently, we have demonstrated that peritoneal lavage in an experimental model of acute pancreatitis not only leads to a decrease in serum levels of TNF-α and IL-6 but also results in an increase in serum levels of IL-10.[33] (Table 4). We have also demonstrated in the pancreatic tissue a reduction in cycloxygenase-2 and inducible nitric oxide synthase expression.[33] (Table 5)

	Serum TNF-α (pg/ml)	Serum IL-6 (pg/ml)	Serum IL-10 (pg/ml)
AP Non-treated	32 ± 10	258 ± 46	39 ± 8
AP Peritoneal lavage-treated	7 ± 5*	141 ± 26*	149 ± 46*

Date are expressed of mean ± SEM * $p<0.05$

Table 4. Effect of peritoneal lavage on systemic inflammation in acute pancreatitis (AP).

	COX-2	iNOS
Sham	100 ± 0	100± 0
AP Non-treated	454 ± 38 *	609 ± 104 *
AP Peritoneal lavage-treated	304 ± 25 #	410 ± 63 #

Data are expressed of mean ± SEM *,# $p<0.05$

Table 5. Effect of peritoneal lavage on the expression of COX-2 and iNOS (Western blot analysis) in the pancreas in acute pancreatitis (AP).

We concluded that peritoneal lavage has an anti-inflammatory effect in acute pancreatitis. It is possible that a special subset of peritoneal macrophages with anti-inflammatory properties is preserved or activated during peritoneal lavage.[24]
It has been demonstrated that CO_2 pneumoperitoneum decreases TNF-α and interleukin IL-6 production while increasing the production of IL-10.[34]
Indeed peritoneal macrophages exposed to CO2 in vitro have a significant decrease of TNF-α production when stimulated with LPS.[35] CO2 pneumoperitoneum pretreatment alters acute-phase response[36] and increases survival in an experimental model of lipopolysaccharide (LPS)-contaminated laparotomy.[37]

It has been suggested that the local tissue acidification due to CO2 pneumoperitoneum decreases the production of cytokines by peritoneal macrophages.[36] Recently, we have demonstrated that CO_2 abdominal insufflation decreases pancreatic inflammation and systemic inflammatory response in an acute pancreatitis model.[38] (Tables 6-8).

	Ascitic Fluid (ml)	TNF-α (pg/ml ascitic fluid)	Peritoneal cells ($x10^6$)
AP Non-treated	4.2 ± 0.4	534 ± 129	21 ± 2
AP CO_2-treated	2.4 ± 0.4*	188 ± 47*	14 ± 2*

Date are expressed of mean ± SEM * $p<0.05$

Table 6. Effect of CO_2 insufflation on the peritoneal inflammation induced by acute pancreatitis (AP).

	Serum TNF-α (pg/ml)	Serum IL-6 (pg/ml)	Serum IL-10 (pg/ml)	Serum IL-10/TNF- α ratio
AP Non-treated	228 ±92	92 ±19	40 ±5	0.18
AP CO2-treated	34 ±16*	42 ±12*	37 ± 9	1.09*

Date are expressed of mean ± SEM * $p<0.05$

Table 7. Effect of CO_2 insufflation on the systemic inflammation induced by acute pancreatitis (AP).

	COX-2	iNOS
Sham	100 ± 0	100± 0
AP Non-treated	545 ±159 *	446 ±85*
AP CO_2-treated	198 ±31	132 ±5

Data are expressed of mean ± SEM * $p<0.05$

Table 8. Effect of CO_2 insufflation on the expression of COX-2 and iNOS (Western blot analysis) in the pancreas in acute pancreatitis (AP).

In this study we also demonstrated that CO_2 abdominal insufflation not only reduces the serum levels of proinflammatory cytokines but did not changed the serum levels of IL-10. The ratio of IL-10 over TNF-α demonstrates a clear anti inflammatory effect of CO_2 pneumoperitoneum.[38] The CO_2 pneumoperitoneum also decreases the inflammation in the peritoneal cavity reducing the volume of ascitic fluid and the total content of TNF- α.[38] It is conceivable that if an endoscopic procedure for stone retrieval has to be performed it should be done during the laparoscopic cholecystectomy to decrease the inflammatory response secondary to acute pancreatitis. These results suggested that peritoneal macrophages play an important role on the outcome of acute pancreatitis and should be considered an important target for therapeutic management in acute pancreatitis. However, peritoneal macrophages are also important in the defense against infection in the peritoneal cavity. In a large experience in the surgical treatment of acute pancreatitis we have observed that even draining pancreatic abscess through the abdominal cavity we rarely observed bacterial peritonitis. It seems that peritoneal macrophages priming by pancreatic enzymes are more effective to protect peritoneal cavity from bacterial infection.[27]

3. Conclusion

In spite to be a small fraction of body population peritoneal macrophages have an important role in the pathophysiology of acute pancreatitis and should be object of future clinical trials and probably a target for the modulation of systemic inflammatory response in acute severe pancreatitis.

4. References

[1] Pitchumoni CS, Patel NM, Shah P. Factors influencing mortality in acute pancreatitis: can we alter them? J *Clin Gastroenterol*, 2005; 39: 798-814.

[2] Frossard JL, Steer ML, Pastor CM. Acute pancreatitis. *Lancet*, 2008; 12; 371: 143-152.

[3] Bhatia M, Wong FL, Cao Y, Lau HY, Huang J, Puneet P et al. Pathophysiology of acute pancreatitis. *Pancreatology*, 2005; l5: 132-144.

[4] Granger J, Remick D. Acute pancreatitis: models, markers, and mediators. *Shock*, 2005; 1: 45-51.

[5] Elfar M, Gaber LW, Sabek O, Fischer CP, Gaber AO. The inflammatory cascade in acute pancreatitis: relevance to clinical disease. *Surg Clin North Am*, 2007; 87: 1325-1340.

[6] Bhatia M. Acute pancreatitis as a model of SIRS. *Front Biosci*, 2009; 14: 2042-2050.

[7] Malleo G, Mazzon E, Siriwardena AK, Cuzzocrea S. Role of tumor necrosis factor-alpha in acute pancreatitis: from biological basis to clinical evidence. *Shock*, 2007; 28: 130-140.

[8] Liang T, Liu TF, Xue DB, Sun B, Shi LJ. Different cell death modes of pancreatic acinar cells on macrophage activation in rats. *Chin Med J*, 2008; 121: 1920-1924.

[9] Gea-Sorlí S, Closa D. Role of macrophages in the progression of acute pancreatitis. *World J Gastrointest Pharmacol Ther*, 2010; 1: 107-111.

[10] Shrivastava P, Bhatia M. Essential role of monocytes and macrophages in the progression of acute pancreatitis. *World J Gastroenterol*, 2010; 16: 3995-4002.

[11] Hirota M, Nozawa F, Okabe A, Shibata M, Beppu T, Shimada S et al. Relationship between plasma cytokine concentration and multiple organ failure in patients with acute pancreatitis. *Pancreas,* 2000; 21: 141-146

[12] Zhang Q, Ni Q, Cai D, Zhang Y, Zhang N, Hou L. Mechanisms of multiple organ damages in acute necrotizing pancreatitis. Chin Med J (Engl), 2001; 114: 738-742.

[13] Shi C, Zhao X, Lagergren A, Sigvardsson M, Wang X, Andersson R. Immune status and inflammatory response differ locally and systemically in severe acute pancreatitis. *Scand J Gastroenterol,* 2006; 41: 472-480.

[14] Dugernier TL, Laterre PF, Wittebole X, Roeseler J, Latinne D, Reynaert MS et al. Compartmentalization of the inflammatory response during acute pancreatitis: correlation with local and systemic complications. Am J *Respir Crit Care Med,* 2003; 68: 148-157.

[15] Mosser DM, Edwards JP. Exploring the full spectrum of macrophage activation. *Nat Rev Immunol,* 2008; 8: 958-969.

[16] Sakorafas GH, Tsiotou AG. Etiology and pathogenesis of acute pancreatitis: current concepts. *J Clin Gastroenterol,* 2000; 30: 343-356.

[17] Machado MC, Coelho AM, Pontieri V, Sampietre SN, Molan NA, Patzina RA, et al. Local and systemic effects of hypertonic solution (NaCl 7.5%) in experimental acute pancreatitis. *Pancreas,* 2006; 32: 80-86.

[18] Matheus AS, Coelho AM, Sampietre S, Jukemura J, Patzina RA, Cunha JE et al. Do the effect of pentoxifylline on inflammatory process and pancreatic infection justify its use in acute pancreatitis? *Pancreatology,* 2009; 9: 687-693.

[19] Coelho AM, Jukemura J, Sampietre SN, Martins JO, Molan NA, Patzina RA et al. Mechanisms of the beneficial effect of hypertonic saline solution in acute pancreatitis. *Shock,* 2010; 34: 502-507.

[20] Oreopoulos GD, Bradwell S, Lu Z, Fan J, Khadaroo R, Marshall JC et al. Synergistic induction of IL-10 by hypertonic saline solution and lipopolysaccharides in murine peritoneal macrophages. *Surgery,* 2001; 130: 157-165.

[21] Cuschieri J, Gourlay D, Garcia I, Jelacic S, Maier RV. Hypertonic preconditioning inhibits macrophage responsiveness to endotoxin. *J Immunol,* 2002; 168: 1389-1396.

[22] Stein M, Keshav S, Harris N, Gordon S. Interleukin 4 potently enhances murine macrophage mannose receptor activity: a marker of alternative immunologic macrophage activation. *J Exp Med,* 1992; 176: 287-292.

[23] Gordon S. Alternative activation of macrophages. *Nat Rev Immunol,* 2003; 3: 23-35.

[24] Fadok VA, Bratton DL, Konowal A, Freed PW, Westcott JY, Henson PM. Macrophages that have ingested apoptotic cells in vitro inhibit proinflammatory cytokine production through autocrine/paracrine mechanisms involving TGF-beta, PGE2, and PAF. *J Clin Invest,* 1998; 101: 890-898.

[25] Lundberg AH, Eubanks JW 3rd, Henry J, Sabek O, Kotb M, Gaber L et al. Trypsin stimulates production of cytokines from peritoneal macrophages in vitro and in vivo. *Pancreas,* 2000; 21: 41-51.

[26] Heath DI, Wilson C, Gudgeon AM, Jehanli A, Shenkin A, Imrie CW. Trypsinogen activation peptide (TAP) concentration in the peritoneal fluid of patients with acute

pancreatitis and their relation to the presence of histologically confirmed pancreatic necrosis. *Gut,* 1994; 35,: 1311-1315.

[27] Sameshima N, Kei S, Mori K. The role of tumor necrosis factor alpha in the aggravation of cerulein-induced pancreatitis in rats. *Int J Pancreatol,* 1993; 14: 107-115.

[28] Ranson JH, Spencer FC. The role of peritoneal lavage in severe acute pancreatitis. *Ann Surg,* 1978; 187: 565-575.

[29] Coticchia JM, Lessler MA, Carey LC, Gower WR, Mayer AD, McMahon MJ. Peritoneal fluid in human acute pancreatitis blocks hepatic mitochondrial respiration. *Surgery,* 1986; 100: 850 856.

[30] Takeyama Y, Nishikawa J, Ueda T, Hori Y, Yamamoto M, Kuroda Y. Involvement of peritoneal macrophage in the induction of cytotoxicity due to apoptosis in ascitic fluid associated with severe acute pancreatitis. *J Surg Res,* 1999; 82: 163-171.

[31] Mikami Y, Takeda K, Shibuya K, Qiu-Feng H, Shimamura H, Yamauchi J et al. Peritoneal inflammatory cells in acute pancreatitis: Relationship of infiltration dynamics and cytokine production with severity of illness. *Surgery,* 2002; 132: 86-92.

[32] Mikami Y, Takeda K, Shibuya K, Qiu-Feng H, Shimamura H, Yamauchi J et al. Do peritoneal macrophages play an essential role in the progression of acute pancreatitis in rats? *Pancreas,* 2003; 27: 253-260.

[33] Souza LJ, Coelho AM, Sampietre SN, Martins JO, Cunha JE, Machado MC. Anti-inflammatory effects of peritoneal lavage in acute pancreatitis. *Pancreas,* 2010; 39: 1180-1184.

[34] Hanly EJ, Bachman SL, Marohn MR, Boden JH, Herring AE, De Maio A et al. Carbon dioxide pneumoperitoneum-mediated attenuation of the inflammatory response is independent of systemic acidosis. *Surgery,* 2003; 137: 559-566.

[35] West MA, Baker J, Bellingham J. Kinetics of decreased LPS-stimulated cytokine release by macrophages exposed to CO2. *J Surg Res,* 1996; 63: 269-274.

[36] Are C, Talamini MA, Murata K, De Maio A. Carbon dioxide pneumoperitoneum alters acute-phase response induced by lypopolysaccharide. *Surg Endosc,* 2002; 16: 1464-1467.

[37] Fuentes JM, Hanly EJ, Aurora AR, De Maio A, Shih SP, Marohn MR et al. CO2 abdominal insufflation pretreatment increases survival after a lipopolysaccharide-contaminated laparotomy. *J Gastrointest Surg,* 2006; 10: 32-38.

[38] Machado MC, Coelho AM, Martins JO, Sampietre SN, Molan NA, Patzina RA et al. CO2 abdominal insufflation decreases local and systemic inflammatory response in experimental acute pancreatitis. *Pancreas,* 2010; 39: 175-181.

9

Molecular Biology of Acute Pancreatitis

Francisco Soriano and Ester C.S. Rios
University of São Paulo, Medical School,
Brazil

1. Introduction

In the Acute Pancreatitis the pancreatic enzymes are activated locally, causing a tissue injury followed by a pancreatic inflammation, characterized by edema, leucocyte infiltration, hemorrhage and necrosis.

The etiology of the pancreatitis presents as major cause of this disease, the alcoholism and the gallstone. These risk factors are common in the actual society and are determining to the increase pancreatitis incidence.

Despite the default in the establishment of the initializing mechanism of the acute pancreatitis, experimental studies suggest a disturbance in the intracellular calcium levels as a first event of the process.

Following this idea, a duct obstruction or alcohol exposure could modify the calcium release, leading to a migration of exocytosis machinery from the apical area of the membrane to the basolateral area. The relocation of the enzyme vesicles and the release of the content in the inter membrane space are the starter of pancreatic auto-digestion.

Experimental pancreatitis studies have shown that the membrane permeability (disruption) of the acinar cell is crucial to the calcium disorders and consequent pathologic mechanisms, resulting in the release of cytoplasmic proteins. However, the understanding of the deficiency remains unclear, i.e., if it is a disturbance of the plasmatic membrane or a delay in the calcium-dependent mechanisms for cell membrane resealing.

Actually, the membrane exocytosis machinery can be disturbed under the exposition to different stimulation. It has been reported a blockade apical granule fusion after stimulus with cholecystokinin (CCK) and carbachol, for example.

The fusion of zymogen granules occurs in a very limited apical region of surface membrane to increase the effectiveness of pancreatic content delivering. This efficiency is due to the protein machinery that control the direct fusion of the zymogen granules with the membrane as well as the granule-to-granule fusion of the distant granules to the most apically located. This granule-granule fusion remains occurring despite of the apical releasing blockade and could be responsible to aggravate the basolateral exocytosis, the event possibly responsible by the pancreatitis starting.

The definition of initial cause of the acute pancreatitis is decisive to the control of late complication in this disease. However, the knowledge about the exact mechanism among a variety of etiologies still remains controversial.

Despite the alcoholism be often associated with a chronic pancreatitis, there are several reports of bouts of acute pancreatitis resulting of alcohol abuse. This could be due to the association of the raised gut permeability with alcohol intake and the concomitant endotoxemia. In other view, the pancreatic stellate cells could be activated by the alcohol consumption. The role of these cells in pancreatic injury is similar to the liver injury during alcoholism, with the fibrosis establishment. Thence, the mechanism related to these cells is more evident in the chronic pancreatitis.

The molecular mechanism of biliary acute pancreatitis is Ca^{2+} mediated. Several authors suggested that the increase in bile acids preventing reuptake of Ca^{2+} by a PI3K-dependent mechanism.

The molecular mechanism of gallstone - associated pancreatitis seems to be simpler. The pancreatic duct obstruction confine the zymogen and lysosomal granules causing the condensing vacuoles and impeding the acinar exocytosis. Consequently, the trypsinogen is activated to trypsin and triggers the cascade of enzyme activation leading to the pancreatic injury.

Pancreatitis induced by hypertriglyceridemia is associated to amylase release and the cell injury due to the free acids released because its detergent properties.

2. Molecular biology of multiple organ failure during acute pancreatitis

The local and systemic complications during pancreatitis aggravate the prognostic of the disease. The morbidity and the mortality pancreatitis-associated occur due the systemic inflammation and the multiple organ dysfunctions, mainly lung, liver and kidney.

The intra and extra pancreatic events of the acute pancreatitis are responsible by the complexity of the disease. Initially, there is the local activation of the trypsinogen. Subsequently, the trypsine activates other enzymes those turn begin to digest the pancreatic tissue, whose content leaks into the abdominal cavity, causing cytokine release, activation of the immune system, coagulation and fibrinolysis.

The cytokines activates the inflammatory pathway, resulting in the increase of adhesion molecules, neutrophils infiltrate, production of Reactive Oxygen Species (ROS) and several inflammatory molecules such as Prostaglandin E2 (PGE2), Tromboxan A2 (TXA2), Platelet Activating Factor (PAF). On the other hand, the release of these mediators leads to Systemic Inflammation Response Syndrome (SIRS).

The ascitic fluid released in response to pancreatic inflammation could lead to activation of Kupffer Cells that will produce cytokines and others mediators, such protelytic enzymes, establishing the hepatic inflammation. The lung is often a target of these mediators and the dominant cause of mortality.

It has been shown that severe acute pancreatitis correlates with the incidence of hepatic injury. Although the liver is known to be a primary target of cytokines released in pancreatic blood, the liver itself releases inflammatory substances, such as reactive oxygen species, thereby leading to the injury of distant organs.

The oxidative stress is important in the early stages of the systemic inflammation that occurs in pancreatitis and the liver is a target of this event. Also, the liver is a source of oxidative stress. Multiple hepatic cells, including hepatocytes, Kupffer cells, stellate cells, endothelial cells can generate nitric oxide, superoxide, and peroxynitrite. On the other hand, these oxygen and nitrogen - derived species might lead to the early Hepatic Stellate Cells (HSC) activation, which leads to alteration in the extracellular matrix components and involves as much degradation as fibrogenesis. The extracellular matrix degradation could be responsible by the amplification of the inflammatory mediators release and the systemic inflammation (Figure 1). Moreover, the oxidative and nitrative stress are responsible by the alteration in the mitochondrial respiration and the consequent apoptosis induction.

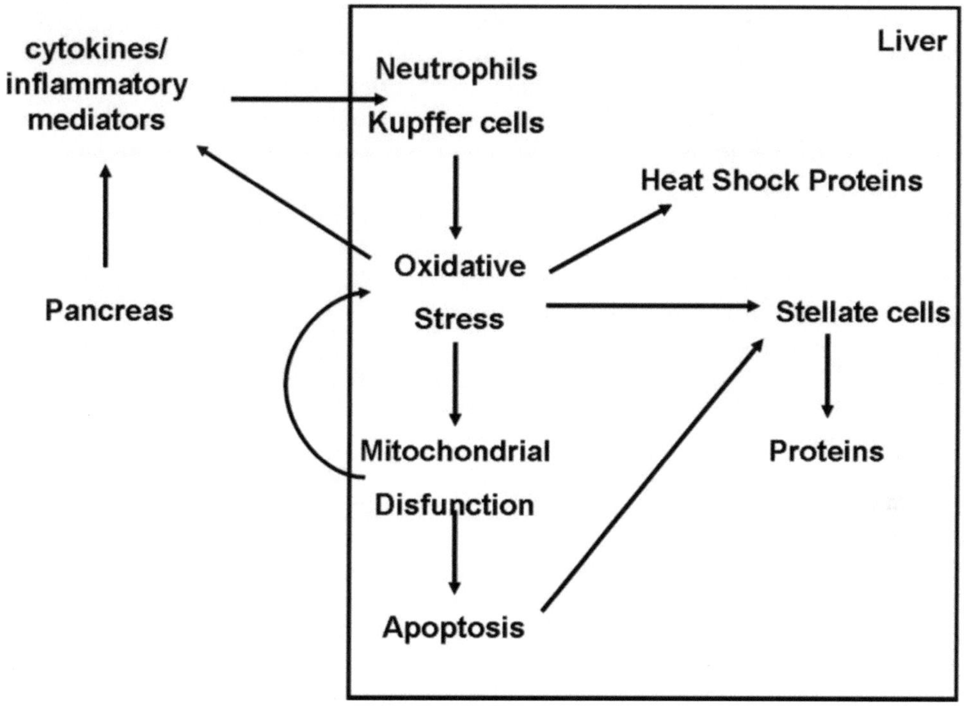

Fig. 1. The hepatic injury involved in the multiple organ failure during pancreatitis. The liver is both a source and target of the inflammatory mediators systemically released during pancreas inflammation. These mediators activate several hepatic cells causing oxidative stress, mitochondrial dysfunction and consequently apoptosis and synthesis of inflammatory proteins that will aggravate the involvement of distant organs.

3. Molecular signaling of the oxidative stress

Despite the initial cause of pancreatitis, the oxidative stress is the mainly contributing factor to the destruction of the pancreatic tissue. Moreover, the dysbalance redox participates of hepatocellular injury as well as the pulmonary lesion.

Among the effects of the pancreatitis in the liver it was demonstrate the reduction of oxygen consume by the mitochondria in animals that received samples of ascitic fluid from rats with acute pancreatitis.

Reactive oxygen species (ROS) activates necrosis and modify the production of cytokine and adhesion molecules. Furthermore, lipid peroxidation products are chemotactic and might lead to amplification of the inflammation process.

It is known that the Nitric Oxide Synthases exhibit different profiles during the pancreatic inflammation. The Reactive Nitrogen Species (RSN), produced constantly, are responsible by the regulating the exocrine secretion of the pancreas. At basal levels, RSN protect against pancreatitis by increasing microcirculatory flow, inhibiting the leukocyte infiltration and suppressing the Catepsine, an important mediator to the activation of trypsinogen.

On the other hand, an increase in the Inducible Nitric Oxide Synthase (iNOS) expression followed by an exacerbated Nitric Oxide (NO) production during Acute Pancreatitis could lead to an activation of the inflammatory pathway, inhibition of the cellular respiration, nitrosylation and nitration of proteins, resulting in cell death by necrosis and apoptosis.
In the mammalian cell, the NO is protective against chemistry agents generating of oxidative stress .This anti-oxidant effect could be important to minimize the tissue injury in the ROS-associated process. Once the NO is accumulated in its activated form, its concentration in the tissues is important to the regulation of immunity by modulation of the protein expression and activity.
Pancreatitis is known to cause a marked increase in superoxide production. The key players in the physiology of inflammatory processes are NO and its products. There is great controversy in the literature as to whether the effects of NO are protective or harmful. There is evidence that NO promotes cell death under conditions of oxidative stress, indicating concurrent superoxide production. However, under resting conditions, NO is protective. Recent studies have shown an increase of lipid peroxidation, which indirectly indicates the release of oxidative products, during pancreatitis. This increase was concomitant to enhance the NO production.
It has been shown that, in the presence of high superoxide levels, peroxynitrite formation becomes dependent on NO production. Peroxynitrite can exert its toxic effect through the nitration of macromolecules or as a selective oxidant, contributing to either necrosis or apoptosis. The formation of nitrotyrosine is a consequence of peroxynitrite activity, and increased nitrotyrosine levels have been detected in human diseases associated with oxidative stress. There are various ways in which peroxynitrite-induced impairment of endothelial function might contribute to the pathogenesis of organ failure due to circulatory shock: by exacerbating local vasospasm, increasing local neutrophil adhesion, and increasing neutrophil migration into inflamed tissues; by exacerbating platelet activation and aggregation; or by promoting hypoperfusion of certain parts of various organs. During pancreatitis, it was shown that the hepatocytes around the central vein were apparently the most susceptible to aggression. The superoxide anion and NO both react rapidly to form the toxic reaction product, the peroxynitrite anion. Pharmacological studies in a variety of experimental systems have demonstrated that peroxynitrite is more cytotoxic than is NO or superoxide, as well as being able to induce necrosis and apoptosis. Peroxynitrite (endogenous or exogenous) is a potent trigger of DNA single-strand breakage, whereas NO is not. In turn, DNA single-strand breakage activates the nuclear enzyme poly (adenosine diphosphate-ribose) polymerase.
The concentrations of NO and superoxide determine the formation of peroxynitrite, which was demonstrated after pancreatitis induction. This event is correlated to the increase of liver injury during pancreatitis.

4. Molecular biology of cell death in acute pancreatitis

Acute pancreatitis–associated distant organs injury is mediated by inflammatory cytokines that are produced within tissue resident macrophages. These organs, in turn, participate in the systemic inflammation releasing several inflammatory mediators leading to amplification of the injury of distant organs. Substances released systemically during pancreatitis, such as Nitric Oxide (NO) and free radicals can interfere with mitochondrial respiration and induce apoptosis. The apoptotic cell death may play a considerable role in affecting mortality and morbidity in severe acute pancreatitis. Apoptosis pathway, by death receptors or the mitochondrial pathway, activates the final caspase to cell death. Death Receptors signaling has been associated with apoptosis in several hepatic diseases such as ethanol-induced liver injury and cholestatic liver disease. Apoptosis related to the severe acute pancreatitis injury is known to be triggered through the mitochondrial pathway.

Cell death has been seen in both apoptotic and necrotic forms, in clinical as well as experimental acute pancreatitis. Current evidence suggests that the amount and the balance between apoptosis and necrosis influence the severity of acute pancreatitis.

There are two apoptotic pathways: the extrinsic pathway is activated by death receptors and is subjected to caspase-8 activation. The mitochondrial or intrinsic pathway is mediated by caspase-9 activation. Both pathways activate the caspase-3, initializing the programmed cell death.

On the other hand, the pancreatitis can activate directly the caspase-9, which forms a complex with Activator Protease Factor-1 and cytochrome c, priming the mitochondrial pathway.

The mitochondria are the determining factor to modulation of cell death during pancreatitis, defining whether the cell death will occur by necrosis or apoptosis. While the necrosis is often observed in severe pancreatitis, apoptosis is more evident in the pancreatitis of medium gravity.

5. Important proteins signaling during acute pancreatitis

The family of protein associated to the membrane fusion machinery includes receptors bind to proteins attachment to N-ethylmaleimide-sensitive fusion proteins and donor vesicles. Some isoforms of this multiprotein complex are present in the pancreatic acinar cells where they mediated the granule-granule fusion as well as the membrane-granule fusion.

The regulation of these proteins is mediated by other protein family called Munc. Recent studies demonstrated molecular interaction of the isoform 18c of Munc and proteins of SNARE family during CCK or carbachol stimulation. This interaction is mediated by modifying in the calcium release. It is important to mention that this basolateral plasma membrane activity is intermediated by protein kinase C family proteins, which are activated by carbachol stimulation.

It was demonstrated that the pancreatitis could induced the Heat Shock Protein (HSP) gene transcription and, in contrast, reduce the protein levels. This modulation is important due the different physiologic roles of each one of the HSP. HSP60, for example, is involved in toll-like receptors activation and necrosis process. On the other hand, the HSP70 is described as a tissue protector in several disease models.

Recently, heat-shock proteins and their cofactors have been revealed associated to apoptotic and necrotic pathways .Heat shock proteins are molecular chaperones that stabilize and refold damaged intercellular proteins, preventing the intracellular protein aggregation and making the cells resistant to stress-induced cell damage.

In the experimental acute pancreatitis, induced by cholecystokinine, cerulean, arginine and taurocholic acid, there is an increase of the Heat Shock Protein (HSP) -70 expression concurrent to a reduction of the HSP60. On the other hand, some authors suggest that HSP60 could reduce the trypsinogen activation, a basic event to the onset of pancreatitis.

During inflammation, neutrophils connect to tissue areas activated. Throughout the neutrophylic invasion, there is the release of enzymes responsible by the tissue digestion, such as metalloproteinases, which in turn could enhance the injury due the release of signaling molecules after the extracellular matrix digestion.
The local injury during pancreatitis induces the production of proinflammatory cytokines such as tumor necrosis factor-α (TNF-α) and interleukin-1β (IL-1β). These cytokines are released via portal vein and lymph fluid drainage to the circulation. In turn, it occurs the vascular endothelium activation and the leukocyte migration. In the acute pancreatitis, the increase of pro and anti-inflammatory cytokines was correlated to the reduced human leukocyte antigen-DR levels, which characterizes the immunosuppression. This event could explain the multiple organ failure often related to the pancreatitis.

6. Molecular biology in the treatment of the acute pancreatitis

Currently, the treatment of the acute pancreatitis aims the hemodynamic balance, nutrition, control of the pain and complications. However, the major events in the pancreatitis are: Systemic Inflammatory Response Syndrome, microcirculatory disturb and translocation of bacteria.
Several experimental studies demonstrate the efficiency of Nitric Oxide, block of endothelial receptors, antagonists of the PAF-receptors, antibodies against Intercellular Adhesion Molecules. These treatments improved the microcirculatory flow during acute pancreatitis.

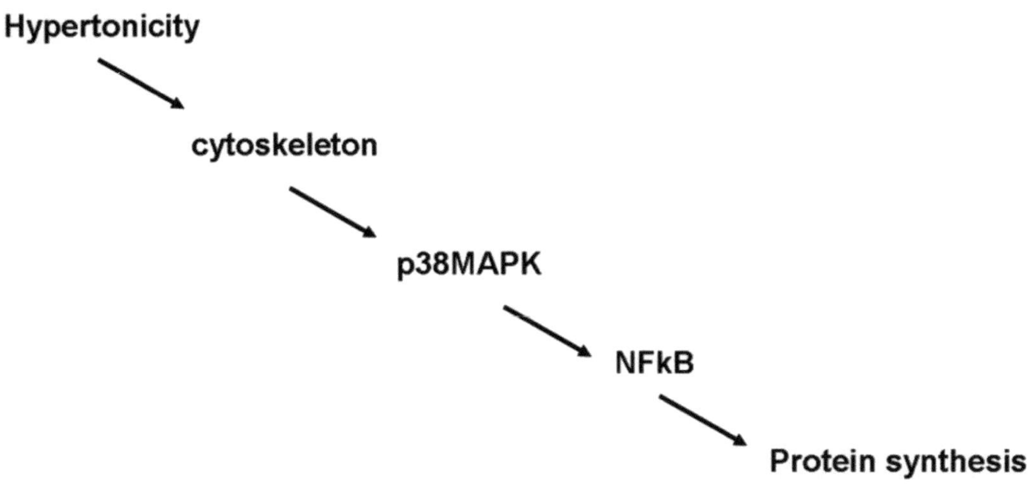

Fig. 2. Molecular effects of the hypertonic solution. The water loss could modify the cytoskeleton structure leading to activation of a protein cascade triggering specific gene transcription.

Fluid resuscitation is a necessary therapeutic intervention in severe pancreatitis. Patients with pancreatitis present volume extravasation to the peritoneum and retroperitoneum, and some have hemodynamic inestability. However, the infusion of large volumes can induce pulmonary interstitial edema and can increase intra-abdominal pressure. Fluid accumulation in the lungs exacerbates respiratory failure and can make mechanical ventilation necessary. Increased abdominal pressure reduces the venous return to the heart, thereby decreasing cardiac output, as well as reducing perfusion of the kidney and gut, all of which can provoke organ damage.

In experimental animal models of pancreatitis, hypertonic saline has been shown to alter circulating plasma volume, reduce trypsinogen levels, prevent acinar necrosis, reduce inflammatory cytokine levels, and avert pancreatic infection, thereby minimizing injury, limiting the local and end-organ and reducing mortality. It has recently been demonstrated that administration of hypertonic saline in a rat model of acute pancreatitis reduces systemic inflammation rather than protecting local (pancreatic) tissue. Hypertonic saline modulates pancreatitis-related injury to the lungs and liver. This effect was attributed to the modulated expression and activity of various proteins, such as metalloproteinase, collagen, and members of the HSP family. Also hypertonicity could modify the gene transcription, expression and function of several proteins, activation of kinases (figure 2), cell adhesion and the ROS and cytokines release. This modifying may be due the alteration in the cytoskeleton because the cell edema diminishing.

7. References

Gaisano HY, Gorelick FS. New insights into the mechanisms of pancreatitis. *Gastroenterology* 2009; 136(7):2040-4.

Khan AS, Latif SU, Eloubeidi MA. Controversies in the etiologies of acute pancreatitis. *JOP.* 2010; 11(6):545-52.

Kylänpää ML, Repo H, Puolakkainen PA. Inflammation and immunosuppression in severe acute pancreatitis. *World J Gastroenterol.* 2010; 16(23):2867-72.

Leung PS, Chan YC. Role of oxidative stress in pancreatic inflammation. *Antioxid Redox Signal* 2009; 11(1):135-65.

Moretti AI, Rios EC, Soriano FG, de Souza HP, Abatepaulo F, Barbeiro DF, Velasco IT. Acute pancreatitis: hypertonic saline increases heat shock proteins 70 and 90 and reduces neutrophil infiltration in lung injury. *Pancreas* 2009; 38(5):507-14.

Odinokova IV, Sung KF, Mareninova OA, Hermann K, Gukovsky I, Gukovskaya AS. Mitochondrial mechanisms of death responses in pancreatitis. J *Gastroenterol Hepatol.* 2008; 23 Suppl 1:S25-30.

Petrov MS, Shanbhag S, Chakraborty M, Phillips AR, Windsor JA. Organ failure and infection of pancreatic necrosis as determinants of mortality in patients with acute pancreatitis. *Gastroenterology.* 2010; 139(3):813-20.

Rios EC, Moretti AS, Velasco IT, Souza HP, Abatepaulo F, Soriano F. Hypertonic saline and reduced peroxynitrite formation in experimental pancreatitis. *Clinics* 2011; 66(3):469-76.

Rios EC, Moretti AI, de Souza HP, Velasco IT, Soriano FG. Hypertonic saline reduces metalloproteinase expression in liver during pancreatitis. *Clin Exp Pharmacol Physiol.* 2010;37(1):35-9.

Shrivastava P, Bhatia M. Essential role of monocytes and macrophages in the progression of acute pancreatitis. *World J Gastroenterol.* 2010; 16(32):3995-4002.

Talukdar R, Vege SS. Recent developments in acute pancreatitis. *Clin Gastroenterol Hepatol.* 2009; 7(11 Suppl):S3-9.

Thrower EC, Gorelick FS, Husain SZ. Molecular and cellular mechanisms of pancreatic injury. *Curr Opin Gastroenterol.* 2010; 26(5):484-9.

Thrower E, Husain S, Gorelick F. Molecular basis for pancreatitis. *Curr Opin Gastroenterol.* 2008; 24(5):580-5.

Vonlaufen A, Wilson JS, Apte MV. Molecular mechanisms of pancreatitis: current opinion. *J Gastroenterol Hepatol.* 2008; 23(9):1339-48.

Zhang XP, Li ZJ, Zhang J. Inflammatory mediators and microcirculatory disturbance in acute pancreatitis. *Hepatobiliary Pancreat Dis Int.* 2009; 8(4):351-7.

Wang GJ, Gao CF, Wei D, Wang C, Ding SQ. Acute pancreatitis: etiology and common pathogenesis. *World J Gastroenterol* 2009; 15(12):1427-30.

10

Oxidative Stress and Antioxidative Status in the Acute Pancreatitis

Andrzej Lewandowski[1], Krystyna Markocka-Mączka[1], Maciej Garbień[2], Dorota Diakowska[1] and Renata Taboła[1]
[1]Department of Gastrointestinal & General Surgery Silesian Piasts, University of Medicine in Wrocław,
[2]Department of General Surgery Railway Hospital in Wrocław, Poland

1. Introduction

Acute pancreatitis is the inflammatory condition of a gland, including an invasion into, to a lesser or greater extent, the surrounding tissues, and also the contiguous or distant organs (Braganza, 2001; Frossard et al., 2008).

The analysis of the processes, occurring in the course of acute pancreatitis, has made it possible to define this disease as the one which comprises of two phases.

Initially, the hyperstimulation of the immunological system with the excessive local activation of the cells of inflammatory focus in the pancreas occurs, and later on, as a result, the systemic response, expressed as Systemic Inflammatory Response Syndrome (SIRS), develops.

Compensatory Anti-inflammatory Response Syndrome (CARS) causes early organic complications (Gamaste, 1994; Toouli et al., 2002; Yousaf & McCallion, 2003).

The intensification of an inflammatory response, hypoxia and the occurrence of oligovolemic shock may result in the clinical development of Multi-Organ Dysfunction Syndrome (MODS), which is defined as the more advanced stage of SIRS. In this period, greater susceptibility to bacterial infections and fungal infections and, consequently, an increased mortality rate, caused by blood poisoning, is observed. Multi-Organ Dysfunction Syndrome requires the application of the powerful methods of supporting the organism of a patient (Song et al., 2003).

Acute pancreatitis is a disease of an unpredictable course. It is, usually, a reversible process, in which the pain ailments of the abdomen undergo regression and the activity of pancreatic enzymes returns to its normal level.

In 70 - 75% of cases, this process becomes subjected to the self-limitation and has the properties of interstitial inflammation. However, in 5 – 15%, a form characterized by severe, necrotic course may develop.

In this case, local complications and multi-organic complications are alike present

The morbidity rate in case of acute pancreatitis in Poland is estimated to be at the level of 240 cases per 1 million in a year.

The mortality rate amounts to 5 - 10% in total. However, in the cases of severe course, it amounts to approximately 35% (Baillie, 1997; Balthazar et al., 2002; Beger et al., 1997; Lund et al., 2006; Munoz, & Katerndahl 2000; Mutinga et al., 2000; Song , 2003). In pathomorphology, the oedemic and the necrotic form of acute pancreatitis, which constitutes an infavourable development of the oedemic form, or is developing as a separate form of the disease from the beginning is observed (Banks & Freeman, 2006; Yousaf et al., 2003).

In Atlanta, in 1992 (Bradley, 1993), an obligatory classification of acute pancreatitis was drawn up; this classification it assumes the division into:

- acute pancreatitis of mild course.
- acute pancreatitis of severe course, which means the occurrence of one of the following states:
- local complications: necrosis, false cyst and abscess,
- organic dysfunction,
- meeting 3 or more criteria on the Ranson scale (Ranson, 1997),
- obtaining 8 or more points on the APACHE II scale II (Lankisch et al., 2002; Song, 2003).

Acute pancreatitis results in the destruction of the alveolar cells, which results in the handicap of the extra-secretory functions of the pancreas. What may also contribute to the damage to the alveolar cells and releasing active proteases and other enzymes into the parenchyma of the pancreas, is the obstruction of the pancreatic ducts and increase in pressure in them connected with that or the intra-cellular activity of chemical substances (Braganza, 2000; Sharma & Howden, 1999).

Nowadays, there is more and more information about the chain of events, occurring after the release of active enzymes into the pancreatic parenchyma. However, the mechanism of the activation of the zymogens at molecular level still remains unknown (Braganza, 2001; Song et al., 2003).

2. Causes of acute pancreatitis

The causes of acute pancreatitis may be divided into: mechanical, toxic, metabolic, infection-related, vascular, genetic and idiopathic (Yadav & Lowenfels, 2006).

2.1 Mechanical causes

The most frequent cause of acute pancreatitis is choledocholithiasis and alcohol.

It is estimated that both of these etiological factors are the cause of as many as 80% of cases of the disease.

In medical literature, the connection between choledocholithiasis and acute pancreatitis was a subject of publication for the first time in 1909 (Song et al., 2003).

Large stones, of the diameter of 20 mm and more, cause increase in the risk of the acute inflammation of the gall bladder.

The risk of acute pancreatitis increases if the diameter of the stones does not exceed 5 mm.

Their being jammed in the duodenal papillae and the occurrence of acute pancreatitis is also made more likely by the shape of concretions if it is similar to that of mulberry fruit.

In 3 hours after getting jammed in the duodenal papillae, inflammatory changes in the pancreas occur. It is assumed upon the basis of estimations that if the obstacle is removed within a 24-hour period, acute pancreatitis of severe course occurs in only as few as 6% cases.

The risk increases to 90% if the obstacle is removed later than within a 48-hour period (Baron et al., 1996).

Damage to the alveolar cells resulting from the inflammatory process of the pancreas, may also occur if the bacterial infection of gall coexists with choledocholithiasis. (Liu et al., 1997). Bacterial endotoxins cause the release of cytokines and the occurrence of SIRS.
Pancreas divisum, which means chronic pancreatitis, may be the cause of the acute, recurrent inflammations of this organ, particularly in case of children.
This developmental variety of the pancreas is revealed in case of approximately of 5% population.
The risk of the occurrence of inflammatory changes is connected with the papillary stenosis of the smaller duodenal papilla.
According to estimations, approximately 3% of the cases of acute pancreatitis, described in literature, is caused by a tumour on the pancreas or duodenal papillae (Fan et al., 1993).
Sphincteritis Oddi stenosans, which means the stenotic inflammation of the duodenal papilla, by means of handicapping the outflow of biliary juice and pancreatic secretion, may result in the occurrence of an incident of acute pancreatitis (Song et al., 2003).
Into the group of the mechanical causes able to cause acute pancreatitis, may also be included penetrative and blunt abdomen injuries.
Endoscopic retrograde cholangiopancreatography (ERCP) is also a described cause of the occurrence of acute pancreatitis. The frequency of such cases reaches 2% (Demols & Deviere, 2003; Folsch et al., 1997).
Accidental damage to the Wirsung duct during an operations is a following mechanical cause of acute pancreatitis.
It most frequently occurs during the fixation of the intestine with the stump of the pancreas in the course of operative procedures (Golub et al., 1998, Vaquero-Raya & Molero-Richard, 2005).
A not very frequent cause of acute pancreatitis may be blocking the pancreatic duct or the biliary duct by a lumbricus (Ascaris lumbricoides hominis).
Duodenal-pancreatic reflux, occurring in the conducting loop syndrome after a resection procedure on the stomach with the application of the B_2 method, may also be a cause of the occurrence of acute pancreatitis (Frossard & Hadengue, 2001, Gamaste, 1994).

2.2 Toxic causes

A frequent factor causing acute pancreatitis is ethyl alcohol (Dufour & Adamson, 2003).
It may cause the oedema of the papillae of Vater, the regurgitation of duodenal contents into the pancreatic ducts and increase in the permeability of the pancreatic ducts.
Ethyl alcohol exerts cytotoxic influence as well because it form the ethyl esters of fat acids, which damage the cells of the pancreas, causing acute alcohol-related pancreatitis (Golub et al., 1998; Schenker & Montalvo, 1998).
It is suspected that some kinds of medications are able to induce acute pancreatitis. This group encompasses: mesalazinum, sulfasalazinum, furosemide, rifampicin, sulphonamides, octreotide, didanozinum, isoniazid, azathioprine, erythromycin, shadowing medications administered in ERCP and others. A rare cause of acute pancreatitis is having been bitten by animals representing venomous species, e.g. by certain species of scorpions.

2.3 Infection-related causes

A cause of the occurrence of acute pancreatitis may be bacterial infection.
As a result of translocation, bacteria reach the tissue of the pancreas on their way from the large intestine.

Those bacteria produce endotoxins, which induce releasing pro-inflammatory cytokines, which as a result causes damage to the pancreatic cells.
Viral infection - a virus of epidemic parotid inflammation and HIV is also a described cause of the occurrence of acute pancreatitis.
In case of patients with developed AIDS, the frequency of the occurrence of acute pancreatitis is several hundred times larger than in case of healthy population.
Acute pancreatitis in course of AIDS may be caused by the virus itself, but also the very occurrence of opportunistic infections generates inflammatory processes.
Patients with AIDS frequently come from the backgrounds abusing alcohol and psychoactive substances, which is an additional factor, able to case acute pancreatitis
This is caused by the co-existence of several factors simultaneously.
Medications administered to patients, for example didanozinum (DDI), may also induce the occurrence of acute pancreatitis.

2.4 Metabolic causes

Increase in the concentration of triglycerides, particularly above 1000 mg%, may be a factor inducing the development of acute pancreatitis.
Such a state is observed in case of patients, suffering from hyperlipidaemies of type I, IV and V.
Hypercalcaemia connected with the hyperacitivity of the parathyroid glands, uremia and the neoplasm of bones also increases the risk of the induction of inflammatory processes in the pancreatic gland (Rau et al., 1997; Schoenberg et al., 1995).

2.5 Vascular causes

The development of acute pancreatitis may occur after cardiac-surgical operations, performed with the use of cardiopulmonary bypass, and after image-based examinations with the use of contrast, for example after abdominal aortography (Niederau & Lüthen, 1997).
In the literature, there are described cases of acute pancreatitis, occurring as a result of the complications of sclerosis such as the block of upper mesenteric artery and the block of the celiac trunk.
In the research conducted in the recent years, changes in pancreatic microcirculation are regarded as the cause of the disease in such cases (Sabater et al., 2004).
The disorders of celiac flow within pancreatic microcirculation occur in the early phase of the disease and precede changes in the digestive duct microcirculation.
The disorders of celiac flow within pancreatic microcirculation are of importance in the transformation of mild (oedemic) form in the necrotic-hemorrhagic one.
Substantial reductions in capillary perfusion and of the saturation of hemoglobin with oxygen occur.
The disorders within pancreatic microcirculation are a complex process, in which the dysfunctions of the cells of endothelial vessels occur.
Free oxygen radicals being released and cytokines participate in this process.
Important mediators causing the inflammatory reactions are: blood platelet activating factor, neoplasm necrosis factor α (TNF-α), cytokines (IL-1, IL- 6, IL-8), interferon γ (INF- γ), thromboxane, leukotrienes and prostaglandins (Lewandowski et al., 2007; Osman & Jensen, 1999; Rau et al. 1997).

2.6 Genetic causes

The course of acute pancreatitis is dependent on one hand on the activity and strength of factors, damaging the pancreas, and, on the other hand, on the genetically-conditioned response of the immunological system.

Depending upon the individual properties, the self-limitation of the inflammatory process may occur, or, alternatively, its intensification and proliferation may occur.

Genetic research has differentiated a disease of the genetically-conditioned mechanism of development: *hereditary pancreatitis* - acute pancreatitis occurring within the family.

The research suggests the existence of mutation N34S in the gene responsible for coding a pancreatic inhibitor, trypsin, defined as PSTI (*pancreatic secrectory trypsin inhibitor*) or SPINK1 (*serine peptidase inhibitor, Kasal type 1*).

This polypeptide constitutes one of the barriers, safeguarding against self-digestion of the cells of the pancreas.

The mutation of the gene results in the earlier activation of trypsinogen inside the cell and its destruction (Karczowski, 2002; Swaroop et al., 2004).

The premature activation of the pancreatic pro-enzymes is still regarded as the essential pathomechanism of self-digestion of the pancreatic gland which occurs in the severe form of acute pancreatitis.

Molecular researches on the mutation of trypsinogen in the course of acute pancreatitis occurring within the family have shown the superior role of the trypsin in the premature activation of proteolithic enzymes (Niederau & Lüthen, 1997; Swaroop et al., 2004).

All it takes to activate them is a small amount of free trypsin remaining in balance with the complex: trypsin-pancreatic secretory trypsin inhibitor (PSTI) (Karczowski, 2002).

In 2000, it was found out that the gene for pancreatic trypsin inhibitor (PSTI) may contribute to the modification of the risk of pancreatitis, particularly in case of mutation N34N PSTI, wherein the risk of the occurrence of acute pancreatitis is increased ten-fold (Karczowski, 2002).

In approximately 10% cases, it proves impossible to determine the cause of acute pancreatitis. Such cases are defined as idiopathic (Kim et al., 2003; Testoni et al., 2008).

3. The clinical record of the acute pancreatitis

Acute pancreatitis of mild course, or, in other words, its oedemic form, does not cause complications.

In some cases, so-called liquid collections of acute phase appear.

This is the state in which effusion liquid is accumulated in the anatomical spaces of the peritoneal cavity.

The cistern of the acute phase does not have a tissue-connecting capsule and, as a rule, it is subject to resorption to four weeks from the beginning of the disease.

Sometimes, however, it is encysted and causes the formation of false cyst of the pancreas (Sabater et al.: 2004, Williford et al., 1983).

Liquid cysterns of the acute phase may occur in the pancreatitis of mild course and the severe one alike (Morgan et al 1997).

Clinical symptoms of acute pancreatitis depend above all on the form (degree of severity), spread of changes and time of the disease duration.

The main symptom of acute pancreatitis is pain.

It is described by the patients as: encircling, and sometimes as radiating to the left or to the both of shoulder blades, and to the spine.

It is frequently felt as the pressure similar to compressing with a girdle.
Initially, it is the pain of celiac character, but after some time it transforms into somatic-celiac (mixed) one.
The individuals are unable to identify its source precisely.
Celiac pain is formed as a result of the irritation of receptors (nociceptors) in a particular organ of the abdominal cavity.
Its cause is the sudden increase of wall tension or the constriction of the smooth muscles of the celiac organs.
The pain is usually dull, less frequently stabbing, with a location that is difficult to define.
It radiates to the areas of the same neural segment, which is affected by the pain of the disease-changed celiac organ.
Frequently, it is accompanied by vegetative symptoms, for example acceleration or slowing down the heart action, vomiting or decrease in arterial blood pressure.
The pain is intensified during rest, and weakens during performing movements - the individuals are restless and motor-activated.
Conducting the stimuli of celiac pain is connected with the autonomous nervous system.
Somatic pain is connected with the irritation of the sensory endings of the core nerves of the parietal peritoneum, mesentery, retriperitoneal space or the walls of the abdominal integuments.
This pain is acute or blunt, but constant, easy to describe and clearly-localized.
It is accompanied by the tension of the muscles, called muscular defense.
The individuals are calm and they avoid movement.
The pain accompanying acute pancreatitis may be of constant intensity, but it may, alternatively, be getting more intensive (Morgan et al., 1997; Dervenis et al., 1999).
In the initial period of the disease, nausea and vomiting, which do not bring about relief, occur.
They are the symptoms of the irritation of the pneumogastric nerve.
These ailments are accompanied by the integuments, excessive hyperhidrosis, increased thirst, accelerated breath and, frequently, decrease in arterial blood pressure.
Disorders for the part of the nervous system, such as anxiety developing into fear, strong psycho-motor excitation, and hallucinations may occur (Dervenis et al 1999).
The position adopted by the individuals and their outsider appearance are frequently characteristic of this disease.
The patients are lying on their side with their lower extremities bent and appear to be suffering a lot.
The initial paleness of the body integuments may be joined by the characteristic erythema of the skin of the face - the Loeffler symptom or marbleness of the skin of the abdomen and the extremities - Halsted symptom.
These are the symptoms of vessel-widening activity of mediators of inflammatory state.
What is also a quite characteristic symptom is abdominal distention, the presence of hepatitis or blue disease.
In case of acute pancreatitis with severe course, as the complication of necrosis of fat subcutaneous tissues, lividness of the skin may occur.
If it is found in the era near the navel, it is described in the literature as Cullen symptom.
If this is found in lumbar region, this is Grey-Turner symptom (Steinberg & Tenner, 1994).
Researching abdominal integuments in a palpative manner, we frequently discover tenderness, muscular defense, peritoneal symptoms and Blumberg symptom.

It is sometimes possible to discover the presence of free liquid in the peritoneal cavity or an effusion on the left pleural cavity - Clairmont symptom

3.1 Diagnostic investigation in the acute pancreatitis

The most frequently performed examination is determining the activity of amylase in the serum.

In order for it to be possible to diagnose acute pancreatitis, the activity of amylase ought to be three-fold larger than the norm. It happens in the course of acute pancreatitis of severe course that the activity of amylase is correct, probably as a result of a massive damage to the parenchyma of the gland.

The most sensitive marker of pancreatitis is the increase in the activity of pancreatic lipase. This is an enzyme, produced only by the pancreatic gland, and therefore the increase in its activity is the most typical of acute pancreatitis. Proinflamatory cytokines play a crucial role in the primary activation of the cells of the immunological system as a result of damage to the pancreas (Lewandowski et al. 2007).

In the x-ray chest, it is possible to ascertain the presence of the liquid in the left pleural cavity. The plain radiological picture of the abdomen is taken as a routine measure in the diagnostics of acute pancreatitis.

Ultrasonography (USG) - possesses as many as 90% of the tenderness in diagnosing acute pancreatitis. It is a non-invasive treatment, which may be repeated several times. Ultrasonography pictures the dynamics of the pathological changes course in pancreatic parenchyma and in the adjacent tissues

Computer tomography (CT) is currently regarded as a diagnostic standard the highest is a sensitivity in terms of acute pancreatitis, Magnetic resonance imagining (MRI) - is a method, alternative to CT.

Endoscopic retrograde cholangiopancreatography (ERCP) - is the most effective method of discovering the cause of acute pancreatitis. It is simultaneously possible to remove the triggering factor.

Endoscopic sphincterotomy performed within the first 24 hours after the occurrence of the first symptoms causes alleviating the course of the disease and reduces the risk of complications

Endoscopic ultrasonography (EUS) is a modern method of imagining of the cause of acute pancreatitis, however, without a possibility of procedural intervention.

4. Oxidative stress and antioxidative status in acute pancreatitis

Oxidative stress was defined by Sies in 1985 as a state of relative balance in a living organism between the prooxidation activity, which means the production of free oxygen radicals and antioxidative processes, which means the deactivation of free radicals (Braganza et al., 1995; Kikuchi et al., 1997; Sies H & Cadenas, 1985).

Free oxygen radicals are substances possessing one non-paired electron, or more.

Such a chemical structure determines high instability of these chemical compositions and tendency to become involved in violent biochemical reactions parts, leading to damaging cellular structures (Matkovics et al., 1995; Schulz et al., 1999).

Contemporarily, instead of the notion free oxygen radicals theRreactive Oxygen Form (ROF) is more frequently used.

The best researched ROFs are: hyper-oxygen radical, hydrogen-oxygen radical, hyper-oxide radical, hydrogen hyper-oxygen radical and nitrogen oxide (Schulz et al., 1999; Song et al., 2003; Petrov, 2010).

Non-radical form also include non-radical type substances, the derivatives of oxygen, displaying similar impact as radicals, e.g. hydrogen peroxide, hypochlorous acid, ozone or singleton oxygen (Abu-Zidan et al., 2000; Braganza et al., 1995).
The sources of ROFs are the reactions of oxidation and reduction, mainly occurring in mitochondria and cellular membranes, including the cells of the vessel perithelium.
The source of ROFs is also the process of oxidizing hypoxanthine by xanthine oxidase, and also by the reaction in which the ions of some metals, mainly iron and copper, participate (Chmiel et al., 2002).
The formation of the reactive form of oxygen takes place, among others, in the chain of changes of arachidonic acid.
Large amounts of ROFs are formed in the course of inflammatory processes.
The source of them are the cells, directly participating in immunological response and pathogens, for example bacteria (Park et al., 2003).
The oxidation of organic substances, such as proteins and lipids, is also the source of the
ROFs display strong toxic impact in relation to the cells of a human organism. The effect of their impact is damaging structural proteins, enzymatic structures, lipids of cellular membranes, breaking up the threads of DNA, damage to chromosomes, degeneration of the cytoskeleton of the cell, disorders of the synthesis of collagen and neoplasm transformation, which consequently leads to the death of a cell, which is preceded by a substantial damage and disordering its functions (Winterbourn et al., 2003).
In the course of inflammatory process in the pancreas, the local accumulation of activated phagocytes occurs; these phagocytes are producing chemotactic factors, which cause the migration of new leukocytes to the area, invaded by inflammation.
The activated phagocyte cells release proteolithic enzymes, which damage the tissues and are the secondary source of new ROF (Wereszczyńska-Siemiatowska et al., 1998, 2004).
Pathogenetic factors, causing handicapping of blood flow through the pancreas are the cause of ischaemia and hypoxia of the cells of this organ.
Ischaemia is a reversible and temporary process.
After this period, reperfusion occurs.
An increase in the concentration of oxygen in the blood results in the production of a very active and cytotoxic hydrogen oxide radical, regarded as the main cause of the damage to the cells of the pancreas.
As a result of reperfusion, occurring after ischaemia, deepening the damage to the endothelium of the blood vessels and activation of the components of the complement system, the activation of the mast cells, the intensification of the aggregation of blood platelets, which consequently leads to the formation of micro-thromboses occur.
The activated cells of the immunological system secondarily cause the intensified production of the reactive form of oxygen, damaging the adjacent tissues (Sweiry & Mann 1996; Telek et al., 2001).
In turn, antioxidants counteract the reactive form of oxygen in an organism.
Their function is to maintain the balance between the processes of oxidation and reduction (Curran et al., 2000; Dabrowski et al., 1999; Johnson, 2007; Satinder et al., 2011).
There are two essential defense mechanisms - non-enzymatic and enzymatic.
Non-enzymatic defense anti-oxidation system is composed of substances, so-called „sweepers", reacting directly with the reactive form of oxygen.
They include: vitamin E, vitamin C, beta- carotene, uric acid, ceruloplasmin and glutation.

The most important enzymatic anti-oxidants include: hyperoxide dismutase (SOD), the system of glutation peroxidases (GPX) and the system of catalases (Tsai et al.; Vaquero-Raya &Molero-Richard, 2005).
The disturbance of balance between the oxidation and anti-oxidation factors in case of patients with acute pancreatitis leads to oxidation stress.
The level of its intensification has a direct influence on the severity of the course of disease, the risk of complications and prognosis.

5. The aim of the work

The aim of the work was to examine the dynamics of oxidative (8-OhdG) and antioxidative status (TAS) in patients with mild and severe form of acute pancreatitis.
The profiles of exchanged parameters, the degree of the correlation among them and the degree of statistical significance can give certain information relating to prognose of the course of the acute pancreas, as also he can give therapeutic and prognostic instructions.

6. The principles of the work

Forty patients admitted to the clinic with the symptoms of acute pancreatitis were subjected to the assessment.
All patients expressed their consent to perform the research.
Consent of the Regionale Commission of Research Ethics was obtained.
In all patients, apart from a routine examination, the following data were determined for the blood serum and the urine:

1. Oxidative activity of peroxide DNA 8- hydroxyl – 2 – deoxyguanosine (8-OhdG) in I, III, V, VII day of hospitalization.

and in the blood serum:

2. Total antioxidative status in I, III, V, VII day of hospitalization.

The patients were divided in two groups: with mild and severe form of acute pancreatitis.
In both of the groups, the dynamics of the processes of oxidation (8-OhdG) and antioxidation (TAS) were assessed; moreover, it was assessed, whether there was a correlation between separate parameters.
The obtained results were subjected to statistical analysis and the influence of the disease process on the level of the researched parameters was assessed.

7. Material and methods

7.1 Clinical material

Material for the research was obtained by means of collecting the venous blood and urine from the patients, admitted to the Department of Gastrointestinal & General Surgery Silesian Piasts` University of Medicine in Wrocław and the Department of General Surgery Railway Hospital in Wrocław during the emergency service because of acute pancreatitis between 2004 and 2006 years.
The samples of blood and urine were collected in I, III, V and VII day of hospitalization.
The research on the following parameters: 8-OhdG and TAS included patients with the acute pancreatitis of severe course and, randomly selected, with the acute pancreatitis of mild course.

In all patients, the quantitative markings of 8-OhdG and TAS respectively in I, III, V, VII day of stay at the hospital were conducted.
The patients were qualified into a research group upon the basis of the typical symptoms of acute pancreatitis.
In the group with the mild form, dominated the pain ailments of the abdomen of various intensity, bad general mood, nausea, vomiting and other symptoms.
The ailments abated most frequently after 3-4 days after the application of intravenous liquid-based therapy and treatment with analgesic and antispasmodic drugs.
This group included 20 of thepatients.
In the group with the severe form, the symptoms were more serious.
The dominating ones were the pain ailments of the abdomen and the symptoms of Systemic Inflammatory Response Syndrome (SIRS), connected with the hyperstimulation of the immunological system.
In the patients, the temperature of the body increased, the action of the heart was accelerated, and the level of leukocytosis grew, while the diuresis per hour decreased.
As a result of the outflow of liquid and protein from the vascular bed, the cardiac-vascular failure, kidney failure, the respiratory system failure, necrotic changes in the parenchyma of the pancreas (visible thanks to computer tomography), thrombotic complications and enzymatic toxemia occurred.
This group encompassed 20 patients.
Altogether, 40 patients were researched in the course of the research.
Among the researched, there were 7 women and 33 men.

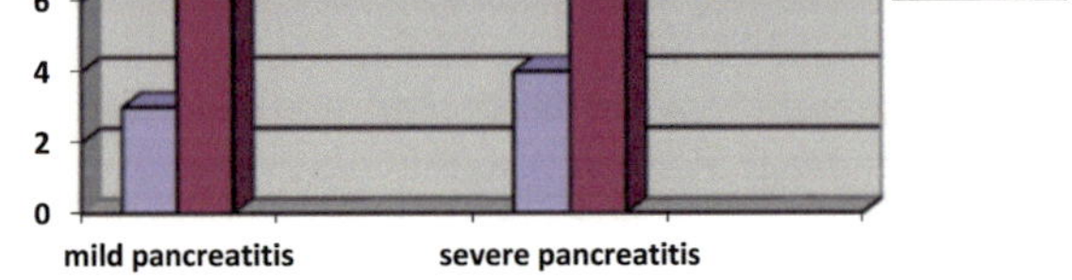

Fig. 1. Clinical material

In the group of the patients with the mild course, there were 3 women and 17 men.
In the group of the individuals with the severe course, there were 4 women and 16 men.
The oldest group member was 76 years old, whilst the youngest one 26 years old.
The average age of the patients was 51 years.
In the researched group with acute pancreatitis, women constituted 17.5%, while men 82.5%.
In the group with the mild pancreatitis, women constituted 15 %, while men 85%.
In the group with the severe pancreatitis, women constituted 20 %, whilst men 80%.
The lowest incidence rate was observed in the age groups 26-35 and 36-45.
The highest incidence rate was observed in the age groups 46-55 and 66-75.

7.2 Laboratory methods

7.2.1 Marking oxidation activity in the serum and urine in case of the patients with acute pancreatitis

Oxidation activity was marked in the serum and in urine upon the basis of marking 8-hydroxydeoxyguanosine (8-OhdG) with the Elis method.
The research was conducted in strict accordance with the procedure, determined by the producer - bioxtech 8-OhdG-eia kit-oxis.
The results were expressed in ng/ml.
The range of detection rate 8-OhdG in accordance with the applied methods amounted to 0.125-200 ng/ml.
The results for 8-OhdG in urine were expressed in relation to creatinine.
The norms marked in case of 15 healthy volunteers at the age of 19 to 50 years are within the range 0.00 - 0.8 ng/ml in serum and between 0,00 - 0,3 ng/ml/g/creatinine in urine.

7.2.2 Marking total antioxidation ability in the serum in case of the patients with acute pancreatitis

The principle of marking according to the set produced by the Random Laboratories Company - the strict application of the regulations of the producer.
The norm marked in the serum of 30 health volunteers at the age of 20 to 65 years is within the range 1.30 - 1.75 mmol/l, and corresponding to the standard of Trolox - a substance with antioxidative properties.

8. The results of the serearch

8.1 Clinical analisis

Taking under consideration the aetiological factor in the entire group, the patients with biliary acute pancreatitis constituted 50% of the patients (20 patients).
The patients with alcoholic acute pancreatitis constituted 35% (14 patients).
In case of 15% (6 patients), it proved impossible to determine the causes of acute pancreatitis.
These cases were diagnosed as idiopathic.
In the group with the mild pancreatitis, patients with biliary pancreatitis constituted 40% (8 patients), with alcoholic pancreatitis constituted 35% (7 patients), while with idiopathic pancreatitis constituted 25% (5patients).
In the group with the severe pancreatitis, patients with biliary pancreatitis constituted 60% (12 patients), with alcoholic pancreatitis constituted 30%(6 patients), while with idiopathic pancreatitis constituted 10% (2 patients).
The treatment of the patients with acute pancreatitis encompassed actions in accordance with established therapeutic
principles depending on the severity of the course of the disease.
In case of 20 patients with the mild pancreatitis, conservative treatment was applied. That consisted in: fasting, intravenous liquid-based therapy, pumping out the stomach contents with a pro-bang, inserted through the nose, treatment of pain, monitoring the activity of the kidneys, monitoring the pressure of the peripheral blood, monitoring arterial blood gas values and thrombotic prophylaxis.
In case of 2 patients, with biliary pancreatitis, after several weeks, cholecystectomy was performed.

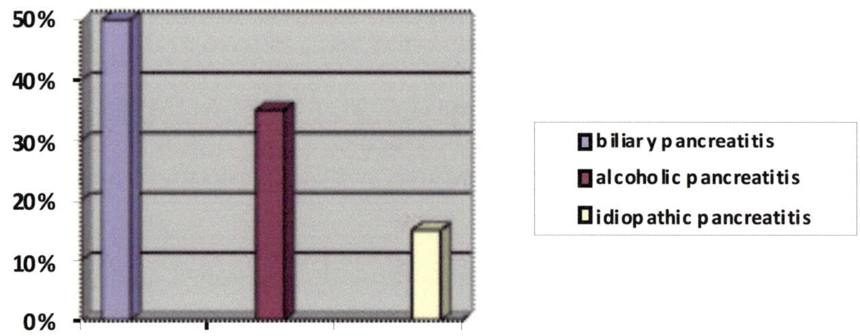

Fig. 2. The cause of the acute pancreatitis

In one patient, after 8 weeks, junction cyst of the pancreas with the jejunum was performed.
In the group of patients with the mild course, the longest stay amounted was 12 days and the shortest 5 days.
Twenty patients with the severe form were divided into two sub-groups.
In the sub-group of 7 patients, ERCP with sphincteroctomy was performed.
However, in one of case after three weeks an operative drainage of the abscess of the pancreas was performed.
In the sub-group of 13 patients with the severe course of acute pancreatitis, surgical procedure was required.
In case of 7 patients, cholecystectomy with the lavage of the peritoneal cavity was performed.
In case of 6 patients, the lavage of the peritoneal cavity with laparostomy was performed; in this group, in two cases- lavage was performed twice, in two cases- three times, while two other cases- four times.
In the course of further lavages, pancreatic necrectomy was performed.
All the patients were receiving antibiotics of a wide spectrum, intravenous liquid-based therapy and an analgesic drugs.
Moreover, the following were applied: gastric suction, and thrombolytic prophylaxis.
The functioning of the kidneys, the pressure of the peripheral blood and acid-alkaline economy were monitored.
Sixteen patients were fed parenterally with the supplementation of microelements.
In case of four patients, a nutritional microjejunostomy was making.
In case of 1 patient, a complication in the form of cerebrovascular accident occurred, while in case of 2 patients, the course of acute pancreatitis was made more complicated by atrial fibrillation.
These patients were treated within the framework of Intensive Care Unit.
After obtaining the stabilization of the blood circulation system, the patients returned to the surgical ward.
In one patient, massive hemorrhage from the upper digestive tract occurred, and, in spite of interventional endoscopy, the patient died.
Two other patients' death as a result of the complications of multi-organic failure.
Out of the group of 20 patients with the severe course, 3 persons died, therefore, the mortality rate in this group amounted to 15%.
The longest stay amounted to 57 days, the shortest 7 days.

The average time of hospitalization was 8 days for cases with the mild course and 18 days for the cases with the severe course (Fig. 3).

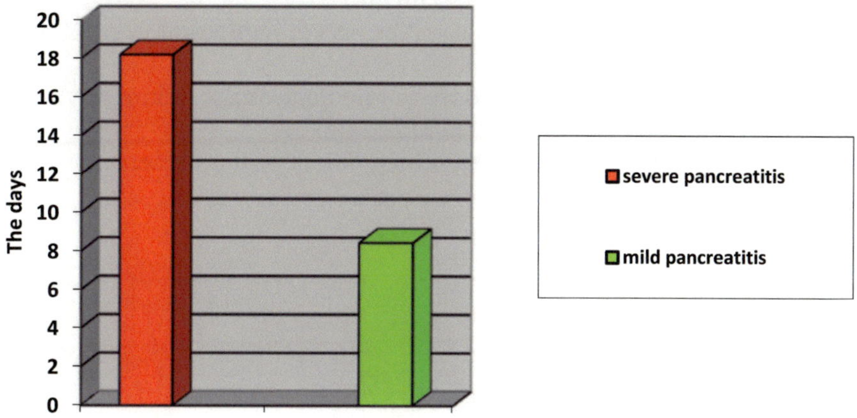

Fig. 3. The average time of hospitalization

8.2 Oxidation activity measured by the amount of 8-OhdG in the blood serum in patients with the mild and severe pancreatitis

In both groups of the patients, quantitative marking of 8-OhdG in the blood serum was performed.

As it is made clear by the data presented in Fig. 4, in case of the patients with the mild course of acute pancreatitis, the average value of 8-OhdG was decreasing along with the time of stay at hospital.

Therefore, on I day it amounted to, on average, 2.49 ng/ml SD±1,51, on III day 2.13 ng/ml SD±1,52, on V day 1.71 ng/ml SD±0,43, and on VII day to 1.59 ng/ml SD±0,29.

In case of the patients with the severe form of acute pancreatitis, the average value of 8-OhdG was two times higher and was growing with the time of stay at hospital.

On I day, the level of 8-OhdG amounted to, on average, 4.77 ng/ml SD±2,65, on III day 5.97 ng/ml SD±3,01, on V as much as 6.68 ng/ml SD±4,01, and on VII day 6.21 ng/ml SD±3,74, Fig. 4.

In case of the patients, in whom multi-organic complications (the abscesses of the peritoneum, circulation-respiratory failure, septic shock, thrombolytic complications) occurred, a high concentration of 8-OhdG was noticeable These were patients from the group with the severe course of acute pancreatitis.In the group with the severe course of acute pancreatitis, the highest concentration of 8-OhdG were observed in case of the patients with complications in the form of the abscesses of the peritoneum.

For a male, aged 63, with the abscess of the peritoneum, value of 8-OhdG on V day of hospitalization amounted to 16.5 ng/ml.

For a male, aged 28, also with the abscess of the peritoneum, value of 9-OhdG on III day amounted to 16 ng/ml.

For a female, aged 69, value 8-OhdG on V day amounted to 15 ng/ml.

For a female, aged 60, value of 8-OhdG on III day amounted to 9.5 ng/ml.

In the group of patients with the severe course with other complications, for example with circulation-respiratory failure, the values of 8-OhdG were lower.
For a male, aged 33, with acute respiratory failure, requiring the use of an endotracheal tube - the value of 8-OhdG amounted to 2.8 ng/ml on V Day.
For a male, aged 70, treated at the Intensive Care Ward with respiratory failure, the value of 8-OhdG on V day amounted to 3 ng/ml.
For a male, aged 48, with acute respiratory failure and cardiac failure (rhythm disturbance) on III day, the value of 8-OhdG amounted to 7.82 ng/ml.
A male, aged 70, with circulation-respiratory failure - the value of 8-OhdG on V day amounted to 2.8 ng/ml.

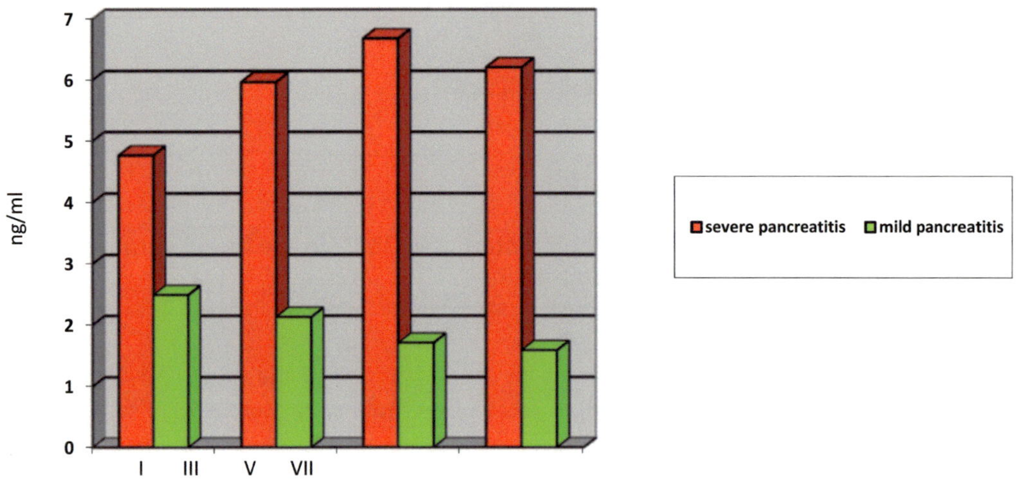

Fig. 4. The average values of 8-OhdG in the blood serum in patients with acute pancreatitis.

8.3 Oxidation activity measured with the amount of 8-OhdG in urine in patients with the mild and severe pancreatitis

In case of the patients with the severe form of acute pancreatitis, the average values of 8-OhdG were several times higher than in case of the patients with the mild form of acute pancreatitis.
In case of the patients with the mild form of acute pancreatitis, on I day the average value of 8-OhdG amounted to 2.69 ng/ml SD±1, 30, on III day amounted to 2.14 ng/ml SD±0, 66, on V day only as little as 1.87 ng/ml SD±0, 53, and on VII day it amounted to 1.62 ng/ml SD±0, 47 (Fig. 5).
In case of patients with the severe form of acute pancreatitis, the average value of 8-OhdG on I day amounted to 7.99 ng/ml SD±9, 75, on III day it increased to 8.68 ng/ml SD±7, 16, on V day it amounted to as much 9.51 ng/ml SD±7, 90, on VII day it reached the value of 7.55 ng/ml SD±4, 31 (Fig. 5).

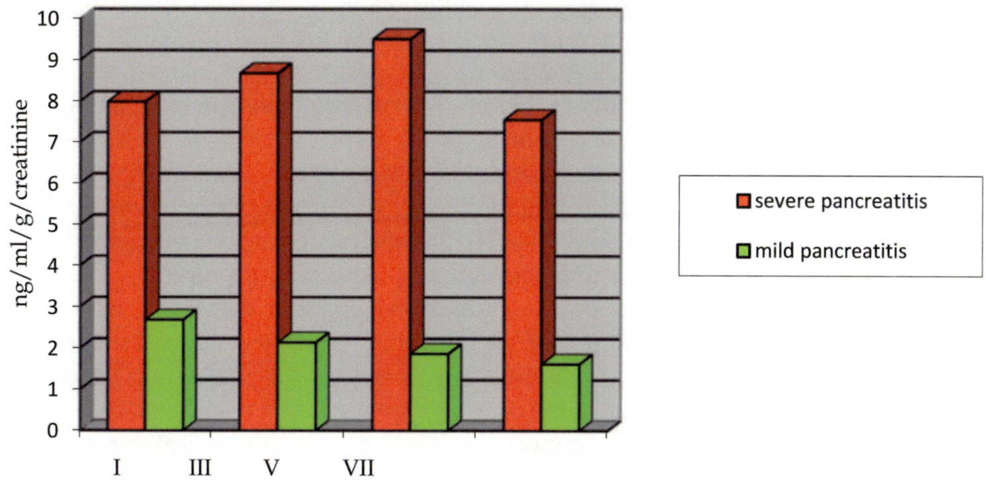

Fig. 5. The average values of 8-OhdG in urine in patients with acute pancreatitis.

8.4 Results of total antioxidation ability in the blood serum in patients with the mild and severe pancreatitis

In case of the patients with the mild form of acute pancreatitis on I day of hospitalization, the average total antioxidation activity measured with the TAS, amounted to 1.19 mmol/l SD±0, 10, on III day it amounted to respectively 1.26 mmol/l SD±0, 12, on V day it insignificantly increased to 1.27 mmol/l SD±0, 10, and on VII day it reached the value of 1.26 mmol/l SD±0, 14 (Fig.6). In case of the patients with the severe form of acute pancreatitis, the average values of TAS amounted respectively to: on I day - 1.27 mmol/l SD ± 0,21, on III day - 1.27 mmol/l SD ± 0,21, on V day - 1.31 mmol/l SD ±0,16, and on VII day - 1.32 mmol/l SD±0,17 (Fig. 6).

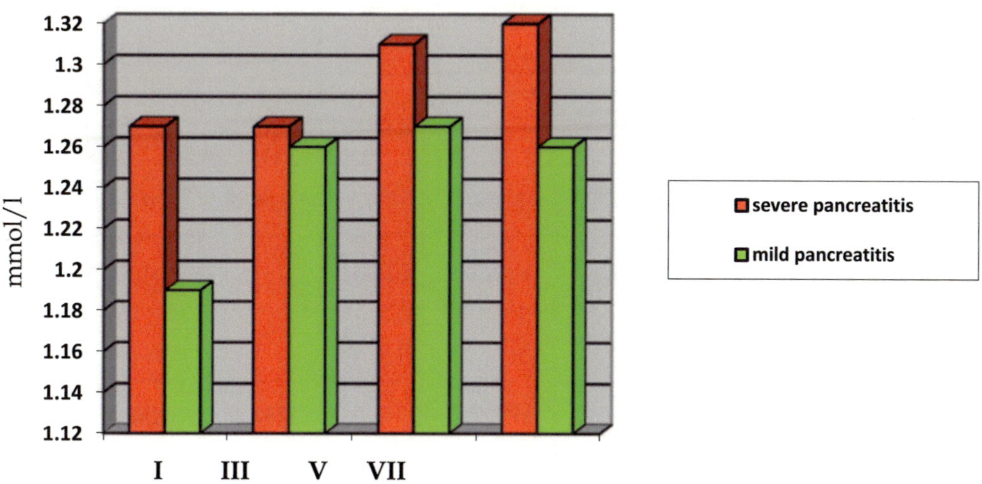

Fig. 6. The average values of TAS in case of the patients with acute pancreatitis.

8.5 Statistical analysis

Statistical analysis applies to the interpretation of the results of laboratory research and their mutual connections with a clinical image in case of the selected group of 40 patients, suffering from acute pancreatitis.

The analysis encompassed the results of the research on oxidation potential, anti-oxidation potential, interleukin-6 and the protein of acute phase. In this manner, the values making it possible to assess the level of advancement of the disease process and the risk of possible complications were obtained. The results of the research are the indicator of the dynamics of acute pancreatitis. In the course of the research, the analysis encompassed the influence of selected clinical parameters on the dynamics of the inflammatory process, and what was attempted, was the interpretation of the correlations between these parameters. These parameters were assessed in terms of their usefulness in the diagnostics and prognostics of the course of acute pancreatitis. At the separate stages of hospitalization, causal-result interdependencies between the researched parameters were determined. A so-called level of significance (p) was subjected to analysis. The levels of significance (p) for a group of patients with the mild form of pancreatitis are presented in Table 1, while for a group of patients with the severe form in Table 2.

The results of the research were correlated in both of the groups of patients, with the mild and severe forms of acute pancreatitis. The analysis of the degree of dependence of parameters was presented with the use of correlation co-efficient. Table 3 illustrates the correlations for a group of patients with the mild course of acute pancreatitis, while Table 4 for a group of patients with the severe course.

	8-OhdG I	8-OhdG III	8-OhdG V	8-OhdG VII	8-OhdG I urine	8-OhdG III urine	8-OhdG V urine	8-OhdG VII urine
8-OhdG I		0,0016	0,4371	0,1364	0,0177	0,4419	0,9263	0,9061
8-OhdG III	0,0016		0,2048	0,0859	0,0049	0,0167	0,3057	0,7938
8-OhdG V	0,4371	0,2048		0,0639	0,4399	0,0288	0,3732	0,6942
8-OhdG VII	0,1364	0,0859	0,0639		0,9844	0,4258	0,9106	0,5278
8-OhdG I urine	0,0177	0,0049	0,4399	0,9844		0,0001	0,0564	0,0696
8-OhdG III urine	0,4419	0,0167	0,0288	0,4258	0,0001		0,0013	0,1426
8-OhdG V urine	0,9263	0,3057	0,3732	0,9106	0,0564	0,0013		
8-OhdG VII urine	0,9061	0,7938	0,6942	0,5278	0,0696	0,1426	0,0088	

A group of patients with the mild form of pancreatitis.

Table 1. The levels of significance (p) for intra-group correlations.

	8-OhdG I	8-OhdG III	8-OhdG V	8-OhdG VII	8-OhdG I urine	8-OhdG III urine	8-OhdG V urine	8-OhdG VII urine
8-OhdG I		0,0081	0,1213	0,0254	0,0059	0,0044	0,0000	0,0148
8-OhdG III	0,0081		0,0066	0,0345	0,0612	0,0097	0,0032	0,0126
8-OhdG V	0,1213	0,0066		0,0000	0,9842	0,8771	0,2748	0,3124
8-OhdG VII	0,0254	0,0345	0,0000		0,5568	0,9066	0,1522	0,4137
8-OhdG I urine	0,0059	0,0612	0,9842	0,5568		0,0017	0,0002	0,1536
8-OhdG III urine	0,0044	0,0097	0,8771	0,9066	0,0017		0,0002	0,0004
8-OhdG V urine	0,0000	0,0032	0,2748	0,1522	0,0002	0,0002		0,0002
8-OhdG VII urine	0,0148	0,0126	0,3124	0,4137	0,1536	0,0004	0,0002	

A group of patients with the severe form of acute pancreatitis.

Table 2. The levels of significance (p) for intra-group correlations.

	8-OhdG I	8-OhdG III	8-OhdG V	8-OhdG VII	8-OhdG I urine	8-OhdG III urine	8-OhdG V urine	8-OhdG VII urine
8-OhdG I	1,00	0,74	0,24	0,62	0,55	0,21	-0,03	-0,05
8-OhdG III		1,00	0,38	0,69	0,73	0,61	0,34	0,10
8-OhdG V			1,00	0,73	-0,26	-0,60	-0,32	-0,17
8-OhdG VII				1,00	0,01	-0,36	0,07	-0,29
8-OhdG I urine					1,00	0,88	0,65	0,67
8-OhdG III urine						1,00	0,84	0,53
8-OhdG V urine							1,00	0,92
8-OhdG VII urine								1,00

Marked correlations are significant, with $p < 0.05$.

Table 3. Intra-group correlations of a group of patients with the mild form of pancreatitis.

	8-OhdG I	8-OhdG III	8-OhdG V	8-OhdG VII	8-OhdG I urine	8-OhdG III urine	8-OhdG V urine	8-OhdG VII urine
8-OhdG I	1,00	0,57	0,36	0,54	0,69	0,67	0,86	0,68
8-OhdG III		1,00	0,59	0,51	0,51	0,62	0,71	0,69
8-OhdG V			1,00	0,89	0,01	-0,04	0,30	0,32
8-OhdG VII				1,00	0,19	0,03	0,42	0,26
8-OhdG I urine					1,00	0,76	0,83	0,49
8-OhdG III urine						1,00	0,81	0,85
8-OhdG V urine							1,00	0,89
8-OhdG VII urine								1,00

Marked correlations are significant, with $p < 0.05$.

Table 4. Intra-group correlations of a group of patients with the severe form of acute pancreatitis.

9. Discussion

Acute pancreatitis is a disease of moderate-to-severe or severe course.
In terms of anatomy, it is characterized by the reversible damage to the pancreas and the tissues adjacent to the pancreas in the form of oedema and necrosis, but sometimes by multi-organic complications as well.
Acute pancreatitis still constitutes a major problem for contemporary medicine.
It results from the fact of diagnosis-related difficulties and from the lack of an effective therapy of the severe course of acute pancreatitis.
The pathogenesis of acute pancreatitis still remains unknown.
Many researches has proved that the origins of anatomical changes, occurring in the course of the pancreatic gland, are connected with micro-circulation disorders.
What has also been confirmed is the participation of many mediators in the development of the changes of this type.
The direct factors of changes causing acute pancreatitis are: the activation of pancreatic enzymes and micro-circulation disorders.
In the cases of severe acute pancreatitis with multi-organic complications, micro-circulation disorders, mainly afflicting the lungs, liver, the digestive tract and the circulation system occur, accompanied by the development of Systemic Inflammatory Response Syndrome (SIRS) and Multi-Organ Dysfunction Syndrome (MODS).
The research showed that the increase in the value of 8-OhdG, particularly within the fifth days, was connected with the severe pancreatitis with multi-organic complications.

The increase in the values, particularly of 8-OhdG, in the serums and urine, in case of the individuals with the severe form of acute pancreatitis, may be associated with the spread and intensification of inflammatory process, damaging the cellular structures.
Those results are compatible with the research of (Szulz et al.1999 and of Wereszczyńska-Siemiątkowska et al 2003, 2004), who emphasize the role of oxidation stress in the processes of destruction of factors connected with them in the forecasting of acute pancreatitis.
8-OhdG is defined as a marker of the living cell DNA damage.
The reactive form of oxygen, produced in oxidation stress, may attack the biological structures of DNA and destroy them, this being the result of the oxidation of chemical compounds, contained in it.
Damage to nucleic bases or breaking up the bounds, connecting nucleotides, occur.
Lower values of 8-OhdG and reduced dynamics of its increase in the course of disease were found in the case of the individuals with the mild form of acute pancreatitis.
Those results suggest that the values of 8-OhdG reflect the activity of disease process and may be useful in the assessment of the severity of disease, as well as in the forecasting in the course of treatment.
The review of the literature (Rahman et al., 2004; Roth et al., 2004; Virlos et al., 2003) shows that the perfect antioxidation ability, marked in blood serums, in case of the individuals with the severe form of acute pancreatitis, is lowered as compensative mechanisms are being exhausted.
Therefore, TAS, as one of methods of marking the anti-oxidation properties, is a useful forecasting marker, and lowering its value may signal transfer from the mild form of acute pancreatitis into the severe form.
Own research provided no evidence for the claim that there were any substantial differences in terms of the value of TAS in the case of the individuals with the severe and mild form of acute pancreatitis.
Both in case of the severe and mild form of acute pancreatitis, no TAS growth or TAS fall tendency in separate markings of the conducted research was noticed, either.
Such results, when confronted with the research of others authors (Dziurkowska-Marek et al., 2004; Modzelewski, 2005; Rahman et al., 2004), in which lowering of the value of antioxidation potential in the individuals with acute pancreatitis - may result from the method of marking.
In own research, the behaviour of the TAS values at similar level in separate markings may be connected with the administered treatment, for it is known that some medicines may show antioxidation properties.
According to the research of (Scott et al., 1993), such is the action of vitamin C.
Anti-oxidation action of beta-carotene, vitamin A (retinol) and vitamin E (tocopherol) was confirmed by (Curran et al., 2000) in their work.
Similar reports were received from (Virlos et al., 2003), researching the properties of vitamin C, selenium and acetylcysteine (Dejong et al., 2001).
In own material, all the patients with the severe pancreatitis, apart from operational treatment, required intensive treatment.
All the patients were provided with extra-intestinal or intra-intestinal feeding (in 4 cases, with the use of microjejunostomy) with the supply of elementary diets and of micro- and macro-elements.

The Vitalipid preparation was administered; this preparation contains, among others, vitamin A (retinol) and vitamin E (tocopherol).
As an additive to industrial diets, enriching intravenous drip, among others, with vitamin C, folic acid, biothin and pantothenic acid.
Oxidation processes exert a destructive influence on many important functions of the organism and may constitute an additional, apart from other inflammatory factors, property, destroying the cellular and tissue structures of the organism.
The potential of oxidation activity may, therefore, constitute an indication of intensified inflammatory reactivity.
Antioxidation potential (TAS) may inform about the efficiency of the systems antioxidation systems, significant in the neutralization of the intensified oxidation processes.
Currently, the pharmacological attempts of alleviating the results of acute pancreatitis are made (Curran et al., 2000; Vaquero-Raya & Molero-Richard, 2005; Virlos et al., 2003).
In the light of the most up-to-date knowledge, certain pharmacological impacts provide hope for the application of a new, effective strategy, which may significantly improve the results of the treatment of the severe pancreatitis.
The improvement in the blood flow in organs is achieved by means of using isovolemic haemo-dilution.
In this method, intravenous drips, such as 0,9% NaCl, Dextran 40 000, 10% HES and albumins, are
The application of heparin, as an anticoagulation factor, may result in the improvement in the blood saturation of organs, too.
Application of the antagonists of receptors of bradykinin B_2 and gabexate mesylate exerts a beneficial influence on microcirculation.
Cleansed beef hemoglobin turned out to be a safe substitute of the blood and to improve, as an oxygen carrier, the saturation of the tissues with oxygen (Panek et al., 2007).
The application of oxidizing agents, so-called plasma oxygen carriers, is currently a new strategy in the treatment of the severe pancreatitis.
Upon the basis of own research, it was determined that the high values of 8-OhdG in the serum of peripheral blood and urine alike in case of the patients with acute pancreatitis, indicate these tests may reflect the severity of the course of acute pancreatitis, as well as serve for predicting the occurrence of multi-organic complications to a degree greater than that in case of other biochemical tests.

10. Conclusion

1. As performed examinations show, 8-OhdG parameter, marked by means of Elisa method in the serum and urine is the sensitive parameter of acute pancreatitis inflammatory activity.
2. High values of 8-OhdG are characteristic for acute pancreatitis with severe course and are the indicator of oxidative stress. They inform also about the risk of multiorganic complications.
3. Total antioxidative status (TAS) is similar in both groups of patients and its decrease is not statistically significant for the severe form of acute pancreatitis.

11. References

Braganza, J. Towards a novel treatment strategy for acute pancreatitis. 1. Reappraisal of the evidence on aetiogenesis. *Digestion* 2001; Vol.63: pp.69-91.

Frossard, J.; Steer, M. & Pastor, C. Acute pancreatitis. *Lancet*. 2008; Vol.371: pp.143-152.

Gamaste, V. Diagnostic tests for acute pancreatitis. *Gastroenterologist* 1994; Vol.2: pp.119-30. Toouli, J.; Brooke-Smith, M.; Bassi, C.; Carr-Locke, D.; Telford, J.; Freeny, P.; Imrie, C. & Tandon, R. Guidelines for the management of acute pancreatitis. *J Gastroenterol Hepatol*. 2002; Vol.17: pp. 15-39. Yousaf, M.; McCallion, K. & Diamond, T. Management of severe acute pancreatitis. *Br J Surg*. 2003; Vol.90: pp. 407-20.Song, J; Lim, J.; Kim, H.; Morio, T. & Kim, K. Oxidative stress induces nuclear loss of DNA repair proteins Ku70 and Ku80 and apoptosis in pancreatic acinar AR42J cells. *J. Biol. Chem*. 2003; Vol.278: pp. 532-41.

Baillie, J. Treatment of acute biliary pancreatitis *N. Engl. J. Med.* 1997; Vol.336: pp.286-7.

Balthazar, E. Acute pancreatitis: assessment of severity with clinical and CT evaluation. *Radiology*. 2002; Vol.223: pp.603-13.

Beger, H.; Rau, B.; Mayer, J. & Pralle, U. Natural course of acute pancreatitis. World J. Surg. 1997; Vol.21: pp. 130-35.

Lund,H.; Tønnesen, H.; Tønnesen, M.; & Olsen,O. Long-term recurrence and death rates after acute pancreatitis. *Scand J Gastroenterol*. 2006; Vol. 41: pp.234-38.

Munoz, A. & Katerndahl, D. Diagnosis and management of acute pancreatitis *Am. Fam. Physician*. 2000; Vol.62: pp. 164-74.

Mutinga,M.; Rosenbluth, A.;Tenner, S.; Odze,R.; Sica,G. & Banks, P. Does mortality occur early or late in acute pancreatitis? *Int J Pancreatol*. 2000; Vol.28: pp. 91-95.

Banks P & Freeman M. Practice guidelines in acute pancreatitis. *Am J Gastroenterol* . 2006; Vol.101: pp. 2379–400.

Bradley, E. 3rd. A clinically based classification system for acute pancreatitis: *Arch.Surg*. 1993; Vol.128: pp.586-90. Ranson, J. Diagnostic standards for acute pancreatitis. *World J. Surg*. 1997; Vol.21: pp.136-42

Lankisch, P.;Warnecke,B.;Bruns,D.;Werner, H.; Grossman, F.; Struckmann,G.; Brinkmann,G.; Maisonneuve,P.& Lowenfels,A. The APACHE II score is unreliable to diagnose necrotizing pancreatitis on admission to hospital. *Pancreas*. 2002; Vol.24: pp.217-22.

Braganza, J. Mast cell: pivotal player in lethal acute pancreatitis: *QJM* . 2000; Vol.93: pp.469-76

Sharma, V. & Howden, C. Metaanalysis of randomized controlled trials of endoscopic retrograde cholangiography and endoscopic sphincterotomy for the treatment of acute biliary pancreatitis. *Am J Gastroenterol*. 1999; Vol.94: pp. 3211-4. Yadav, D. & Lowenfels, A. Trends in the epidemiology of the first attack of acute pancreatitis: a systematic review. *Pancreas*. 2006; Vol.33: pp.323-30.

Baron, T.; Thaggard, W.; Morgan, D. & Stanley R. Endoscopic therapy for organized pancreatic necrosis. *Gastroenterology*. 1996; Vol.111: pp. 755-764.

Liu, C.; Lo C. & Fan S. Acute biliary pancreatitis: diagnosis and management. *World J Surg*. 1997; Vol.21: pp.149-54.

Fan, S., Lai, E., Mok, F., Lo, C., Zheng, S. & Wong J. Early treatment of acute biliary pancreatitis by endoscopic papillotomy. *N Engl J Med*. 1993; Vol.328: pp.228-32.

Demols, A & Deviere, J. New frontiers in the pharmacological prevention of post-ERCP pancreatitis: the cytokines. *Journal of Pancreas*. 2003; Vol.4: pp. 21-57.

Folsch, L., Nitsche, R. &Ludtke, R. Early ERCP and papillotomy compared with conservative treatment for acute biliary pancreatitis. *N Engl J Med*. 1997; Vol.336: pp.237-42.

Golub, R.; Siddiqi, F. & Pohl, D. Role of antibiotics in acute pancreatitis. *J Gastrointest Surg.* 1998; Vol.2: pp. 496-503. Vaquero-Raya, E. & Molero-Richard, X. Reactive oxygen species in inflammatory diseases of the pancreas. A possible therapeutic target? *Gastroenterol. Hepatol.* 2005; Vol.28: pp.473-84.

Frossard, J. & Hadengue,A. Acute pancreatitis: new physiopathological concepts. *Gastroentérol.Clin. Biol.* 2001; Vol. 25: pp. 352-356.

Dufour, M. & Adamson, M. The epidemiology of alcohol-induced pancreatitis. *Pancreas.* 2003; Vol.27: pp.286-90. Schenker, S. & Montalvo, R. Alcohol and the pancreas. *Recent Dev. Alcohol.* 1998; Vol.14: pp.41- 65.

Rau ,B.; Steinbach, G.; Gansauge, F.; Mayer, J.; Grünert, A. & Berger, H. The potential role of procalcitonin and interleukin 8 in the prediction of infected necrosis in acute pancreatitis. *Gut.* 1997; Vol.41: pp. 832-40.

Schoenberg, M.; Büchler, M.; Pietrzyk, C.; Uhl, W.; Birk, D.; Eisele, S.; Marzinzig M. & Beger, H. Lipid peroxidation and glutathione metabolism in chronic pancreatitis. *Pancreas.* 1995; Vol.10: pp.36-43.

Niederau, C. & Lüthen, R. Current aspects in the pathogenesis of acute pancreatitis. *Praxis.* 1997; Vol.86: pp. 385-391. Sabater, L.; Pareja, E.; Aparisi, L.; Calvete, J.; Camps, B.; Sastre,J.;Artiques,E.; Oviedo,M.; Trullenque,R. & Liedó S. Pancreatic function after severe acute biliary pancreatitis: the role of necrosectomy. *Pancreas.* 2004; Vol. 28: pp. 65-68. Lewandowski, A.; Kopeć, W.; Diakowska, D.& Garbień, M. Proinflammatory cytokines IL-6, IL-8 and C-reactive protein in acute pancreatitis-the role of IL-8 in prognosing complications. *Gastroenterol.Pol.* 2007; Vol.14: pp.165-69 Osman,M. & Jensen, S. Acute Pancreatitis: the pathophysiological role of cytokines and integrins; New trends for treatment? Dig.Surg. 1999; Vol.16: pp. 347-62.

Karczowski, B. Dziedziczne zapalenie trzustki. *Gastroenterol Pol.* 2002; Vol.3: pp. 321-325.

Swaroop, V.; Chari, S. & Clain J. Severe Acute Pancreatitis. *JAMA.* 2004; Vol.291: pp. 2865-68.

Kim, H.; Kim, M.; Bae, J.; Lee, S.; Seo, D. & Lee, S. Idiopathic acute pancreatitis. *J.Clin. Gastroenterol.* 2003; Vol. 37: pp. 238-50.

Testoni, P.; Mariani, A.; Curioni, S.; Zanello, A. & Masci, E. MRCP-secretin test-guided management of idiopathic recurrent pancreatitis: long-term outcomes. *Gastrointest Endosc.* 2008; Vol.67: pp. 1028–34.

Williford, M.; Foster, W.; Halvorsen, R. & Thompson, W. Pancreatic pseudocyst: comparative evaluation by sonography and computed tomography. *Am. J. Roentgenol.* 1983; Vol.140: pp. 53-57.

Morgan, D.; Baron, T.; Smith J.; Robbin, M. & Kenney,P. Pancreatic fluid collections prior to intervention. *Radiology.*1997; Vol.203: pp.773-7 8.

Dervenis, C., Johnson, C. & Bassi, C. Diagnosis, objective assessment of severity, and management of acute pancreatitis. *lnt J Pancreatol.* 1999; Vol.25: pp. 195-210.

Steinberg, W. & Tenner, S. Acute pancreatitis. *N Engl J Med.* 1994; Vol.330: pp. 1198-1210.

Braganza J.; Scott P; Bilton D; Schofield D; Chaloner C; Shiel N; Hunt LP & Bottiglieri T. Evidence for early oxidative stress in acute pancreatitis. Clues for correction. *Int. J.Pancreatol.* 1995; Vol.17: pp. 69-81.

Kikuchi, Y.; Shimosegawa,T.; Moriizumi, S.; Kimura, K.; Satoh, A.; Koizumi, M.; Kato, I.; Epstein, C.& Toyota, T. Transgenic copper/zinc-superoxide dismutase ameliorates caerulein-induced pancreatitis in mice. Biochem. Biophys. Res. Commun. 1997; Vol.233: pp. 177-81

Sies, H. & Cadenas, E. Oxidative stress: damage to intact cells and organs. *Philos Trans R.Soc.LondB.Biol.Sci.* 1985; Vol.311: pp. 617-31.

Matkovics, B.; Novák, Z.; Varga, I. & Takács, T. Hemo-rheologic and antioxidant changes in acute human pancreatitis. *Orv Hetil.* 1995; Vol. 136: pp. 1663-65.

Schulz, H.; Niederau, C.; Klonowski-Stumpe H.; Halangk, W.; Luthen, R. & Lippert, H. Oxidative stress in acute pancreatitis. *Hepatogastroenterology.*1999; Vol.46: pp.2736-50.

Petrov,M. Therapeutic implications of oxidative stress in acute and chronic pancreatitis. *Curr.Opin.Clin.Nutr.Metab.Care.* 2010; Vol.13: pp.562-68.

Abu-Zidan, F.; Bohnam, M. & Windsor J. Severity of acute pancreatitis: a multivariate analisis of oxidative stress markes and modified Glasgow criteria. *Br.J.Surg.* 2000; Vol.87: pp.1019-23.

Chmiel, B; Grabowska-Bochenek, R; Piskorska, D; Skorupa, A; Cierpka, L & Kuśmierski, S. Red blood cells deformability and oxidative stress in acute pancreatitis. *Clin.Hemorheol.Microcirc.* 2002; Vol.27: pp.155-62.

Park, B.; Chung J,; Lee, J.; Suh, J.; Park, S.; Song, S.; Kim, H.; Kim, K. & Kang J. Role of oxygen free radicals in patients with acute pancreatitis. *World J. Gastroenterol.* 2003; Vol. 9: pp. 2266-69.

Winterbourn, C.; Bonham, M.; Buss, H.; Abu-Zidan, F. & Windsor J. Elevated protein carbonyls as plasma markers of oxidative stress in acute pancreatitis. *Pancreatology.* 2003; Vol.3: pp. 375-82.

Wereszczyńska-Siemiatkowska, U.; Dabrowski, A.; Jedynak, M. & Gabryelewicz A. Oxidative stress as an early prognostic factor in acute pancreatitis (AP): its correlation with serum phospholipase A2 (PLA2) and plasma polymorphonuclear elastase (PMN-E) in different-severity forms of human AP. *Pancreas.* 1998; Vol.17: pp. 163-68.

Wereszczynska-Siemiatkowska, U.; Mroczko, B.; Siemiatkowski, A.; Szmitkowski, M.; Borawska, M. & Kosel, J. The importance of interleukin 18, glutathione peroxidase, and selenium concentration changes in acute pancreatitis. *Dig. Di. Sci.* 2004; Vol.49: pp. 642-50.

Sweiry, J. & Mann, G. Role of oxidative stress in the pathogenesis of acute pancreatitis. *Scand. J. Gastroenterol.* 1996; Vol.219: pp. 10-15.

Telek, G.; Regöly-Mérei, J.; Kovács, G.; Simon, L.; Nagy, Z.; Hamar, J. & Jakab, F. The first histological demonstration of pancreatic oxidative stress in human acute pancreatitis. *Hepatogastroenterology.* 2001; Vol. 48: pp. 1252-58.

Curran, F; Sattar, N; Talwar, D; Baxter, J & Imrie, C. Relationship of carotenoid and vitamins A and E with the acute inflammatory response in acute pancreatitis. *Br.J.Surg.* 2000; Vol.87: pp.301-5.

Dabrowski, A; Konturek, S; Konturek, J & Gabryelewicz, A. Role of oxidative stress in the pathogenesis of caerulein-induced acute pancreatitis. *Eur. J. Pharmacol.* 1999; Vol.377: pp. 1-11.

Johnson, C. Antioxidants in acute pancreatitis. *Gut.* 2007; Vol.56: pp. 1344-45

Satinder, Kaur.; Verma, I.; Narang,A.; Chinna, R.; Singh, P. & Aggarwal,S. Assessment of total antioxidant status in acute pancreatitis and prognostic Significance *Int J Biol Med Res.* 2011; Vol.2: pp. 575-76

Tsai, K.; Wang, S.; Chen, T.; Kong, C.; Chang, F.; Lee, S. & Lu. F. Oxidative stress: an important phenomenon with pathogenetic significance in the progression of acute pancreatitis. *Gut.* 1998; Vol.42: pp. 850-55.

Wereszczynska-Siemiatkowska, U.; Dabrowski, A.; Siemiatkowski, A.; Mroczko, B.; Laszewicz, W. & Gabryelewicz, A. Serum profiles of E-selectin, interleukin-10, and interleukin-6 and oxidative stress parameters in patients with acute pancreatitis and nonpancreatic acute abdominal pain. *Pancreas* 2003; Vol.26: pp. 144-52.

Rahman, S.; Ibrahim, K.; Larvin, M.; Kingsnorth, A. & McMahon, M. Association of antioxidant enzyme gene polymorphisms and glutathione status with severe acute pancreatitis. *Gastroenterology* 2004;Vol. 126: pp. 1312-22.

Roth, E.; Manhart, N. & Wessner, B. Assessing the antioxidative status in critically ill patients. *Curr. Opin. Clin. Nutr. Metab. Care.* 2004; Vol.7: pp. 161-68.

Virlos, I.; Mason, J.; Schofield, D.; McCloy, R.; Eddleston, J. & Siriwardena, A. Intravenous n-acetylcysteine, ascorbic acid and selenium-based anti-oxidant therapy in severe acute pancreatitis. *Scand. J. Gastroenterol.* 2003; Vol.38: pp. 1262-67. Dziurkowska-Marek, A.,; Marek, T., Nowak, A., Kacperek-Hartleb, T., Sierka, E. & Nowakowska-Duława, E. The dynamics of the oxidant-antioxidant balance in the early phase of human acute biliary pancreatitis. *Pancreatology.*200; Vol.4: pp. 215-222.

Modzelewski, B. Serum anti-oxidative barrier in acute pancreatitis. *Pol. Merkur. Lekarski* . 2005; Vol.18: pp.418-20.

Scott, P.; Bruce, C.; Schofield, D.; Shiel, N.; Braganza, J. & McCloy R. Vitamin C status in patients with acute pancreatitis. *Br. J. Surg.* 1993; Vol. 80: pp. 750-4.

Dejong, C; Greve, J & Soeters, P. Nutrition in patients with acute pancreatitis. *Curr Opin. Crit Care.* 2001; Vol.7: 251-56. Panek, J.; Zasada, J. & Pożniaczek, M. Microcirculatory disturbance in the course of acute pancreatitis. *Przegl. Lek.* 2007; Vol.64: pp. 435-37.

11

Microcirculatory Disturbances in the Pathogenesis of Acute Pancreatitis

Dirk Uhlmann
2nd Department of Surgery, University of Leipzig
Germany

1. Introduction

In acute pancreatitis, reductions in blood flow and alterations of microvascular integrity resulting in impaired tissue oxygenation play an important part in the progression and possibly the initiation of the disease. Independently of the initial noxa, the intra-pancreatic activation of trypsinogen to trypsin is the crucial trigger of acute pancreatitis. The central events for the further course are the release of local mediators (cytokines, vasoactive substances, free oxygen radicals) and subsequently the development of microcirculatory disturbances and the activation of leukocytes and their infiltration into the tissue. At present, the deterioration of microcirculation is seen as the most important pacemaker in the progression to a necrotizing pancreatitis. In addition to its potentiatory role, severe pancreatic ischemia can play a pathogenetic role in the initiation of acute pancreatitis. The acute edematous pancreatitis is characterized by an increased and homogeneous microperfusion. The experimental necrotizing pancreatitis shows a progredient decrease of capillary perfusion despite stable macrohemodynamics.

There is increasing evidence that ischemia alone may be the primary cause of pancreatitis or may be the exacerbating promotor for the progression from edematous to necrotizing pancreatitis. In clinical studies there was evidence, that ischemia during cardiopulmonary bypass triggered acute pancreatitis and acute pancreatitis was found in up to 25% of autopsies of patients dying after shock. In animal models severe pancreatitis could be induced by obstruction of terminal pancreatic arterioles. The study by Mithöfer et al. [1] demonstrates, that temporary hemorrhagic hypotension in rats per se initiates acute pancreatitis.

The hypothesis, that the manifestation of microvascular injury in acute pancreatitis involves ischemia/reperfusion(I/R)-associated events, is supported by the study of Menger et al. [2], who analyzed the pancreatic microcirculation of rats during postischemic reperfusion by use of intravital fluorescence microscopy (Fig. 1, 2). In this investigation, post-ischemic reperfusion was characterized by a significant reduction of functional capillary density (no-reflow) and by a marked increase of the permanently adherent leukocytes in postcapillary venules (reflow paradox) (Fig. 3). In addition, the functional and histomorphological alterations in this study were similar to the alteration seen in edematous pancreatitis. Postischemic activation of leukocytes has been reported to determine the outcome of I/R injury. Kusterer et al. [3] have demonstrated that sodium taurocholate-induced pancreatitis is characterized by early arteriolar vasoconstriction with ischemia, followed by arteriolar vasodilation with reestablishment of blood flow (reperfusion). Increased leukocyte-endothelial cell interactions in postcapillary venules - mimicking the I/R event - were observed during vasodilation. The concept of I/R-induced pancreatitis is mostly reflected in the clinical situation of post-transplant pancreatitis. Experimental studies using the model of syngeneic pancreas transplantation in rats show microcirculatory disturbances and cellular damages similar to those seen in the beginning of an acute pancreatitis [4]. Pancreatitis after hemorrhagic shock or hypotension with hypoxia, but not complete ischemia/anoxia may also involve pathomechanisms associated with ischemia/reperfusion. A recent study demonstrates, that hemorrhagic hypotension in rats induces intermittent capillary perfusion, which is characterized by periods of normal blood flow followed by periods of complete cessation of blood flow [5]. This type of regional ischemia and reperfusion may contribute to the manifestation of pancreatitis, independent of the etiology.

2. Cell-cell interactions

By means of intravital microscopy (Fig. 1-3) in conjunction with technique of selected cell-labeling, direct impairments of pancreatic microcirculation induced by controlled haemorrhage or interruption of arterial blood supply to the pancreas in the early phase of acute pancreatitis have been observed [6], suggesting the pancreatic microcirculation being highly susceptible to ischemia [7-9]. The nature of blood cell-endothelium, especially leukocyte-endothelium, interactions as an early step in the inflammatory response has been characterized in experimental pancreas transplantation and in models of I/R-induced acute pancreatitis [4, 10].

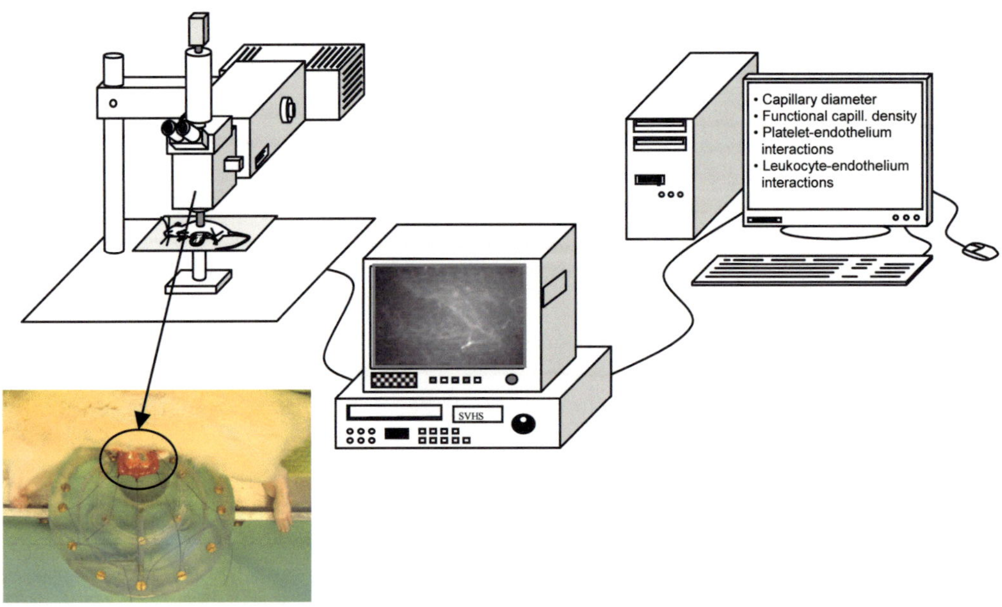

Fig. 1. Processing of intravital microscopy of the rat pancreas.

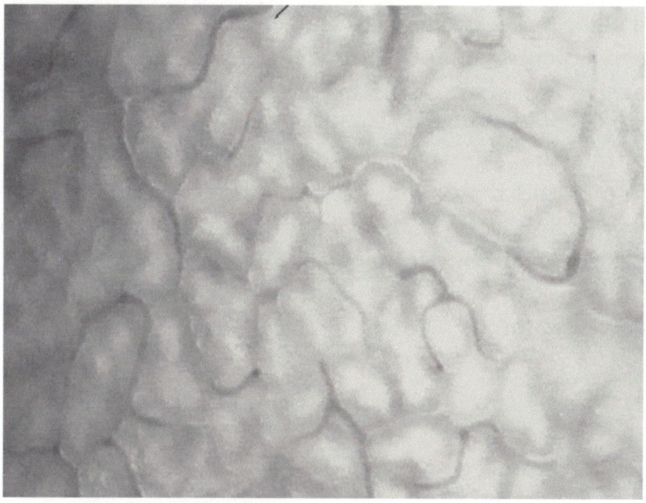

Fig. 2. In-vivo microscopic image of pancreas microcirculation.

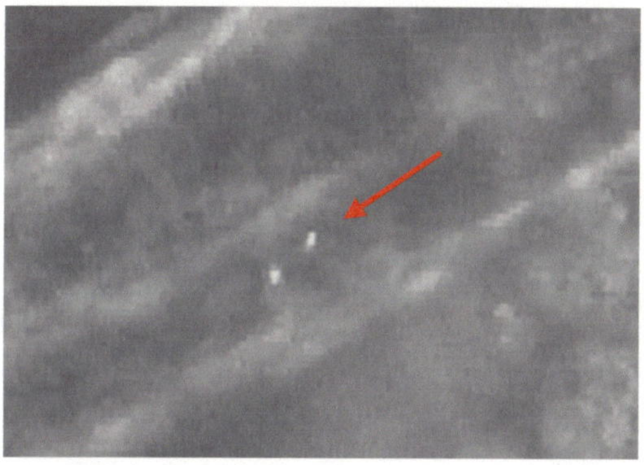

Fig. 3. In-vivo microscopic image of sticking platelets in a postcapillary venule of a post-ischemic rat pancreas.

2.1 Leukocytes

The neutrophils play a central part in the inflammatory process of acute pancreatitis. Their activation and that of the endothelium by cytokines (IL-6, TNFa, IL-8, IL-1b and others) and of proinflammatory mediators (platelet-activating factor (PAF), free radicals and others) will allow a narrow interaction between them that will result in a significant concentration of neutrophils activated in the interstitium [11-14]. This interaction takes place in three parts: a weak adhesion of the neutrophils to the endothelium, followed by a stronger adhesion and, finally, the neutrophil migration (Fig. 4). Three families of adhesion molecules are implicated: selectins, b2-integrins and immunoglobulins (Table 1). The selectins are surface glycoproteins implicated in weak adhesion. The L-selectin, expressed by the endothelial cells and the neutrophils, plays a part at the beginning of reperfusion. It interacts with the P-selectin on the neutrophils and a specific ligand present on the membrane of the neutrophil, the E-selectin-specific ligand-1 (ESL-1) [15]. Endothelial P-selectin will be expressed later from the Weibel–Palade bodies after activation of the endothelium by reactive oxygen species (ROS), hypercalcaemia, complement or thrombin. Its peak of expression occurs 10–20 min after the beginning of reperfusion [14]. It interacts with P-selectin glycoprotein ligand-1 (PSGL-1) expressed by the neutrophils. These interactions are very weak, giving the neutrophils a weak, transitory, reversible adhesion known as 'leukocyte rolling'. This phase prepares the neutrophil and the endothelium for the following stage. A more important stowing of neutrophils in the endothelium utilizes other leukocyte and endothelium proteins that have a stronger affinity for each other.

Leukocyte adhesion receptor	**Endothelial ligand**	**Function**
a4b7 (unactivated)	MadCAM-1	Rolling
a4b1 (unactivated)	VCAM-1	Rolling
PSGL-1	P-selectin	Capture, Rolling
L-selectin	P-selectin Peripheral node addressin (PNAd) E-selectin MadCAM-1	Capture Rolling
a4b7 (activated)	VCAM-1/MAdCAM-1	Firm adhesion
a4b1 (activated)	VCAM-1	Firm adhesion
CD11a /CD18 (LFA-1)	ICAM-1, ICAM-2	Firm adhesion, Emigration
CD11b/CD18 (Mac-1)	ICAM-1	Firm adhesion, Emigration
PECAM-1	PECAM-1	Emigration

Table 1. Leukocyte-endothelium interactions. Adhesion receptors and their ligands on activated endothelial cells. Modified from [17].

The ROS, PAF and leucotriene (LTB4) stimulate the expression by neutrophils of b2-integrins from the intracellular granules. This family of membrane proteins consists of CD11a/CD18, CD11b/CD18 and CD11c/ CD18 and interacts with the ICAM-1 endothelial protein whose expression is enhanced by TNFa and IL-1 [16, 17]. This interaction fastens the neutrophil to the surface of the endothelial cell and allows the next stage. ICAM-1 and PECAM-1 are adhesion molecules belonging to the superfamily of immunoglobulins which take part and orchestrate the transfer of the neutrophils towards the interstitium. The leukocyte extravasation utilizes many stages, not all of which are yet clear. Nevertheless, it seems that PECAM-1, localized at the level of the intercellular endothelial junctions, is necessary to allow neutrophil migration [18]. This transfer is facilitated by the inflammation mediators, the connection of CD11/CD18–ICAM-1 and the ROS making the endothelial barrier receptive by decreasing the expression of cadherin and phosphorylation of vascular endothelial cadherin and cathenin, components of the intercellular junctions [19, 20].

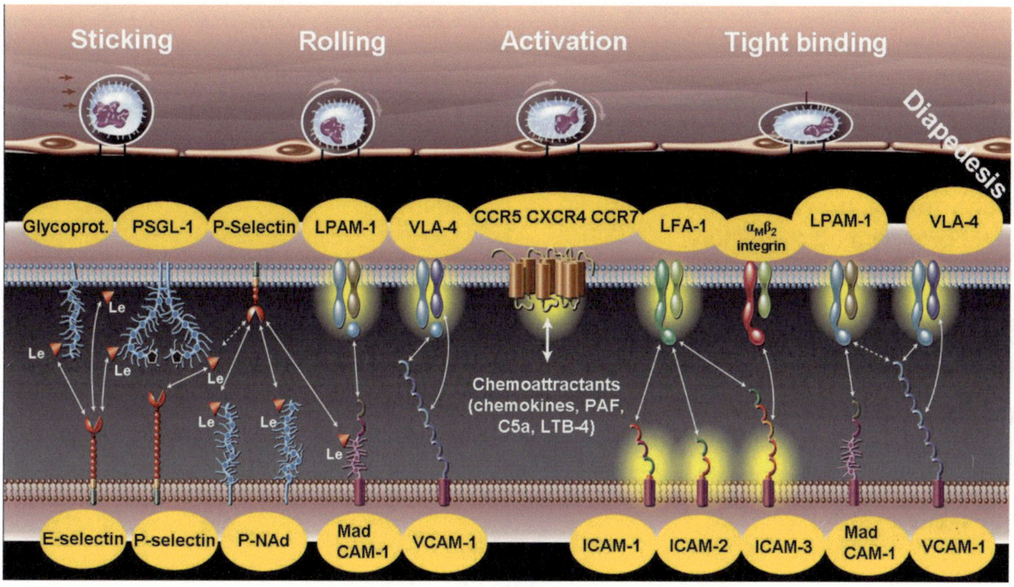

Fig. 4. Multistep adhesion cascade of leukocyte-endothelium interactions. Modified from [183].

Arriving at the interstitium, the activated neutrophil will cause considerable damage to a tissue, which has already suffered from hypoxia. These lesions are mainly related to the massive ROS production, to the release of the contents of the neutrophilic granules and to the metabolites of arachidonic acid. The last, metabolized by phospholipase A2, generates PAF and LTB4, two powerful chemoattractive components that stimulate the adhesion of neutrophils to the endothelium and their degranulation in the interstitium. The neutrophilic granules, filled with proteases, collagenases, elastases, lipooxygenases, phospholipases and myeloperoxidases, will digest and disorganize the protein network of extracellular matrix (Table 2). The proteic network of extracellular matrix is important in healing while being used to guide tissue formation. The inflammation induced by reperfusion is a major cause of the lesions observed after restoration of blood flow in an ischemic organ. The massive production of cytokines, the activation of the complement and a complex choreography of the neutrophils are the key factors and are therefore being examined in research to modulate the inflammatory reaction.

2.2 Platelets

Considerable evidence has accumulated that platelets can also contribute to I/R injury in several organs, such as the heart [21], lung [22], and pancreas [23]. Upon activation, platelets are able to generate reactive oxygen species and nitric oxide (NO) and can release pro-inflammatory mediators, such as chemokines, cytokines, growth factors, and cytotoxic proteases [24]. Therefore, platelets can potentially contribute to the manifestation of pancreatitis after normothermic I/R injury. In the liver of a rat model, Khandoga et al. [25] have demonstrated that platelets interact with the hepatic endothelium after 90 min of warm ischemia and 20 min of reperfusion and evoke the development of hepatic microvascular and hepatocellular injury.

Leukocytes	Platelets
Cytokines/chemokines IL-1, IL-2, IL-6, IL-8, IL-12 IFN-a, IFN-b TNF-a, TNF-b Transforming growth factor-b Monocyte chemotactic factor-1 *Reactive oxygen species* Superoxide Hydrogen peroxide *Proteases* Cathepsin-G Elastase Collagenase *Oxidases* Myeloperoxidase *Lipid mediators* Leukotrienes B4, C4 Platelet activating factor *Miscellaneous* Cationic proteins Histamine VEGF	*Cytokines/chemokines* IL-1, IL-7, IL-8 RANTES TNF-b CD40 ligand *Reactive oxygen species* Superoxide Hydrogen peroxide *Growth factors* PDGF Transforming growth factor-b VEGF *Lipid mediators* Thromboxane A2 12-HETE *Procoagulants* Thrombin ADT and ATP Platelet factor-4 Polyphosphates

Table 2. Activation products released by leukocytes and platelets that may impair endothelial barrier function. Modified from [18].

Platelet activation was accompanied by leukocyte activation in a study of Hackert et al. [7]. An interaction between these two cell types has been demonstrated by different authors in the past [26-28]. Among others, P-selectin seems to be one of the most important adhesion molecules, which links the inflammatory and procoagulatory cascades and has the potency to activate leukocytes and platelets as the cellular elements of either pathway [27-30]. Besides their adherence to endothelial cells, activated platelets form stable aggregates with leukocytes. This results in a combined inflammatory and coagulatory contribution to thrombus formation and is also mediated by P-selectin and beta-integrins [31, 32]. Especially, the formation of microthrombotic vessel occlusion with microcirculatory perfusion failure and consequent ischemia, hypoxia, and tissue necrosis promote organ damage.

2.3 Lymphocytes

Recent studies have implicated peripheral blood lymphocytes in Ag-independent inflammatory-mediated injury following organ reperfusion [33-36]. The contributory role of lymphocytes in I/R is likely a multifactorial one.

Evidence is mounting on the importance of T cells in mediating both short- and long-term damage during I/R injury, which in turn could explain why I/R contributes to poor late allograft function [37, 38]. The demonstration that systemic immunosuppression (CsA, FK506) attenuates hepatocellular injury following I/R implies the involvement of T lymphocytes in the pathophysiology of the injury [39, 40], data supported by Shen et al. in T-cell-deficient (nude) mice [41, 42], as well as in rats in which treatment with FTY720 prevented hepatic I/R insult in parallel with massive redistribution of recirculating T cells from host peripheral blood into the lymph node compartment [43]. The adherence of lymphocytes in hepatic sinusoids occurs early duringreperfusion and impairs liver function following prolonged cold ischemic times [44]. Recent data have also shown that circulating CD4+ T lymphocytes may act as a cellular mediator in subacute PMN recruitment following hepatic I/R injury [38] (Table 3).

Platelet receptors	Ligand	Function
P-selectin	PSGL-1	Rolling, adhesion, RANTES deposition
PSGL-1	P-selectin	Rolling, adhesion and P/L interactions
GP1b*a*	vWF P-selectin Mac-1	Aggregation, rolling, adhesion and P/L interactions
GPIIb/IIIa	GPIIb/IIIa ICAM-1 (via fibrinogen) a*v* b3 Mac-1	Aggregation and adhesion
JAM-A	PSD95/ZO-1	Aggregation and adhesion
PECAM-1	PECAM-1	Aggregation and adhesion

Table 3. Platelet–endothelium interactions: Potential molecular determinants. Modified from [157]

JAM-A junctional adhesion molecule-A
PECAM platelet endothelial cell adhesion molecule-1
PSGL-1 P-Selectin glycoprotein ligand-1
vWF von Willebrand factor
ZO-1 zona occludens protein-1

3. Adhesion molecules

A variety of adhesion molecules are implicated in the progression of disease. Intercellular adhesion molecule, platelet endothelial cell adhesion molecule 1 and endothelial leukocyte adhesion molecule 1 (ELAM-1) are up-regulated, expression of P- and E-selectin enhanced, and leukocytes become CD18 positive in acute pancreatitis [11].

3.1 Intercellular Adhesion Molecule-1 (ICAM-1)

ICAM-1, a single-chain transmembrane glycoprotein with a molecular weight of 80-110 KDa, consists of five Ig-like domains, a hydrophobic transmembrane domain and a short cytoplasmic C-terminal domain [45]. Its ligand includes lymphocyte function- associated antigen-1 (LFA-1) and macrophage antigen-1 (Mac-1) [46]. ICAM-1 is an immunoglobulin molecule mainly expressed in vascular endothelial cells, and plays an important role especially in the process of inflammation. Under normal circumstances, it will not be expressed or just with low expression in most vessels. However, when its expression increased, it can interact with integrin on the surface of granular cells. Therefore, it can cause leukocyte migration through capillary endothelial barriers to inflammatory regions, and then cause excessive architectonic inflammatory response [47]. Experiments show that ICAM-1 high expression may cause leukocyte adhesion through endothelial cells - leukocyte interaction, increase capillary permeability, reduce capillary blood flow velocity, cause pancreatic microcirculation disorder [48-50]. ICAM-1 expression correlates with histological severity and leukocyte infiltration [51], and can be upregulated by trypsin in vivo and in vitro [49]. This upregulation is mirrored by increased tissue infiltration of leukocytes and increased endothelium-leukocyte interaction.
Whereas the binding of endothelial ICAM is directly to CD18 on the leukocyte surface, the binding of platelets to the endothelium is possible via the following mechanism. I/R leads to fibrinogen deposition on microvascular endothelial cells and a corresponding accumulation of firmly adherent platelets. Experimental interventions (i.e., anti-fibrinogen antibody or ICAM-1 deficiency) that reduce the I/R-induced fibrinogen accumulation also blunt the accumulation of adherent platelets in both arterioles and venules, suggesting that the binding of fibrinogen to endothelial cell ICAM-1 creates a scaffold on the vessel wall onto which platelets can adhere using GPIIb/IIIa [52] (Table 3).

3.2 Platelet–endothelial cell adhesion molecule (PECAM)-1

The pancreatic circulation during acute experimental edematous pancreatitis may also be influenced by the expression of platelet-endothelial cell adhesion molecule on polymorphonuclear leukocytes. PECAM-1 expression was up-regulated in the peripheral circulation and down-regulated in the pancreatic microcirculation, suggesting that inhibition of PECAM-1 expression may improve the pathological changes associated with acute edematous pancreatitis in rats [53, 54].

3.3 P-selectin

P-selectin is normally stored in granular structures of both platelets (α-granules) and endothelial cells (Weibel–Palade bodies), from which it can be rapidly mobilized to the cell surface upon endothelial cell activation. Some vascular beds (e.g., intestine) exhibit significant basal expression of P-selectin [55], with little basal expression on inactivated circulating platelets. Several studies have addressed the contributions of platelet vs. endothelial cell P-selectin to the platelet adhesion induced by stimuli such as I/R [56, 57], [58], endotoxin [59], and TNF-α [60]. In I/R models of platelet adhesion, it appears that those models that elicit a rapid adhesion response in both venules and arterioles are entirely dependent on endothelial P-selectin [56], while I/R models exhibiting slow, time-dependent platelet adhesion only in venules involve both platelet and endothelial cell P-selectin [57]. A blocking mAb directed against PSGL-1, a ligand for P-selectin that is expressed on leukocytes and platelets [61], is also effective in attenuating the I/R-induced platelet adhesion observed hours after reperfusion, which further supports a role for platelet-derived P-selectin [57].

Influenced Paramter	Treatment	Effect	References
Leukocytes	Neutrophil depletion Diannexin Tacrolimus Anti-fibrinogen antibody Erythropoeitin	+ + +	[57] [42] [158, 7] [159] [160, 161]
Platelets	Platelet depletion, anti-platelet serum	+	[162]
Lymphocytes	FTY720 Tacrolimus	+ +	[43, 163, 33] [158, 7]
ICAM-1	Anti-ICAM-1 antibody ICAM-1-deficiency Phloretin Erythropoeitin	+ + +	[51, 164, 165] [52] [166] [160, 161]
P-selectin	CP-96,345 Statins	+ +	[167] [168-170]
ET	ET_A receptor antagonist	+	[79, 171-173]
NO	L-arginine Sodium nitroprusside	+	[174-176]
TNF-α	Receptor antagonist Knockout mice Polyclonal antibody	+ + +	[177] [178] [90]
IL-1	Receptor antagonist Knockout mice	+ +	[177] [178]
IL-10	IL-10 administration	+	[108, 109].
PAF	PAF antagonist	+	[179], [180], [111]
Serotonin	5HT2 receptor antagonists	+	[119], [118]
Bradykinin	Bradykinin B2 receptor antagonist	++	[181], [132]
TXA2	TXA2 receptor blocker	+	[182]
VEGF	tyrosinekinase inhibitor PTK787/ZK222584	+	[146]
COX2	Inhibition, depletion	+	[136, 137]

Table 4. Therapeutic approaches to prevent or treat microcirculatory disturbances in acute pancreatitis.

The platelet adhesion elicited by bacterial endotoxin also appears to involve endothelial P-selectin [59]. However, glycoprotein (GP) Ibα is the platelet ligand that appears to mediate this interaction. This glycoprotein and PSGL-1 are two platelet ligands that have been implicated in P-selectin-mediated platelet interactions (primarily rolling) with venular endothelial cells. Platelet GPIbα also exhibits the capacity to bind to endothelial cells in a P-selectin-independent manner. vWF, which is released from Weibel–Palade bodies during endothelial cell activation, can bind to GPIbα. vWF–GPIbα interactions have been implicated in the platelet recruitment in mouse mesenteric venules stimulated with either calcium ionophore, A23187, or histamine [62, 63].

4. Vasoactive mediators

4.1 Endothelin

Endothelin-1 (ET-1) is a potent vasoconstrictor of the pancreatic microcirculation mainly produced by endothelial cells. The intact microvasculature is balanced by the constricting action of ET-1 and the dilating features of nitric oxide (NO), made constitutively by endothelial nitric oxide synthase (eNOS). It has been shown that ET-1 production is controlled at the transcriptional level. Up-regulation of prepro-ET-1 mRNA can be induced by numerous factors such as cytokines, angiotensin, thrombin, and TGF-β [64]. Released from endothelial cells, ET-1 mediates transient vasodilation followed by a profound and longlasting vasoconstriction. Furthermore, ET-1 is able to induce an inflammatory response in human vascular smooth muscle cells by stimulating the synthesis and release of pro-inflammatory cytokines such as interleukin-6 [65]. ET-1 does not only mediate local injury, but also systemic disease.

ET affects microcirculation by:

- constriction of arterioles and venules [66, 67]
- release of prostaglandine E2, IL-6 and IL-8 from monocytes [68]
- stimulation of phospholipase A2 [69]
- reinforced formation of free oxygen radicals in neutrophiles [70]
- expression of adhesion molecules [71, 72]
- stimulation of catecholamine release [73]

Beside its vasoconstrictive effects endothelin as multifunctional cytokine modulates the motility and secretion of the intestinum, stimulates mitogenesis and acts as a growth factor.

Several investigators have shown that the pancreas is especially susceptible to ET-1 [74], [75]. The study of Hildebrand et al. showed that the rat pancreatic acini possess ET_A and ET_B receptors [76]. At doses of 100 to 1000 pmol/kg via intravenous injection, endothelins cause sustained reduction in pancreatic blood flow in the rabbit and dog of up to 80 % [75, 77]. In a study in rats, intravenous infusion of endothelin-1 or alcohol significantly reduced pancreatic capillary blood flow. The deterioration of capillary blood flow was more pronounced when alcohol and ET-1 were combined [78]. Liu et al. observed a decrease of pancreatic blood flow and a reinforcement of morphological changes after application of endothelin to rats with cerulein-induced edematous pancreatitis [47]. Foitzik et al. found in transgenic rats with an overexpression of endothelin receptors a more severe course of a necrotizing pancreatitis, which could be moderated by the application of a selective ET_A receptor antagonist [79]. Plusczyk et al. showed that topical ET-1 application leads to a decrease in blood flow in the pancreas [80]. In intravital microscopy a strong heterogeneity of erythrocyte velocity, a decrease in the number of perfused capillaries and a reduction of the capillary width were seen. This group suggests that high local ET concentrations can cause complex microcirculatory disturbances, leading to acinar cell necrosis and therefore to the development of necrotizing pancreatitis [80]. There is some evidence that endothelins also increase pancreatic capillary permeability [74, 81], though this might be explained by the resulting portal venous vasoconstriction.

4.2 Nitric oxide

Nitric oxide (NO) is synthetized through NO synthases from the amino acid L-arginine. For the first time, this pathway was described in endothelial cells [82], but it is also found in platelets, macrophages and in cells of the pancreas [68, 69]. NO causes a relaxation of vascular smooth muscle cells, depression of platelet aggregation and adhesion and reduces the leukocyte activation in vitro [72, 83]. Reduced NO formation reinforces leukocyte adhesion and migration [84-87]. These effects are regulated by the activation of the soluble guanylatcyclase which leads to increased concentrations of cGMP in the effector cells [86]. NO may also act as scavanger of oxygen free radicals [88]. However, also cytotoxic effects are described [89]. The overproduction of NO by inducible NO synthetase is an important factor in the hemodynamic disturbances of several inflammatory states.

5. Cytokines

During acute pancreatitis, some inflammatory cells and pancreatic tissues release inflammatory mediators and cytokines, which influence the whole process of inflammation. The most important cytokines are tumor necrosis factor-a (TNF-a), interleukins (IL) and transforming growth factor (TGF).

5.1 TNF-α

Lipsett [90] and Hirota et al. [91] independently proved that the levels of inflammatory cytokines always increase during acute pancreatitis and that the degree of the increase is closely linked to the severity of the disease. Many other studies have reported that self-tissue injured with over-activated neutrophil leucocytes is an important causal factor of systemic complications [92-94]. One proposal is that the neutrophilic granulocyte may generate and release inflammatory cytokines such as TNF-α following inflammatory stimulation [95, 96]. TNF-α is an important species of inflammatory cytokines that participates in the pathomechanism during pancreatitis. Hughes et al. [97] found that injecting TNF-α antibody into rats can markedly improve the state and survival of rats with necrotizing pancreatitis, thereby indicating the important role of TNF-α in the onset and progression of the disearse. A number of mechanisms have been proposed for TNF-α-induced pancreatic injury. TNF-α can directly injure pancreatic duct cells and cause microthrombus, pancreatic acinus ischemia, hemorrhage, necrosis, inflammation and edema [6]. When the quantity of produced TNF-α exceeds that of the tissue TNF receptor, the excessive free TNF-α will enter the blood circulation, activate neutrophilic granulocytes and cause their aggregatione. It then stimulates the release of cytokines, such as IL-1b, IL-8 and IL-6 [98], causing a cytokine cascade reaction that promotes the local and systemic injury. The continuous existence of TNF-α may enhance the expression of endothelium adhesion molecules, which is necessary for the aggregation of inflammatory cells. Numerous granulocytes invade the pancreatic and renal tissues, increase granulocyte phagocytosis and degranulation, generate oxygen-derived free radicals, lysosomes, elastin enzyme, among others, and cause cell metabolic disturbances and renal failure [99].

5.2 IL-1

Interleukin (IL) IL-1 is a pro-inflammatory cytokine generated by the pancreas that plays an important role in the early stage of severe acute pancreatitis. In a animal model, the IL-1 receptor antagonist (IL-1r) has been found to decrease case fatality by 30% [100]; in addition, the IL-1 receptor can markedly lower the concentrations of IL-6 and TNF-α [101]. Fink et al. [102] administered the IL-1 receptor antagonist before inducing the pancreatitis model and found that the IL-1 receptor block markedly lowered the release of amylopsin and pancreatic necrosis in a dose-dependent manner.

The generation of IL-1b formed from IL-1 through the mediation of IL-1 convertase (ICE). IL-1β and TNF-a have many of the same biological activities, including pyrogen functions, the promotion of cell catabolism, the production of protein in the acute reaction period, effecting the secretion of PGI2 by epithelial cells and platelet activating factor, among others, that will cause the expansion of the inflammation area and increase the levels of inflammatory mediators, destructive enzymes and ROS secretion. IL-1b can interact with TNF-a to induce or aggravate organ injury. It also has chemotaxis and activating effects on granulocyte and can stimulate the production of other inflammatory mediators, such as IL-8, IL-6 and other inflammatory cytokines, through autocrine or paracrine mechanisms.

5.3 IL-6

IL-6 is mainly generated by mononuclear macrophages, which have extensive inflammation-promoting effects, such as promoting the activation and proliferation of B cells and their final differentiation into plasmocytes, increasing immunoglobulin synthesis, promoting T cell differentiation and proliferation, promoting the acute period reaction and injuring tissue. The level of IL-6 in the serum can reflect the state of necrotizing acute pancreatitis. There are marked differences between acute pancreatitis patients without complications and severe acute pancreatitis patients with complications in terms of IL-6 levels. When present at levels of over 40 μl, IL-6 is considered to be an indication index of severe acute pancreatitis [103]. Relevant data show that IL-1 and IL-6 can act on endothelial cells, causing them to lower their thrombomodulin activity, aggravate renal ischemia, form thrombus [104] and activate inflammatory cells to release NO and ROS to directly cause renal injury.

5.4 IL-8

IL-8 is a potent neutrophilic granulocyte chemotatic factor and activating factor that is mainly generated by neutrophilic granulocytes. Generated by mononuclear/ macrophages and endothelial cells, it can activate and induce T and B cell differentiation, enhance NK cells for killing target cells, promote phagocytosis and play an important role in tissue injury mediated by neutrophilic granulocytes. It is currently believed that most inflammatory reactions induced by TNF-a, IL-1 and IL-6 are realized by inducing the generation of chemotactic factors, mainly IL-8. Studies have shown that during necrotizing acute pancreatitis the levels of IL-6 and IL-8 always increase concurrently and that these positively correlate with the state of severe acute pancreatitis [105].

5.5 Transforming growth factor (TGF)

Kimura et al. [106] studied the expression of TGF-b1 by means of immune electron microscopy and found that a marked effusion of the polymorphonuclear leukocyte and deposition of fibronectin and TGF-b1 among pancreatic lobules and inside lobules within

12–24 h after inducing pancreatitis. They therefore believed that this kind of change at the early stage of pancreatitis is related to the generation of fibronectin and type III collagen in the extracellular matrix during the reparative process of pancreatic tissues. Konturek et al. [107] proposed that TGF-b can induce non-inflammatory apoptosis to repair injured pancreatic tissues.

5.6 IL-10

Interleukin-10 (IL-10) is an anti-inflammatory cytokine. Its plasma levels are elevated in animal models of endotoxemia and inhibit the release of pro-inflammatory cytokines (i.e. IL-1β, IL-6 and TNF-α) from monocytes/macrophages thus preventing subsequent tissue damage. IL-10 also stimulates production of naturally occurring IL-1 receptor antagonist (IL-1ra) and release of soluble p75 TNF receptor [108]. IL-10 is believed to have a protective role in acute pancreatitis. Administration of IL- 10 in experimental acute pancreatitis reduces the local inflammatory response and subsequent mortality [108, 109].

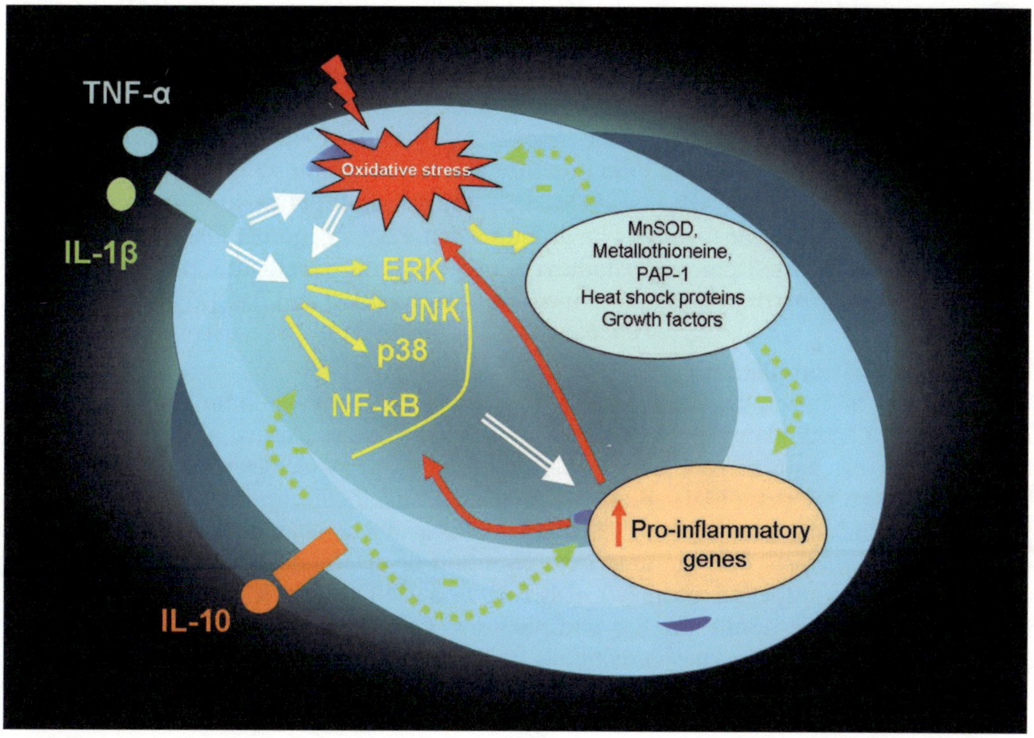

Fig. 5. Interaction between cytokines and oxidative stress in the inflammatory response in acute pancreatitis (IL-1β: interleukin-1β; IL-10: interleukin 10; MnSOD: Mn-superoxide dismutase; PAP-I: pancreatitis-associated protein I; TNF-: tumor necrosis factor α; NF-kB: nuclear factor kappaB; ERK: extracellular signal regulated kinases; JNK: c-jun N-terminal kinases; p38: p38 kinase). Modified from [184].

6. Other mediators

6.1 Platelet activating factor (PAF)

PAF, 1-O-octadecyl-2-acetyl-sn-glycero-3-phosphocholine, is a potent inflammatory mediator produced by endothelial cells, platelets, monocytes, neutrophils, and basophils. It is considered to be the key inflammatory mediator in severe acute pancreatitis external secretion and local/systemic inflammatory reactions [110].

PAF has been shown to be released into the peritoneal fluid as well as the bloodstream and the lung after the induction of acute experimental pancreatitis. Locally, PAF acts on microvascular diameter, permeability and platelet and leukocyte rolling, adhesion and migration through different mechanisms, including synthesis and release of NO and arachidonic acid metabolites, and up-regulated expressions of ICAM-1 and CD11/CD18. Secondary actions include the elevation of adhesion factor b2-integrin, changes in the endothelial cell skeleton, increases in capillary permeability, massive effusion of plasma, increase in blood viscosity and a slowdown of blood flow. It also participates in I/R injury and stimulates other vasoactive substances, including the generation of cytokine and inflammatory mediators. In acute pancreatitis, PAF levels rise due to the cytokine cascade reaction activated by elevated levels of TNF-a [98]. On the one hand, PAF promotes granulocyte aggregation and aggravates inflammatory reactions; on the other hand, it increases capillary permeability and aggravates renal tubule injury. The imbalance between PAF and vasoactive substances can initiate a vicious cycle that leads to a series of chain reactions and amplifying reactions—the cascade reaction. This reaction can increase tissue and organ injury, cause systemic inflammatory reaction syndrome (SIRS) and, eventually, multiple organ dysfunction syndrome (MODS) and/or multiple organ failure (MOF), or even death [98], [48]. Clinical studies have found that PAF antagonist Lexipafant has clear treatment effects on multiple organ failure of severe acute pancreatitis patients and also lowers the serum levels of inflammatory mediators such as IL-8 and IL-6 [111].

6.2 Activation of complement

I/R activates the complement and the formation of many inflammatory mediators, including the anaphylatoxins C3a, C4a and C5a. These recruit and stimulate the inflammatory cells and increase the expression of adhesion molecules such as vascular cell adhesion molecule-1 (VCAM-1), ICAM-1, E-selectin and P-selectin on the surface of the endothelium and the neutrophils [112, 113]. C5a is a chemotactic factor that directly stimulates the synthesis and the leucocyte secretion of cytokines such as IL-1 and 6, the monocytes chemo-attractive protein-1 (MCP-1) and TNFa. The iC3b takes part in the adhesion of the neutrophils on the endothelium. C5b-9, known as the 'final cytolytic membrane attack complex complement', is a powerful chemotactic agent, which causes direct lesions to the endothelial cells, stimulates the endothelial production of IL-8, MCP-1 and ROS and inhibits endothelium-dependent vasodilatation [13, 113, 114].

6.3 Serotonin

Platelet serotonin (hydroxytryptamine; p-5HT) is an index of platelet activation [115, 116]. Furthermore, the administration of human pancreatic fluid caused the release of 5HT in parallel with platelet activation [117]. Several studies showed that the production of 5HT can induce further platelet aggregation and 5HT release [118, 119], a positive feedback that may lead to thrombus formation [120]. Furthermore, 5HT is also a potent vasoconstrictor

[116]. Thus, these proprieties may mean that this bioamine is an aggravating factor for acute pancreatitis. The release of serotonin is considered to be the "gold standard" assay for the detection of platelet activation [121].

6.4 Bradykinin

The neuropeptide bradykinin is well known for its actions as an endothelium-dependent vasodilator. Bradykinin induces relaxation of vascular smooth muscle via stimulation of B2 receptors, which in turn stimulates constitutively expressed endothelial nitric oxide (NO) synthase (eNOS) to produce NO, induces cyclooxygenase-dependent production of prostacyclin and other prostanoids, as well as superoxide, activates charybdotoxin-sensitive K+ channels, and induces the formation of epoxyeicosatrienoic acids by cytochrome P-450 epoxygenase [122-124]. In addition to its actions on arterial and arteriolar vascular smooth muscle, bradykinin also exerts powerful pro-inflammatory effects in postcapillary venules. For example, it generates the release of endothelium-derived mediators from cultured endothelial cells that are chemotactic for neutrophils, eosinophils, monocytes, and pulmonary alveolar macrophages; induces the expression of endothelial adhesion molecules; and provokes leukocyte and platelet adherence to endothelial monolayers and postcapillary venules [125-129].

The specific mechanisms of bradykinin in the pancreas can be listed as follows: bradykinin can promote the synthesis and release of NO, bradykinin influences the pancreatic microcirculation by stimulating the formation of reactive oxygen species, PAF, ET, and different inflammatory mediators.

6.5 Thromboxane A2 (TXA2)

TXA2 is a potent capillary vasoconstrictor substance and platelet aggregation promoter that is able to induce platelet release and secretion, cause local and/or systemic disturbance of hemorrhage blood coagulation and destroy the cell-protection mechanism [130, 131]. Effected by increased phospholipase during acute pancreatitis condition, the cell membrane phospholipids decompose arachidonic acid, evoke TXA2 increase, lead to platelet aggregation, thrombosis, induce platelet deformation, adhesion, result in coagulation dysfunction, precipitate pancreatic ischemia and microcirculation, and increase pancreatic pathology injury [132]. In addition, it can promote neutrophil cell activation, release ROS, injure capillary endothelial cells, result in increased capillary permeability, and plasma extravasation [133].

6.6 Cyclooxygenase (COX)

COX, the key enzyme for prostaglandin synthesis, exists in two isoforms as COX-1 and COX-2. COX-1 is constitutively expressed in most tissues and has been suggested to mediate the synthesis of prostaglandins required for physiological functions and maintenance of organ integrity. COX-2 is undetectable in most tissues in normal condition, but is highly inducible by cytokines, mitogens, and endotoxins, and is responsible for an increased production of prostaglandins during inflammation [134, 135]. The role of COX-2 in pancreatic pathology is unclear. Studies performed by Song et al. [136], and Ethridge et al. [137], with mice have shown that pharmacological inhibition of COX-2 or COX-2 gene disruption reduces the severity of pancreatitis and pancreatitis-associated lung injury.

Furthermore, Foitzik et al. [138], found some beneficial systemic effects of COX-2 inhibition on acute pancreatitis, such as an improvement of renal and respiratory function, but they have not observed any significant effect of COX-2 inhibition on histological score of pancreatic damage or plasma level of trypsinogen activation peptides. Warzecha et al. [135] investigated the role of the blockade of COX-1 or COX-2 and found a significantly reduction of serum lipase and serum poly-C ribonuclease activity, as well as decreased pancreatic edema and inflammatory infiltration in morphological features in animals with cerulein-induced pancreatitis.

6.7 Prostaglandin I2 (PGI_2)

PGI2 is also one of the arachidonic acid metabolites with a strong vasodilator effect. The main influence on pancreatic microcirculation in pancreatitis can be listed as follows: expansion of the pancreatic bed to increase pancreatic blood supply, improvement of pancreatic microcirculation, and increase of pancreatic blood flow by inhibiting platelet aggregation, adhesion and deformation. Furthermore, PGI_2 can also stabilize lysosomalmembrane to prevent cytokine release and attenuate inflammatory response [139], [140].

6.8 Nuclear factor-kappa B (NF-kappa B)

NF-kappa B is a multi-purpose nuclear transcription factor, mainly involved in the regulation of expression referring to immune and inflammatory molecules [141]. Under the normal physiological circumstances, the NF-kappa B exists in the cytoplasm of other cells in the form of inactivity. When it is activated, it will promote a variety of cytokines gene transcription, and it plays an important role in cytokine-mediated infection, inflammation, oxidative stress, cell proliferation and apoptosis, the process of microcirculation and so on. Shi et al. showed that NF-kappa B activation can aggravate acute pancreatitis microcirculation disorder and gradually reduce the amplitude of pancreatic blood flow, and slow down blood flow velocity with the gradual increase of NF-kappa B P65 expression. The possible acting mechanism of NF-kappa B is that the excessive expression of NF-kappa B induces inflammatory cells' excessive secretion of nitric oxide, and then causes dysfunction of endothelial cells and smooth muscle cells, and capillary tension disorders, and leads to capillary pathological expansion, increase in capillary permeability due to endothelial cell injury, and plasma extravasation, which eventually leads to reduction of effective blood volume, pancreatic tissue hypoperfusion, and induces increases microcirculation disorder [142].

6.9 Vascular endothelial growth factor (VEGF)

VEGFs are endogenous vascular peptides that result in angiogenesis, vasodilatation and increased microvascular permeability in vivo [143]. Induction of VEGF mainly occurs in response to hypoxia [144]. Warzecha et al. found an increase in the immunohistochemical expression of VEGF even in the early course of I/R-induced acute pancreatitis [145]. Using the novel tyrosinekinase inhibitor PTK787/ZK222584, von Dobschuetz et al. observed a significant decrease of macromolecular permeability and a slightly increased functional capillary density with reduced leukocyte–endothelium interactions in the treatment group supporting a beneficial effect of this approach [146].

6.10 Role of endotoxin

Endotoxin, which is mainly produced by Gram-negative bacteria, is a component of the lipopolysaccharide present in cell walls. Clinical studies show that endotoxemia occurs in acute pancreatitis and particularly in severe acute pancreatitis, and that it is closely related to the onset, progression and complication of multiple organ failure in severe acute pancreatitis. Windsor et al.'s [147] study demonstrated the link between endotoxin and the state of pancreatitis. Other researchers studying the relation between plasma endotoxin levels of acute pancreatitis patients and multiple organ injury have found that endotoxin has an important promoting effect during the progression of multiple organ injury. As the most potent stimulant of endothelin, endotoxin can elevate the endothelin level in vivo and in blood, potently contracting medium-sized arteries and arterioles. Increased endothelin levels will also aggravate ischemia in other tissues, enhance bacterial translocation, raise blood endotoxin and renin-angiotensin levels and form a vicious cycle chain of tissue ischemia and endothelin that aggravates tissue ischemia endlessly [148].

6.11 Influence of reactive oxygen species (ROS)

The ROS is an oxygen-containing chemical group with high chemical reaction activities, mainly those involving the peroxide anion-free radical (O_2^-) and the hydroxy radical (OH⊙). By causing lipid oxidation, it can increase mucosa permeability, further enhance phagocyte activity, generate more ROS and finally cause histiocyte injury. Scott et al. [149] demonstrated that in the pathological state, excessive ROS can cause tissue and cell injury. ROS can also participate in the formation of acute pancreatitis pancreatic edema and, possibly, in pancreatic necrosis and mediate leukocytes and platelets activated by TNF-α in all organs to

6.12 Toll-like receptor-4 (TLR4)

In the early stage, acute pancreatitis mainly manifests as a chemical inflammation, which is a pancreatic nonspecific inflammatory process resulting from the action of a variety of factors. This inflammatory process is an inflammatory cascade reaction dominated by the body's innate immune system. Toll-like receptors are a kind of protein that can trigger this inflammatory cascade reaction. It is currently thought that TLRs might play a central role in the recognition of endogenous or exogenous antigen in the immune system and in the initiation of signal transduction in the process of inflammatory reaction during acute pancreatitis. Therefore, investigating the tissue-specific expression of TLRs (mainly TLR4) in pancreas and exploring their roles have great significance for understanding the pathogenesis of acute pancreatitis. A report has indicated that in the early stage of acute pancreatitis, the expression levels of TLR4, TNF-α, and IL-6 in pancreas of acute pancreatitis patients are significantly higher than those in the control ones, the level of plasma TNF-α in acute pancreatitis patients increases subsequently, and the increase of plasma TNF-α level is positively correlated with the expression of TLR4, suggesting that the up-regulation of TLR4 expression on the surface of peripheral blood monocytes in patients with early acute pancreatitis might be associated with the activation of the innate immune system in the early stage of the disease [150]. Results of animal experiments have shown that TLR4 messenger RNA is also up-regulated in the pancreas of rats with cerulein-induced edematous pancreatitis in the early stage, the serum levels of cytokines such as TNF-α are subsequently elevated, and the two phenomena are correlated [151].

Some researchers believe that TLR4 may play an important role in the synthesis and release of pro-inflammatory cytokines, and the up-regulation of the TLR4 gene may be related with the development and progression of organ injury during acute pancreatitis [152, 153]. Some studies have indicated that when severe acute pancreatitis is stimulated by LPS, the expressions of cytokines and cell adhesion molecules are significantly up-regulated in pancreas, thereby promoting the accumulation of excessive neutrophils in inflammatory region and leading to the injury of pancreas and other organs [154, 155]. Although it has been known that the translocation of intestinal bacteria and endotoxins is a key to secondary bacterial infection in necrotic pancreatic tissue, the mechanism of how multiple organ failure develops during pancreatitis has not yet been fully clarified [156].

7. Conclusions

Recent advances in experimental research have helped witness the pathophysiology of acute pancreatitis. The phenomena of microcirculatory changes observed in acute experimental pancreatitis during the past few years gradually underlie the disturbance of the local microcirculation in acute pancreatitis, but several challenges remain. Still some questions remain unexplained concerning the mechanisms: (1) Which is the first event in the pathogenesis of acute pancreatitis? (2) Which factor determines the edematous or necrotizing pancreatitis in a given experimental or clinical situation? (3) What is the role of impaired distribution of blood supply in early steps of acute pancreatitis? The potential mediators responsible for the progression of the disease severity and suggestions for therapeutic intervention have largely remained subjecting to speculation and debate.

Further research may help to find sufficient therapeutic approaches, eventually by affecting microcirculatory mechanisms, to influence development and progression of this disease.

8. References

[1] Mithofer K, Fernandez-del CC, Frick TW, Foitzik T, Bassi DG, Lewandrowski KB et al. Increased intrapancreatic trypsinogen activation in ischemia-induced experimental pancreatitis. Ann Surg 1995;221: 364-371.

[2] Menger MD, Bonkhoff H, Vollmar B. Ischemia-reperfusion-induced pancreatic microvascular injury. An intravital fluorescence microscopic study in rats. Dig Dis Sci 1996;41: 823-830.

[3] Kusterer K, Poschmann T, Friedemann A, Enghofer M, Zendler S, Usadel KH. Arterial constriction, ischemia-reperfusion, and leukocyte adherence in acute pancreatitis. Am J Physiol 1993;265: G165-G171.

[4] Mayer H, Schmidt J, Thies J, Ryschich E, Gebhard MM, Herfarth C et al. Characterization and reduction of ischemia/reperfusion injury after experimental pancreas transplantation. J Gastrointest Surg 1999;3: 162-166.

[5] Vollmar B, Preissler G, Menger MD. Hemorrhagic hypotension induces arteriolar vasomotion and intermittent capillary perfusion in rat pancreas. Am J Physiol 1994;267: H1936-H1940.

[6] Klar E, Schratt W, Foitzik T, Buhr H, Herfarth C, Messmer K. Impact of microcirculatory flow pattern changes on the development of acute edematous and necrotizing pancreatitis in rabbit pancreas. Dig Dis Sci 1994;39: 2639-2644.

[7] Hackert T, Pfeil D, Hartwig W, Gebhard MM, Buchler MW, Werner J. Platelet function in acute experimental pancreatitis induced by ischaemia-reperfusion. Br J Surg 2005;92: 724-728.
[8] Zhou ZG, Gao XH. Morphology of pancreatic microcirculation in the monkey: light and scanning electron microscopic study. Clin Anat 1995;8: 190-201.
[9] Zhou Z, Zeng Y, Yang P, Cheng Z, Zhao J, Shu Y et al. [Structure and function of pancreatic microcirculation]. Sheng Wu Yi Xue Gong Cheng Xue Za Zhi 2001;18: 195-200.
[10] von DE, Bleiziffer O, Pahernik S, Dellian M, Hoffmann T, Messmer K. Soluble complement receptor 1 preserves endothelial barrier function and microcirculation in postischemic pancreatitis in the rat. Am J Physiol Gastrointest Liver Physiol 2004;286: G791-G796.
[11] Zhou ZG, Chen YD. Influencing factors of pancreatic microcirculatory impairment in acute panceatitis. World J Gastroenterol 2002;8: 406-412.
[12] Vinten-Johansen J. Involvement of neutrophils in the pathogenesis of lethal myocardial reperfusion injury. Cardiovasc Res 2004;61: 481-497.
[13] Gourdin MJ, Bree B, De KM. The impact of ischaemia-reperfusion on the blood vessel. Eur J Anaesthesiol 2009;26: 537-547.
[14] Sluiter W, Pietersma A, Lamers JM, Koster JF. Leukocyte adhesion molecules on the vascular endothelium: their role in the pathogenesis of cardiovascular disease and the mechanisms underlying their expression. J Cardiovasc Pharmacol 1993;22 Suppl 4: S37-S44.
[15] Hidalgo A, Peired AJ, Wild MK, Vestweber D, Frenette PS. Complete identification of E-selectin ligands on neutrophils reveals distinct functions of PSGL-1, ESL-1, and CD44. Immunity 2007;26: 477-489.
[16] Gu Q, Yang XP, Bonde P, DiPaula A, Fox-Talbot K, Becker LC. Inhibition of TNF-alpha reduces myocardial injury and proinflammatory pathways following ischemia-reperfusion in the dog. J Cardiovasc Pharmacol 2006;48: 320-328.
[17] Granger DN, Senchenkova E. 2010.
[18] Rodrigues SF, Granger DN. Role of blood cells in ischaemia-reperfusion induced endothelial barrier failure. Cardiovasc Res 2010;87: 291-299.
[19] Alexander JS, Alexander BC, Eppihimer LA, Goodyear N, Haque R, Davis CP et al. Inflammatory mediators induce sequestration of VE-cadherin in cultured human endothelial cells. Inflammation 2000;24: 99-113.
[20] Allingham MJ, van Buul JD, Burridge K. ICAM-1-mediated, Src- and Pyk2-dependent vascular endothelial cadherin tyrosine phosphorylation is required for leukocyte transendothelial migration. J Immunol 2007;179: 4053-4064.
[21] Flores NA, Goulielmos NV, Seghatchian MJ, Sheridan DJ. Myocardial ischaemia induces platelet activation with adverse electrophysiological and arrhythmogenic effects. Cardiovasc Res 1994;28: 1662-1671.
[22] Okada Y, Marchevsky AM, Zuo XJ, Pass JA, Kass RM, Matloff JM et al. Accumulation of platelets in rat syngeneic lung transplants: a potential factor responsible for preservation-reperfusion injury. Transplantation 1997;64: 801-806.
[23] Kuroda T, Shiohara E, Homma T, Furukawa Y, Chiba S. Effects of leukocyte and platelet depletion on ischemia--reperfusion injury to dog pancreas. Gastroenterology 1994;107: 1125-1134.

[24] Weyrich AS, Elstad MR, McEver RP, McIntyre TM, Moore KL, Morrissey JH et al. Activated platelets signal chemokine synthesis by human monocytes. J Clin Invest 1996;97: 1525-1534.
[25] Khandoga A, Biberthaler P, Messmer K, Krombach F. Platelet-endothelial cell interactions during hepatic ischemia-reperfusion in vivo: a systematic analysis. Microvasc Res 2003;65: 71-77.
[26] Yeo EL, Sheppard JA, Feuerstein IA. Role of P-selectin and leukocyte activation in polymorphonuclear cell adhesion to surface adherent activated platelets under physiologic shear conditions (an injury vessel wall model). Blood 1994;83: 2498-2507.
[27] Kuijper PH, Gallardo Torres HI, Lammers JW, Sixma JJ, Koenderman L, Zwaginga JJ. Platelet and fibrin deposition at the damaged vessel wall: cooperative substrates for neutrophil adhesion under flow conditions. Blood 1997;89: 166-175.
[28] Salter JW, Krieglstein CF, Issekutz AC, Granger DN. Platelets modulate ischemia/reperfusion-induced leukocyte recruitment in the mesenteric circulation. Am J Physiol Gastrointest Liver Physiol 2001;281: G1432-G1439.
[29] Shebuski RJ, Kilgore KS. Role of inflammatory mediators in thrombogenesis. J Pharmacol Exp Ther 2002;300: 729-735.
[30] Bouchard BA, Tracy PB. Platelets, leukocytes, and coagulation. Curr Opin Hematol 2001;8: 263-269.
[31] Yokoyama S, Ikeda H, Haramaki N, Yasukawa H, Murohara T, Imaizumi T. Platelet P-selectin plays an important role in arterial thrombogenesis by forming large stable platelet-leukocyte aggregates. J Am Coll Cardiol 2005;45: 1280-1286.
[32] Dole VS, Bergmeier W, Mitchell HA, Eichenberger SC, Wagner DD. Activated platelets induce Weibel-Palade-body secretion and leukocyte rolling in vivo: role of P-selectin. Blood 2005;106: 2334-2339.
[33] Martin M, Mory C, Prescher A, Wittekind C, Fiedler M, Uhlmann D. Protective effects of early CD4(+) T cell reduction in hepatic ischemia/reperfusion injury. J Gastrointest Surg 2010;14: 511-519.
[34] Matsuda T, Yamaguchi Y, Matsumura F, Akizuki E, Okabe K, Liang J et al. Immunosuppressants decrease neutrophil chemoattractant and attenuate ischemia/reperfusion injury of the liver in rats. J Trauma 1998;44: 475-484.
[35] Le MO, Louis H, Demols A, Desalle F, Demoor F, Quertinmont E et al. Cold liver ischemia-reperfusion injury critically depends on liver T cells and is improved by donor pretreatment with interleukin 10 in mice. Hepatology 2000;31: 1266-1274.
[36] Martin M, Mory C, Prescher A, Wittekind C, Fiedler M, Uhlmann D. Protective effects of early CD4(+) T cell reduction in hepatic ischemia/reperfusion injury. J Gastrointest Surg 2010;14: 511-519.
[37] Takada M, Chandraker A, Nadeau KC, Sayegh MH, Tilney NL. The role of the B7 costimulatory pathway in experimental cold ischemia/reperfusion injury. J Clin Invest 1997;100: 1199-1203.
[38] Zwacka RM, Zhang Y, Halldorson J, Schlossberg H, Dudus L, Engelhardt JF. CD4(+) T-lymphocytes mediate ischemia/reperfusion-induced inflammatory responses in mouse liver. J Clin Invest 1997;100: 279-289.

[39] Suzuki S, Toledo-Pereyra LH, Rodriguez FJ, Cejalvo D. Neutrophil infiltration as an important factor in liver ischemia and reperfusion injury. Modulating effects of FK506 and cyclosporine. Transplantation 1993;55: 1265-1272.
[40] Matsuda T, Yamaguchi Y, Matsumura F, Akizuki E, Okabe K, Liang J et al. Immunosuppressants decrease neutrophil chemoattractant and attenuate ischemia/reperfusion injury of the liver in rats. J Trauma 1998;44: 475-484.
[41] Shen XD, Ke B, Zhai Y, Gao F, Anselmo D, Lassman CR et al. Stat4 and Stat6 signaling in hepatic ischemia/reperfusion injury in mice: HO-1 dependence of Stat4 disruption-mediated cytoprotection. Hepatology 2003;37: 296-303.
[42] Shen XD, Ke B, Zhai Y, Amersi F, Gao F, Anselmo DM et al. CD154-CD40 T-cell costimulation pathway is required in the mechanism of hepatic ischemia/reperfusion injury, and its blockade facilitates and depends on heme oxygenase-1 mediated cytoprotection. Transplantation 2002;74: 315-319.
[43] Anselmo DM, Amersi FF, Shen XD, Gao F, Katori M, Lassman C et al. FTY720 pretreatment reduces warm hepatic ischemia reperfusion injury through inhibition of T-lymphocyte infiltration. Am J Transplant 2002;2: 843-849.
[44] Clavien PA, Harvey PR, Sanabria JR, Cywes R, Levy GA, Strasberg SM. Lymphocyte adherence in the reperfused rat liver: mechanisms and effects. Hepatology 1993;17: 131-142.
[45] Bella J, Kolatkar PR, Marlor CW, Greve JM, Rossmann MG. The structure of the two amino-terminal domains of human intercellular adhesion molecule-1 suggests how it functions as a rhinovirus receptor. Virus Res 1999;62: 107-117.
[46] Sun W, Watanabe Y, Wang ZQ. Expression and significance of ICAM-1 and its counter receptors LFA-1 and Mac-1 in experimental acute pancreatitis of rats. World J Gastroenterol 2006;12: 5005-5009.
[47] Liu XM, Liu QG, Xu J, Pan CE. Microcirculation disturbance affects rats with acute severe pancreatitis following lung injury. World J Gastroenterol 2005;11: 6208-6211.
[48] Steer ML. Relationship between pancreatitis and lung diseases. Respir Physiol 2001;128: 13-16.
[49] Hartwig W, Werner J, Warshaw AL, Antoniu B, Castillo CF, Gebhard MM et al. Membrane-bound ICAM-1 is upregulated by trypsin and contributes to leukocyte migration in acute pancreatitis. Am J Physiol Gastrointest Liver Physiol 2004;287: G1194-G1199.
[50] Keck T, Friebe V, Warshaw AL, Antoniu BA, Waneck G, Benz S et al. Pancreatic proteases in serum induce leukocyte-endothelial adhesion and pancreatic microcirculatory failure. Pancreatology 2005;5: 241-250.
[51] Werner J, Z'graggen K, Fernandez-del CC, Lewandrowski KB, Compton CC, Warshaw AL. Specific therapy for local and systemic complications of acute pancreatitis with monoclonal antibodies against ICAM-1. Ann Surg 1999;229: 834-840.
[52] Khandoga A, Biberthaler P, Enders G, Axmann S, Hutter J, Messmer K et al. Platelet adhesion mediated by fibrinogen-intercelllular adhesion molecule-1 binding induces tissue injury in the postischemic liver in vivo. Transplantation 2002;74: 681-688.
[53] Gao HK, Zhou ZG, Chen YQ, Han FH, Wang C. Expression of platelet endothelial cell adhesion molecule-1 between pancreatic microcirculation and peripheral

circulation in rats with acute edematous pancreatitis. Hepatobiliary Pancreat Dis Int 2003;2: 463-466.
[54] Gao HK, Zhou ZG, Han FH, Chen YQ, Yan WW, He T et al. Differences in platelet endothelial cell adhesion molecule-1 expression between peripheral circulation and pancreatic microcirculation in cerulein-induced acute edematous pancreatitis. World J Gastroenterol 2005;11: 661-664.
[55] Eppihimer MJ, Wolitzky B, Anderson DC, Labow MA, Granger DN. Heterogeneity of expression of E- and P-selectins in vivo. Circ Res 1996;79: 560-569.
[56] Massberg S, Enders G, Leiderer R, Eisenmenger S, Vestweber D, Krombach F et al. Platelet-endothelial cell interactions during ischemia/reperfusion: the role of P-selectin. Blood 1998;92: 507-515.
[57] Cooper D, Chitman KD, Williams MC, Granger DN. Time-dependent platelet-vessel wall interactions induced by intestinal ischemia-reperfusion. Am J Physiol Gastrointest Liver Physiol 2003;284: G1027-G1033.
[58] Nishijima K, Kiryu J, Tsujikawa A, Honjo M, Nonaka A, Yamashiro K et al. In vivo evaluation of platelet--endothelial interactions after transient retinal ischemia. Invest Ophthalmol Vis Sci 2001;42: 2102-2109.
[59] Katayama T, Ikeda Y, Handa M, Tamatani T, Sakamoto S, Ito M et al. Immunoneutralization of glycoprotein Ibalpha attenuates endotoxin-induced interactions of platelets and leukocytes with rat venular endothelium in vivo. Circ Res 2000;86: 1031-1037.
[60] Gong Z, Yuan Y, Lou K, Tu S, Zhai Z, Xu J. Mechanisms of Chinese herb emodin and somatostatin analogs on pancreatic regeneration in acute pancreatitis in rats. Pancreas 2002;25: 154-160.
[61] Frenette PS, Denis CV, Weiss L, Jurk K, Subbarao S, Kehrel B et al. P-Selectin glycoprotein ligand 1 (PSGL-1) is expressed on platelets and can mediate platelet-endothelial interactions in vivo. J Exp Med 2000;191: 1413-1422.
[62] Andre P, Denis CV, Ware J, Saffaripour S, Hynes RO, Ruggeri ZM et al. Platelets adhere to and translocate on von Willebrand factor presented by endothelium in stimulated veins. Blood 2000;96: 3322-3328.
[63] Romo GM, Dong JF, Schade AJ, Gardiner EE, Kansas GS, Li CQ et al. The glycoprotein Ib-IX-V complex is a platelet counterreceptor for P-selectin. J Exp Med 1999;190: 803-814.
[64] Luscher TF, Oemar BS, Boulanger CM, Hahn AW. Molecular and cellular biology of endothelin and its receptors--Part I. J Hypertens 1993;11: 7-11.
[65] McMillen MA, Huribal M, Cunningham ME, Kumar R, Sumpio BE. Endothelin-1 increases intracellular calcium in human monocytes and causes production of interleukin-6. Crit Care Med 1995;23: 34-40.
[66] Filep JG, Clozel M, Fournier A, Foldes-Filep E. Characterization of receptors mediating vascular responses to endothelin-1 in the conscious rat. Br J Pharmacol 1994;113: 845-852.
[67] Spiegel HU, Scommotau S, Uhlmann D, Giersch B. Effect of the endothelin receptor antagonist bosentan on postischemic liver microcirculation. Zentralbl Chir 1996;121: 788-793.

[68] McMillen MA, Huribal M, Kumar R, Sumpio BE. Endothelin-stimulated human monocytes produce prostaglandin E2 but not leukotriene B4. J Surg Res 1993;54: 331-335.

[69] Deacon K, Knox AJ. Endothelin-1 (ET-1) increases the expression of remodeling genes in vascular smooth muscle through linked calcium and cAMP pathways: role of a phospholipase A(2)(cPLA(2))/cyclooxygenase-2 (COX-2)/prostacyclin receptor-dependent autocrine loop. J Biol Chem 2010;285: 25913-25927.

[70] Ishida K, Takeshige K, Minakami S. Endothelin-1 enhances superoxide generation of human neutrophils stimulated by the chemotactic peptide N-formyl-methionyl-leucyl-phenylalanine. Biochem Biophys Res Commun 1990;173: 496-500.

[71] Bauer M, Zhang JX, Bauer I, Clemens MG. ET-1 induced alterations of hepatic microcirculation: sinusoidal and extrasinusoidal sites of action. Am J Physiol 1994;267: G143-G149.

[72] Lopez FA, Riesco A, Espinosa G, Digiuni E, Cernadas MR, Alvarez V et al. Effect of endothelin-1 on neutrophil adhesion to endothelial cells and perfused heart. Circulation 1993;88: 1166-1171.

[73] Yanagisawa M, Masaki T. Molecular biology and biochemistry of the endothelins. Trends Pharmacol Sci 1989;10: 374-378.

[74] Eibl G, Hotz HG, Faulhaber J, Kirchengast M, Buhr HJ, Foitzik T. Effect of endothelin and endothelin receptor blockade on capillary permeability in experimental pancreatitis. Gut 2000;46: 390-394.

[75] Takaori K, Inoue K, Kogire M, Higashide S, Tun T, Aung T et al. Effects of endothelin on microcirculation of the pancreas. Life Sci 1992;51: 615-622.

[76] Hildebrand P, Mrozinski JE, Jr., Mantey SA, Patto RJ, Jensen RT. Pancreatic acini possess endothelin receptors whose internalization is regulated by PLC-activating agents. Am J Physiol 1993;264: G984-G993.

[77] Hof RP, Hof A, Takiguchi Y. Massive regional differences in the vascular effects of endothelin. J Hypertens Suppl 1989;7: S274-S275.

[78] Foitzik T, Hotz HG, Hot B, Kirchengast M, Buhr HJ. Endothelin-1 mediates the alcohol-induced reduction of pancreatic capillary blood flow. J Gastrointest Surg 1998;2: 379-384.

[79] Foitzik T, Faulhaber J, Hotz HG, Kirchengast M, Buhr HJ. Endothelin receptor blockade improves fluid sequestration, pancreatic capillary blood flow, and survival in severe experimental pancreatitis. Ann Surg 1998;228: 670-675.

[80] Plusczyk T, Bersal B, Westermann S, Menger M, Feifel G. ET-1 induces pancreatitis-like microvascular deterioration and acinar cell injury. J Surg Res 1999;85: 301-310.

[81] Lehoux S, Plante GE, Sirois MG, Sirois P, Orleans-Juste P. Phosphoramidon blocks big-endothelin-1 but not endothelin-1 enhancement of vascular permeability in the rat. Br J Pharmacol 1992;107: 996-1000.

[82] Palmer RM, Ferrige AG, Moncada S. Nitric oxide release accounts for the biological activity of endothelium-derived relaxing factor. Nature 1987;327: 524-526.

[83] Masamune A, Shimosegawa T, Satoh A, Fujita M, Sakai Y, Toyota T. Nitric oxide decreases endothelial activation by rat experimental severe pancreatitis-associated ascitic fluids. Pancreas 2000;20: 297-304.

[84] Kubes P, Kanwar S, Niu XF, Gaboury JP. Nitric oxide synthesis inhibition induces leukocyte adhesion via superoxide and mast cells. FASEB J 1993;7: 1293-1299.

[85] Kubes P, Suzuki M, Granger DN. Nitric oxide: an endogenous modulator of leukocyte adhesion. Proc Natl Acad Sci U S A 1991;88: 4651-4655.
[86] Moncada S, Higgs A. The L-arginine-nitric oxide pathway. N Engl J Med 1993;329: 2002-2012.
[87] Niu XF, Smith CW, Kubes P. Intracellular oxidative stress induced by nitric oxide synthesis inhibition increases endothelial cell adhesion to neutrophils. Circ Res 1994;74: 1133-1140.
[88] Rubanyi GM, Ho EH, Cantor EH, Lumma WC, Botelho LH. Cytoprotective function of nitric oxide: inactivation of superoxide radicals produced by human leukocytes. Biochem Biophys Res Commun 1991;181: 1392-1397.
[89] Beckman JS, Crow JP. Pathological implications of nitric oxide, superoxide and peroxynitrite formation. Biochem Soc Trans 1993;21: 330-334.
[90] Lipsett PA. Serum cytokines, proteins, and receptors in acute pancreatitis: mediators, markers, or more of the same? Crit Care Med 2001;29: 1642-1644.
[91] Hirota M, Nozawa F, Okabe A, Shibata M, Beppu T, Shimada S et al. Relationship between plasma cytokine concentration and multiple organ failure in patients with acute pancreatitis. Pancreas 2000;21: 141-146.
[92] de D, I, Perez M, de La MA, Sevillano S, Orfao A, Ramudo L et al. Contribution of circulating leukocytes to cytokine production in pancreatic duct obstruction-induced acute pancreatitis in rats. Cytokine 2002;20: 295-303.
[93] Descamps FJ, Van den Steen PE, Martens E, Ballaux F, Geboes K, Opdenakker G. Gelatinase B is diabetogenic in acute and chronic pancreatitis by cleaving insulin. FASEB J 2003;17: 887-889.
[94] Ammori BJ. Role of the gut in the course of severe acute pancreatitis. Pancreas 2003;26: 122-129.
[95] Cassatella MA. The production of cytokines by polymorphonuclear neutrophils. Immunol Today 1995;16: 21-26.
[96] Ogawa M. Acute pancreatitis and cytokines: "second attack" by septic complication leads to organ failure. Pancreas 1998;16: 312-315.
[97] Hughes CB, Gaber LW, Mohey el-Din AB, Grewal HP, Kotb M, Mann L et al. Inhibition of TNF alpha improves survival in an experimental model of acute pancreatitis. Am Surg 1996;62: 8-13.
[98] Zhang XP, Wang L, Zhou YF. The pathogenic mechanism of severe acute pancreatitis complicated with renal injury: a review of current knowledge. Dig Dis Sci 2008;53: 297-306.
[99] Pohlman TH, Stanness KA, Beatty PG, Ochs HD, Harlan JM. An endothelial cell surface factor(s) induced in vitro by lipopolysaccharide, interleukin 1, and tumor necrosis factor-alpha increases neutrophil adherence by a CDw18-dependent mechanism. J Immunol 1986;136: 4548-4553.
[100] Norman JG, Franz MG, Fink GS, Messina J, Fabri PJ, Gower WR et al. Decreased mortality of severe acute pancreatitis after proximal cytokine blockade. Ann Surg 1995;221: 625-631.
[101] Norman JG, Fink G, Franz M, Guffey J, Carter G, Davison B et al. Active interleukin-1 receptor required for maximal progression of acute pancreatitis. Ann Surg 1996;223: 163-169.

[102] Fink G, Yang J, Carter G, Norman J. Acute pancreatitis-induced enzyme release and necrosis are attenuated by IL-1 antagonism through an indirect mechanism. J Surg Res 1997;67: 94-97.
[103] Kusske AM, Rongione AJ, Reber HA. Cytokines and acute pancreatitis. Gastroenterology 1996;110: 639-642.
[104] Lentz SR, Tsiang M, Sadler JE. Regulation of thrombomodulin by tumor necrosis factor-alpha: comparison of transcriptional and posttranscriptional mechanisms. Blood 1991;77: 542-550.
[105] Gross V, Andreesen R, Leser HG, Ceska M, Liehl E, Lausen M et al. Interleukin-8 and neutrophil activation in acute pancreatitis. Eur J Clin Invest 1992;22: 200-203.
[106] Kimura Y, Torimura T, Ueno T, Inuzuka S, Tanikawa K. Transforming growth factor beta 1, extracellular matrix, and inflammatory cells in wound repair using a closed duodenal loop pancreatitis model rat. Immunohistochemical study. Scand J Gastroenterol 1995;30: 707-714.
[107] Konturek PC, Dembinski A, Warzecha Z, Ceranowicz P, Konturek SJ, Stachura J et al. Expression of transforming growth factor-beta 1 and epidermal growth factor in caerulein-induced pancreatitis in rat. J Physiol Pharmacol 1997;48: 59-72.
[108] Rongione AJ, Kusske AM, Kwan K, Ashley SW, Reber HA, McFadden DW. Interleukin 10 reduces the severity of acute pancreatitis in rats. Gastroenterology 1997;112: 960-967.
[109] Kusske AM, Rongione AJ, Ashley SW, McFadden DW, Reber HA. Interleukin-10 prevents death in lethal necrotizing pancreatitis in mice. Surgery 1996;120: 284-288.
[110] Bhatia M. Acute pancreatitis as a model of SIRS. Front Biosci 2009;14: 2042-2050.
[111] Johnson CD, Kingsnorth AN, Imrie CW, McMahon MJ, Neoptolemos JP, McKay C et al. Double blind, randomised, placebo controlled study of a platelet activating factor antagonist, lexipafant, in the treatment and prevention of organ failure in predicted severe acute pancreatitis. Gut 2001;48: 62-69.
[112] Eltzschig HK, Collard CD. Vascular ischaemia and reperfusion injury. Br Med Bull 2004;70: 71-86.
[113] Arumugam TV, Magnus T, Woodruff TM, Proctor LM, Shiels IA, Taylor SM. Complement mediators in ischemia-reperfusion injury. Clin Chim Acta 2006;374: 33-45.
[114] Thrane AS, Skehan JD, Thrane PS. A novel interpretation of immune redundancy and duality in reperfusion injury with important implications for intervention in ischaemic disease. Med Hypotheses 2007;68: 1363-1370.
[115] Lechin F, van der DB. Platelet aggregation, platelet serotonin and pancreatitis. JOP 2004;5: 237-238.
[116] Barradas MA, Mikhailidis DP. Serotonin, histamine and platelets in vascular disease with special reference to peripheral vascular disease. Braz J Med Biol Res 1992;25: 1063-1076.
[117] Prinz RA, Fareed J, Rock A, Squillaci G, Wallenga J. Platelet activation by human pancreatic fluid. J Surg Res 1984;37: 314-319.
[118] Yoshino T, Yamaguchi I. Possible involvement of 5-HT2 receptor activation in aggravation of diet-induced acute pancreatitis in mice. J Pharmacol Exp Ther 1997;283: 1495-1502.

[119] de CF, David JL, Janssen PA. Inhibition of 5-hydroxytryptamine-induced and -amplified human platelet aggregation by ketanserin (R 41,468), a selective 5-HT2-receptor antagonist. 1982. Agents Actions 1994;43: 225-234.
[120] Marcus AJ. Recent progress in the role of platelets in occlusive vascular disease. Stroke 1983;14: 475-479.
[121] Gobbi G, Mirandola P, Tazzari PL, Ricci F, Caimi L, Cacchioli A et al. Flow cytometry detection of serotonin content and release in resting and activated platelets. Br J Haematol 2003;121: 892-896.
[122] Bagate K, Grima M, Imbs JL, Jong WD, Helwig JJ, Barthelmebs M. Signal transduction pathways involved in kinin B(2) receptor-mediated vasodilation in the rat isolated perfused kidney. Br J Pharmacol 2001;132: 1735-1742.
[123] Fleming I, Bauersachs J, Busse R. Paracrine functions of the coronary vascular endothelium. Mol Cell Biochem 1996;157: 137-145.
[124] Fulton D, Mahboubi K, McGiff JC, Quilley J. Cytochrome P450-dependent effects of bradykinin in the rat heart. Br J Pharmacol 1995;114: 99-102.
[125] Abbott NJ. Inflammatory mediators and modulation of blood-brain barrier permeability. Cell Mol Neurobiol 2000;20: 131-147.
[126] Feletou M, Bonnardel E, Canet E. Bradykinin and changes in microvascular permeability in the hamster cheek pouch: role of nitric oxide. Br J Pharmacol 1996;118: 1371-1376.
[127] Sato E, Koyama S, Nomura H, Kubo K, Sekiguchi M. Bradykinin stimulates alveolar macrophages to release neutrophil, monocyte, and eosinophil chemotactic activity. J Immunol 1996;157: 3122-3129.
[128] Schuschke DA, Saari JT, Miller FN. Leukocyte-endothelial adhesion is impaired in the cremaster muscle microcirculation of the copper-deficient rat. Immunol Lett 2001;76: 139-144.
[129] Shigematsu S, Ishida S, Gute DC, Korthuis RJ. Concentration-dependent effects of bradykinin on leukocyte recruitment and venular hemodynamics in rat mesentery. Am J Physiol 1999;277: H152-H160.
[130] Mao E, Zhang S, Han T. [Pancreatic ischemia: a continuous injury factor in acute necrotic pancreatitis]. Zhonghua Wai Ke Za Zhi 1997;35: 150-152.
[131] Motoyoshi M, Sugiyama M, Atomi Y, Kimura W, Nagawa H. Effect of a selective thromboxane A2 synthetase inhibitor on the systemic changes induced by circulating pancreatic phospholipase A2. J Gastroenterol 2006;41: 1094-1098.
[132] Hoffmann TF, Leiderer R, Waldner H, Messmer K. Bradykinin antagonists HOE-140 and CP-0597 diminish microcirculatory injury after ischaemia-reperfusion of the pancreas in rats. Br J Surg 1996;83: 189-195.
[133] Shi C, Andersson R, Zhao X, Wang X. Potential role of reactive oxygen species in pancreatitis-associated multiple organ dysfunction. Pancreatology 2005;5: 492-500.
[134] Smith WL, DeWitt DL, Garavito RM. Cyclooxygenases: structural, cellular, and molecular biology. Annu Rev Biochem 2000;69: 145-182.
[135] Warzecha Z, Dembinski A, Ceranowicz P, Konturek SJ, Dembinski M, Pawlik WW et al. Ischemic preconditioning inhibits development of edematous cerulein-induced pancreatitis: involvement of cyclooxygenases and heat shock protein 70. World J Gastroenterol 2005;11: 5958-5965.

[136] Song AM, Bhagat L, Singh VP, Van Acker GG, Steer ML, Saluja AK. Inhibition of cyclooxygenase-2 ameliorates the severity of pancreatitis and associated lung injury. Am J Physiol Gastrointest Liver Physiol 2002;283: G1166-G1174.
[137] Ethridge RT, Chung DH, Slogoff M, Ehlers RA, Hellmich MR, Rajaraman S et al. Cyclooxygenase-2 gene disruption attenuates the severity of acute pancreatitis and pancreatitis-associated lung injury. Gastroenterology 2002;123: 1311-1322.
[138] Foitzik T, Hotz HG, Hotz B, Wittig F, Buhr HJ. Selective inhibition of cyclooxygenase-2 (COX-2) reduces prostaglandin E2 production and attenuates systemic disease sequelae in experimental pancreatitis. Hepatogastroenterology 2003;50: 1159-1162.
[139] Dobosz M, Wajda Z, Hac S, Mysliwska J, Bryl E, Mionskowska L et al. Nitric oxide, heparin and procaine treatment in experimental ceruleine-induced acute pancreatitis in rats. Arch Immunol Ther Exp (Warsz) 1999;47: 155-160.
[140] Yucel K, Alhan E, Kucuktulu U, Piri M, Ercin C, Deger O. The effects of prostaglandin E1 on the microperfusion of the pancreas during acute necrotizing pancreatitis in rats. Hepatogastroenterology 2002;49: 544-548.
[141] Gukovsky I, Gukovskaya AS, Blinman TA, Zaninovic V, Pandol SJ. Early NF-kappaB activation is associated with hormone-induced pancreatitis. Am J Physiol 1998;275: G1402-G1414.
[142] Shi C, Zhao X, Wang X, Andersson R. Role of nuclear factor-kappaB, reactive oxygen species and cellular signaling in the early phase of acute pancreatitis. Scand J Gastroenterol 2005;40: 103-108.
[143] Bates DO, Lodwick D, Williams B. Vascular endothelial growth factor and microvascular permeability. Microcirculation 1999;6: 83-96.
[144] Gray MJ, Zhang J, Ellis LM, Semenza GL, Evans DB, Watowich SS et al. HIF-1alpha, STAT3, CBP/p300 and Ref-1/APE are components of a transcriptional complex that regulates Src-dependent hypoxia-induced expression of VEGF in pancreatic and prostate carcinomas. Oncogene 2005;24: 3110-3120.
[145] Warzecha Z, Dembinski A, Ceranowicz P, Dembinski M, Kownacki P, Konturek SJ et al. Immunohistochemical expression of FGF-2, PDGF-A, VEGF and TGF beta RII in the pancreas in the course of ischemia/reperfusion-induced acute pancreatitis. J Physiol Pharmacol 2004;55: 791-810.
[146] von DE, Meyer S, Thorn D, Marme D, Hopt UT, Thomusch O. Targeting vascular endothelial growth factor pathway offers new possibilities to counteract microvascular disturbances during ischemia/reperfusion of the pancreas. Transplantation 2006;82: 543-549.
[147] Windsor JA, Fearon KC, Ross JA, Barclay GR, Smyth E, Poxton I et al. Role of serum endotoxin and antiendotoxin core antibody levels in predicting the development of multiple organ failure in acute pancreatitis. Br J Surg 1993;80: 1042-1046.
[148] Zhang XP, Zhang J, Song QL, Chen HQ. Mechanism of acute pancreatitis complicated with injury of intestinal mucosa barrier. J Zhejiang Univ Sci B 2007;8: 888-895.
[149] Scott P, Bruce C, Schofield D, Shiel N, Braganza JM, McCloy RF. Vitamin C status in patients with acute pancreatitis. Br J Surg 1993;80: 750-754.
[150] Li HG, Zhou ZG, Li Y, Zheng XL, Lei S, Zhu L et al. Alterations of Toll-like receptor 4 expression on peripheral blood monocytes during the early stage of human acute pancreatitis. Dig Dis Sci 2007;52: 1973-1978.

[151] Li Y, Zhou ZG, Xia QJ, Zhang J, Li HG, Cao GQ et al. Toll-like receptor 4 detected in exocrine pancreas and the change of expression in cerulein-induced pancreatitis. Pancreas 2005;30: 375-381.
[152] Wu HS, Zhang L, Chen Y, Guo XJ, Wang L, Xu JB et al. Effect of nitric oxide on toll-like receptor 2 and 4 gene expression in rats with acute lung injury complicated by acute hemorrhage necrotizing pancreatitis. Hepatobiliary Pancreat Dis Int 2005;4: 609-613.
[153] Sharif R, Dawra R, Wasiluk K, Phillips P, Dudeja V, Kurt-Jones E et al. Impact of toll-like receptor 4 on the severity of acute pancreatitis and pancreatitis-associated lung injury in mice. Gut 2009;58: 813-819.
[154] Ueki M, Taie S, Chujo K, Asaga T, Iwanaga Y, Ono J et al. Urinary trypsin inhibitor reduces inflammatory response in kidney induced by lipopolysaccharide. J Biosci Bioeng 2007;104: 315-320.
[155] Vonlaufen A, Xu Z, Daniel B, Kumar RK, Pirola R, Wilson J et al. Bacterial endotoxin: a trigger factor for alcoholic pancreatitis? Evidence from a novel, physiologically relevant animal model. Gastroenterology 2007;133: 1293-1303.
[156] Yasuda T, Takeyama Y, Ueda T, Shinzeki M, Sawa H, Nakajima T et al. Breakdown of intestinal mucosa via accelerated apoptosis increases intestinal permeability in experimental severe acute pancreatitis. J Surg Res 2006;135: 18-26.
[157] Uhlmann D, Lauer H, Serr F, Witzigmann H. Pathophysiological role of platelets and platelet system in acute pancreatitis. Microvasc Res 2008;76: 114-123.
[158] Noto T, Furuichi Y, Ishiye M, Matsuoka N, Aramori I, Mutoh S et al. Tacrolimus (FK506) limits accumulation of granulocytes and platelets and protects against brain damage after transient focal cerebral ischemia in rat. Biol Pharm Bull 2007;30: 313-317.
[159] Khandoga A, Biberthaler P, Enders G, Teupser D, Axmann S, Luchting B et al. P-selectin mediates platelet-endothelial cell interactions and reperfusion injury in the mouse liver in vivo. Shock 2002;18: 529-535.
[160] Liu X, Xie W, Liu P, Duan M, Jia Z, Li W et al. Mechanism of the cardioprotection of rhEPO pretreatment on suppressing the inflammatory response in ischemia-reperfusion. Life Sci 2006;78: 2255-2264.
[161] Contaldo C, Meier C, Elsherbiny A, Harder Y, Trentz O, Menger MD et al. Human recombinant erythropoietin protects the striated muscle microcirculation of the dorsal skinfold from postischemic injury in mice. Am J Physiol Heart Circ Physiol 2007;293: H274-H283.
[162] Zarbock A, Singbartl K, Ley K. Complete reversal of acid-induced acute lung injury by blocking of platelet-neutrophil aggregation. J Clin Invest 2006;116: 3211-3219.
[163] Prescher A, Mory C, Martin M, Fiedler M, Uhlmann D. Effect of FTY720 treatment on postischemic pancreatic microhemodynamics. Transplant Proc 2010;42: 3984-3985.
[164] Foitzik T, Eibl G, Buhr HJ. Therapy for microcirculatory disorders in severe acute pancreatitis: comparison of delayed therapy with ICAM-1 antibodies and a specific endothelin A receptor antagonist. J Gastrointest Surg 2000;4: 240-246.
[165] Frossard JL, Saluja A, Bhagat L, Lee HS, Bhatia M, Hofbauer B et al. The role of intercellular adhesion molecule 1 and neutrophils in acute pancreatitis and pancreatitis-associated lung injury. Gastroenterology 1999;116: 694-701.

[166] Stangl V, Lorenz M, Ludwig A, Grimbo N, Guether C, Sanad W et al. The flavonoid phloretin suppresses stimulated expression of endothelial adhesion molecules and reduces activation of human platelets. J Nutr 2005;135: 172-178.
[167] Lau HY, Bhatia M. Effect of CP-96,345 on the expression of adhesion molecules in acute pancreatitis in mice. Am J Physiol Gastrointest Liver Physiol 2007;292: G1283-G1292.
[168] Pruefer D, Makowski J, Schnell M, Buerke U, Dahm M, Oelert H et al. Simvastatin inhibits inflammatory properties of Staphylococcus aureus alpha-toxin. Circulation 2002;106: 2104-2110.
[169] Zhao JL, Yang YJ, Cui CJ, You SJ, Gao RL. Pretreatment with simvastatin reduces myocardial no-reflow by opening mitochondrial K(ATP) channel. Br J Pharmacol 2006;149: 243-249.
[170] Nomura S, Shouzu A, Omoto S, Nishikawa M, Fukuhara S, Iwasaka T. Losartan and simvastatin inhibit platelet activation in hypertensive patients. J Thromb Thrombolysis 2004;18: 177-185.
[171] Uhlmann D, Gaebel G, Armann B, Ludwig S, Hess J, Pietsch UC et al. Attenuation of proinflammatory gene expression and microcirculatory disturbances by endothelin A receptor blockade after orthotopic liver transplantation in pigs. Surgery 2006;139: 61-72.
[172] Uhlmann D, Gabel G, Ludwig S, Armann B, Hess J, Pietsch UC et al. Effects of ET(A) receptor antagonism on proinflammatory gene expression and microcirculation following hepatic ischemia/reperfusion. Microcirculation 2005;12: 405-419.
[173] Witzigmann H, Ludwig S, Armann B, Gabel G, Teupser D, Kratzsch J et al. Endothelin(A) receptor blockade reduces ischemia/reperfusion injury in pig pancreas transplantation. Ann Surg 2003;238: 264-274.
[174] Werner J, Rivera J, Fernandez-del CC, Lewandrowski K, Adrie C, Rattner DW et al. Differing roles of nitric oxide in the pathogenesis of acute edematous versus necrotizing pancreatitis. Surgery 1997;121: 23-30.
[175] Dobosz M, Hac S, Mionskowska L, Dobrowolski S, Wajda Z. Microcirculatory disturbances of the pancreas in cerulein-induced acute pancreatitis in rats with reference to L-arginine, heparin, and procaine treatment. Pharmacol Res 1997;36: 123-128.
[176] Vollmar B, Janata J, Yamauchi JI, Menger MD. Attenuation of microvascular reperfusion injury in rat pancreas transplantation by L-arginine. Transplantation 1999;67: 950-955.
[177] Christman JW, Sadikot RT, Blackwell TS. The role of nuclear factor-kappa B in pulmonary diseases. Chest 2000;117: 1482-1487.
[178] Orian A, Whiteside S, Israel A, Stancovski I, Schwartz AL, Ciechanover A. Ubiquitin-mediated processing of NF-kappa B transcriptional activator precursor p105. Reconstitution of a cell-free system and identification of the ubiquitin-carrier protein, E2, and a novel ubiquitin-protein ligase, E3, involved in conjugation. J Biol Chem 1995;270: 21707-21714.
[179] Eibl G, Buhr HJ, Foitzik T. Therapy of microcirculatory disorders in severe acute pancreatitis: what mediators should we block? Intensive Care Med 2002;28: 139-146.

[180] Kingsnorth AN, Galloway SW, Formela LJ. Randomized, double-blind phase II trial of Lexipafant, a platelet-activating factor antagonist, in human acute pancreatitis. Br J Surg 1995;82: 1414-1420.
[181] Bloechle C, Kusterer K, Kuehn RM, Schneider C, Knoefel WT, Izbicki JR. Inhibition of bradykinin B2 receptor preserves microcirculation in experimental pancreatitis in rats. Am J Physiol 1998;274: G42-G51.
[182] Hirano T, Hirano K. Thromboxane A2 receptor antagonist prevents pancreatic microvascular leakage in rats with caerulein-induced acute pancreatitis. Int J Surg Investig 1999;1: 203-210.
[183] von Andrian UH, Mackay CR. T-cell function and migration. Two sides of the same coin. N Engl J Med 2000;343: 1020-1034.
[184] Pereda J, Sabater L, Aparisi L, Escobar J, Sandoval J, Vina J et al. Interaction between cytokines and oxidative stress in acute pancreatitis. Curr Med Chem 2006;13: 2775-2787.

Part 3

Diagnosis

12

Endoscopic Retrograde Cholangiopancreatography-Related Acute Pancreatitis – Identification, Prophylaxis and Treatment

Alejandro González-Ojeda[1], Carlos Dávalos-Cobian[2], Elizabeth Andalón-Dueñas[1], Mariana Chávez-Tostado[1], Arturo Espinosa-Partida[1] and Clotilde Fuentes-Orozco[1]

[1]*Surgical Section of the Research Unit in Clinical Epidemiology, Specialties Hospital, Western Medical Center, Mexican Institute of Social Security, Guadalajara, Jalisco,*
[2]*Department of Gastroenterology and Gastrointestinal Endoscopy, Specialties Hospital, Western Medical Center, Mexican Institute of Social Security, Guadalajara, Jalisco, Mexico*

1. Introduction

Pancreatitis is the most common complication of endoscopic retrograde cholangiopancreatography (ERCP) [1–4]. The reported incidence ranges from 1.8% to 7.2% in most prospective series [5–9] but can be up to 30%, depending on the criteria used to diagnose pancreatitis, the type and duration of patient follow-up, and the type of case mix [10]. More commonly, hyperamylasemia occurs in up to 30% of patients undergoing ERCP [11].
As the indications for ERCP have increased, a greater focus on recognizing and preventing complications has emerged. The recognized complications of ERCP include asymptomatic hyperamylasemia, cardiopulmonary depression, hypoxia, aspiration, intestinal perforation, bleeding, cholangitis, adverse medication reactions, sepsis, acute pancreatitis, and death. Post-ERCP pancreatitis (PEP) remains the leading cause of morbidity and mortality after the procedure and is the focus of studies designed to improve procedural outcomes [12,13]. Some studies have suggested that the rates of PEP can be reduced, but the incidence of pancreatitis remains high particularly in at-risk patient populations. Pancreatitis continues to be the major cause of postprocedure morbidity and mortality [14–17].

2. Diagnosis of PEP

PEP was defined initially as the presence of new pancreatic-type abdominal pain associated with at least a threefold increase in serum amylase concentration occurring 24 h after an ERCP, with pain severe enough to require admission to the hospital or to extend an admitted patient's length of stay. This definition was developed in 1991 based upon approximately 15 000 procedures evaluated during a consensus workshop. The severity of PEP was defined according to the length of stay (mild pancreatitis 2–3 d, moderate pancreatitis 4–10 d, and severe pancreatitis >10 d, or intensive care admission or local complications secondary to pancreatitis) [18]. This consensus definition has not been adopted uniformly and many studies published after 1991 have used different criteria to define PEP and to classify its severity. Several studies have challenged the serum amylase threshold of three times the upper limit of normal, arguing that this definition is not always consistent with the clinical and morphological features of pancreatitis [19–25]. Other criteria for serum amylase elevation include twice [23–26], four times [6,27,28] and five times [20,21,28–30] the upper normal limit.

There is also heterogeneity in the criteria used to classify the severity of PEP in published studies. Some authors have used the Atlanta criteria published in 1993 to define severity [31–33]. The Atlanta criteria incorporate systemic complications of PEP by integrating the Acute Physiologic and Chronic Health Evaluation (APACHE) II classification and Ranson's criteria to define the severity [33–35]. An APACHE II score of >8 or a Ranson's score of ≥3 of 11 criteria are defined as severe PEP. Some studies have used the APACHE II classification alone to grade the severity of PEP [36]. Other studies have used combinations of criteria to define the presence and severity of PEP or have established unique definitions [26,31,37–40]. The heterogeneity of criteria in the literature on PEP hinders direct comparison of the published clinical trials.

3. Pathophysiology of PEP

The pathophysiology of PEP is not well understood. Mechanical, hydrostatic, chemical, enzymatic, allergic, thermal, cytokine, oxidative, and microbiological factors have all been proposed as causes [32,41–46]. Many studies suggest that PEP results from mechanical trauma, causing injury to the papilla or pancreatic sphincter and subsequent swelling of the pancreatic duct and obstruction to the flow of pancreatic enzymes. This hypothesis remains controversial, and no consensus about the pathogenesis of PEP has been established.

The cascade of events leading to acute pancreatitis is characterized by three phases. The first phase is characterized by premature activation of trypsin within the pancreatic acinar cells [47]. The second phase is characterized by intrapancreatic inflammation. The third phase is characterized by extrapancreatic inflammation [47]. Inflammation in the second and third phases has been described as a four-step process: (1) activation of inflammatory cells; (2) chemoattraction of activated inflammatory cells; (3) activation of adhesion molecules causing binding of inflammatory cells to the endothelium; and (4) migration of activated inflammatory cells into areas of inflammation [47]. Recent studies have evaluated proinflammatory markers (TNF, interleukin-1 (IL-1), IL-6, IL-8, PAF, and IL-10) in the setting of PEP [48–51]. Although three randomized controlled trials (RCTs) suggested a protective effect of low- or high-dose (4 μg/kg or 20 μg/kg) IL-10 given intravenously 15–30 min before ERCP [52], subsequent studies using similar IL-10 protocols did not support these findings [53,54]. Although not demonstrated at present, modulation of proinflammatory pathways might be an appealing goal for studies evaluating PEP and the systemic inflammatory response.

4. Procedural-related factors associates with PEP

Although the triggers of the inflammatory cascade are not well understood, procedural- and patient-related factors have been clearly associated with the incidence of PEP. ERCP is the most technically difficult endoscopic procedure performed by trainees and experienced endoscopists in both inpatient and outpatient settings. Whereas trauma to the duodenum or papilla during endoscopy without cannulation rarely causes pancreatitis [55], cannulation of the papilla, especially in moderate to difficult cases, is associated with high rates of PEP. Procedures involving multiple (>1–4) or failed attempts at cannulation, multiple pancreatic injections (≥2–5), pancreatic acinarization, and prolonged cannulation time (>10 min) are associated with PEP. The following factors have also been associated with a higher risk for developing PEP: operator experience, ampullary balloon dilation, precut access sphincterotomy, endoscopic sphincterotomy (ES), sphincter of Oddi manometry, distal common bile duct diameters of ≤1 cm, presence of a pancreatic stricture, papillectomy, and procedures not involving stone removal [45,56–59] (Table 1).

Patient related factors	Young age. Female gender. Suspected sphincter of Oddi dysfunction. Recurrent pancreatitis. Prior history of post-ERCP pancreatitis. Patients with normal serum bilirubin.
Procedure related factors	Multiple pancreatic duct injections. Difficult cannulation. Pancreatic sphincterotomy. Precut access. Balloon dilation.
Operator/technical related factors	Inadequate training and/or experience
	Trainee involvement in procedure

Table 1. Factors Increasing the Risk of Post-ERCP Pancreatitis.

4.1 Operator experience

Although there is no established mandate for the procedure volume to develop competence in ERCP, a prospective study published in 1996 evaluated the number of supervised ERCPs a physician must perform to achieve procedural competence and reported that at least 180 procedures are required [60]. In the United States, the American Society for Gastrointestinal Endoscopy and the American College of Gastroenterology have published quality indicators for ERCP. Competent endoscopists are expected to be able to perform sphincterotomy, clear the common bile duct of stones, provide relief of biliary obstruction, and successfully place stents for bile leaks in ≥85% of patients [61].

Few studies have been published on operator experience in ERCP, and this issue remains controversial. A recent study in Austria showed that a case volume of >50 ERCPs per year had higher success and lower overall complication rates [62]. It is generally agreed that the case mix at high volume and in academic referral centers may include a larger proportion of difficult and high-risk cases, which may confound the relationship between experience and complication rates. Although operator experience is felt to be critical for high-quality outcomes, many large prospective and retrospective trials have not shown consistent correlations between inexperience and PEP. Higher rates of bleeding have been reported after endoscopic sphincterotomy with a mean case volume of <1 per wk [14], and trainee involvement was associated with severe or fatal complications in a recent retrospective analysis [63]. However, a large prospective trial found that case volume had no effect on the incidence of PEP [24]. A prospective study of ERCP in the United Kingdom (UK) in 2007 based on self-reported surveys demonstrated that 15% of all credentialed endoscopists performed <50 ERCPs per year compared with 61% of those in training; 11% of deaths occurred after procedures by endoscopists who performed <50 ERCPs per year. Although the rates of PEP were low at 1.5%, the success rates for bile duct stone extraction and biliary stent placement were 62% and 73%, respectively. The authors concluded that in the UK there is a need for fewer operators and greater experience in those performing therapeutic endoscopy [64]. In the same year, a study in France showed no risk associated with operator inexperience [65].

4.2 Cannulation techniques

Cannulation techniques to access the pancreatic and biliary ducts include the use of a sphincterotome or straight or curved catheter with guide wires or contrast injection. When an initial attempt at cannulation fails, access may be achieved after placement of a pancreatic guide wire or stent to help guide the endoscopist toward the common bile duct and away from the pancreatic duct. Precut access papillotomy is used frequently in referral centers when conventional approaches fail. Rare or experimental techniques such as the use of endoscopic scissors or endoscopic dissection with a cotton swab have been reported but are used rarely in clinical practice [66].

Compared with a standard catheter, the use of a sphincterotome may decrease the number of failed attempts to obtain biliary access, the time required to cannulate the common bile duct, and the rate of PEP [67,68]. Selective sphincterotome cannulation with a guide wire may reduce the rate of PEP compared with cannulation with contrast injection [67–71]. In 2008, a large prospective controlled trial randomized 430 patients into sphincterotome plus guide wire versus conventional cannulation arms. The series demonstrated a significantly higher rate of cannulation with guide wires but failed to show a significant difference in the rate of PEP between the two approaches [72]. The authors reported an 8.8%–14.9% increased risk of PEP after >4 attempts at the papilla, highlighting the importance of cannulation with fewer attempts. These findings are consistent with those of previous studies [7,72].

4.3 Pancreatic duct injection

Multiple pancreatic duct injections (≥2–5) [6,7,15,24,58] and pancreatic acinarization [6,12,15,30] are recognized as risk factors for PEP. Differences in the osmolality and ionicity of contrast media have been studied with varying results in terms of impact on PEP [25,28,59,73–75]. A recent meta-analysis of 13 RCTs found no significant difference between high- and low-osmolality contrast media [75]. Earlier studies suggested that there is a decreased risk of PEP with the use of nonionic contrast agents [73], although this has not been demonstrated consistently [74]. One large retrospective analysis of 14 331 ERCPs suggested that less opacification of the pancreatic duct in the head than in the tail produced significantly lower rates of PEP [59]. Despite the variable findings, clinical trial data suggest that hydrostatic pressure may play a role in the development of pancreatitis.

4.4 Pancreatic duct stenting

The theory that PEP is caused by pancreatic duct obstruction is supported by most RCTs, which show a decreased incidence of pancreatitis in high-risk patients after placement of a pancreatic duct stent [76–84]. The three largest published studies to evaluate the rate of pancreatitis with pancreatic duct stent placement reported significant decreases, by 10.4%, 14.8%, and 52.3%, in the rates of PEP in patients treated with stent placement versus those without stent placement [78,79,85]. Although pancreatic duct stenting decreases the risk of PEP, it has not been shown to prevent it. Despite stent placement, pancreatitis occurs in 2.0%–14% of patients [78,79,81,83,84], and some studies have failed to demonstrate a significant protective effect [59,83,84]. Eight RCTs, multiple prospective uncontrolled studies, and five meta-analyses have compared the rates of pancreatitis after ERCP with and without prophylactic pancreatic stent placement [86–90]. Prophylactic stent placement reduces the incidence of PEP, particularly in high-risk patients, and virtually eliminates the risk of severe pancreatitis.

Many studies have criticized the absence of intent-to-treat analysis (i.e., patients with attempted but unsuccessful stent placement were excluded). However, a meta-analysis showed that the four RCTs used intent-to-treat principles by assuming that PEP developed in patients in whom the attempted prophylactic pancreatic stent placement failed, even when the clinical outcome was not stated in the original study. Despite the use of this approach, the odds ratio in the stent group was 0.44 compared with the controls and differed significantly in favor of stent placement [86]. On the basis of these results, prophylactic stent placement can be considered as the single most important advance in the past 15 years for the prevention of PEP in high-risk patients. Despite these findings, questions remain about when to place a prophylactic pancreatic stent, the type of stent to place, and the optimal follow-up period to ensure adequate removal. The incidence of adverse events associated with pancreatic stent placement is around 4% and must be considered in the decision-making process for the placement of a stent [86,91].

4.5 Biliary stone extraction

In the setting of choledocholithiasis, endoscopic papillary balloon dilatation (EPBD), ES, and mechanical lithotripsy are techniques used to extract obstructing stones. Many studies have shown an increased rate of PEP with EPBD; the rates range from 4.9–20% with EPBD versus 0.42–10% with ES [92–95]. Prospective trials support this observation, although it is difficult to generalize the findings given the many factors that contribute to procedural complications [96–100]. Balloon dilation may also be required in some clinical settings. If a patient has had a prior sphincterotomy and has limited remaining tissue for incision, balloon dilation may be necessary to enlarge the bile duct insertion and enable stone extraction.

5. Patient-related risk factors associated with PEP

Given the high risk of PEP in certain populations, identifying a clear indication is critical for reducing the complication rate. ERCP is riskiest in patients who need it the least [101,102].

Large prospective trials have demonstrated that being female, being younger than 60–70 years, and having suspected sphincter of Oddi dysfunction (SOD) or a recurrent or prior PEP are associated with a higher risk of PEP [6,9,15,24,45,87,103,104] (Table 1). However, there is some variability between studies. For example, one smaller trial suggested an age of <50 years as a significant risk factor [104]. A recent large retrospective study of 16 855 patients reported that the highest rates of PEP occurred in patients with SOD, but the rate was not significantly higher in younger patients or in women [63]. Alternatively, a meta-analysis evaluating five patient-related risk factors demonstrated relative risks of SOD of 4.09 (95% CI, 1.93–3.12; P<0.001) and of being female of 2.23 (95% CI, 1.75–2.84; P<0.001) [87]. One study demonstrated a 10-fold increase in the risk of PEP in patients with SOD [105]. Some factors may be protective as well. The absence of chronic pancreatitis [57], presence of obesity [106], older age (>80 years) [107], and a history of alcohol consumption or cigarette smoking may be associated with a lower risk of PEP [108]. Proper patient selection and identification of patients at higher risk are the most effective means for reducing the incidence of PEP.

6. Pharmacological agents evaluated for the prevention or reduction of PEP

The effects of pharmacological agents on PEP have attracted much interest. Preventing cellular injury and pancreatic tissue auto-digestion may involve blocking the premature activation of proteolytic enzymes within the acinar cells [14,45,109–116]. Although conceptually straightforward, the goal of blocking this activation has been difficult to achieve. Multiple trials have been performed with the goal of reducing the incidence or severity of PEP. About 34 pharmacological agents and procedures (e.g., topical application of pharmacological agents injected or sprayed onto the papilla) have been evaluated for their potential to prevent PEP in controlled trials. Most clinical trials have been disappointing, and only a minority of studies has demonstrated benefit (Table 2-5) [26,29,37,39,40,53,54,58,87,117–175].

In two of five prospective trials, allopurinol was shown to decrease the incidence of PEP [119,120]. In these trials showing benefits, allopurinol was given in 300 mg or 600 mg doses 15 h and 3 h before ERCP. When reviewing other studies of allopurinol, these effects were not significant in patients dosed on different 4 h and 1 h regimens and with varying dose concentrations of allopurinol [121–123]. This suggests that both the dose and timing of allopurinol administration are important in reducing the risk of PEP.

Three meta-analyses have been published using data obtained from four prospective, randomized, placebo-controlled studies that compared rectally administered diclofenac or indomethacin at a dose of 100 mg versus placebo [124–126]. No statistical heterogeneity was detected between the studies. Two RCTs evaluated the effect of rectal administration of 100 mg diclofenac immediately after the procedure [39,143], and the other two evaluated rectal administration of 100 mg indomethacin immediately before the procedure [144,145]. Both sets of studies showed similar results. Patients who were considered to be at high risk for PEP were included in both studies. Overall, PEP occurred in 20/456 (4.4%) patients in the treatment groups versus 57/456 (12.5%) patients in the placebo groups. The estimated pooled relative risk was 0.36 (95% CI, 0.22–0.60), and the number needed to treat to prevent one episode of PEP was 15. The administration of nonsteroidal anti-inflammatory drugs (NSAIDs) was associated with a similar decrease in the incidence of PEP regardless of risk. No adverse event attributable to NSAIDs has been reported. A trial evaluating diclofenac 50

Agent	Author	Factor studied	*n*	Overall	Control	Intervention	*P*value
			Rate of post-ERCP pancreatitis (%)				
STEROIDS							
Hydrocortisone							
	Kwanngern[130]	Hydrocortisone 100 mg IV at 1 h before ERCP	120	6.67	11.86	1.64	0.031
	Manolakopoulos[131] MC	Hydrocortisone 100 mg IV at 30 min before ERCP	340	10.00	13.00	7.10	0.380
	De Palma[26]	Hydrocortisone 100 mg IV immediately before ERCP	529	5.30	4.90	5.70	NS
Prednisone							
	Sherman[132] MC	Prednisone 40 mg PO at 15 h and at 3 h before ERCP	1115	15.07	13.60	16.60	0.190
	Budzyńska[123]	Prednisone 40 mg at 15 h; 40 mg at 3 h before ERCP		10.70	7.90	12.00	0.330
Methylprednisolone							
	Dumot[118]	Methylprednisolone 125 mg IV immediately before ERCP	286	NR	8.70	12.40	0.340
NSAID´s							
Diclofenac							
	Khoshbaten[143]	Diclofenac 100 mg PR immediately after ERCP	100	15.00	26.00	4.00	< 0.010
	Cheon[146]	Diclofenac 50 mg PO at 30-90 min before and at 4-6 h after ERCP	207	16.40	16.70	16.20	NS
	Murray[39]	Diclofenac 100 mg PR immediately after ERCP	220	11.00	15.45	6.36	0.049
	Senol[147]	Diclofenac 75 mg IV immediately after ERCP	80	12.5	17.5	7.5	0.176
Indomethacin							
	Sotoudehmanesh[145]	Indomethacin 100 mg PR before ERCP	442	4.98	6.78	3.16	OR 0.4 (0.2 - 1.1)
	Montaño-Loza[144]	Indomethacin 100 mr PR before ERCP	150	10.6	16	5.3	0.034
ANTIOXIDANTS							
Allopurinol							
	Martinez-Torres [119]	Allopurinol 300 mg PO at 15 h; 300 mg PO at 3 h before ERCP	170	6.47	9.40	2.30	0.049
	Romagnuolo[121] MC	Allopurinol 300 mg PO at 1 h before ERCP	586	NR	4.10	5.50	0.440
	Katsinelos[120]	Allopurinol 600 mg PO at 15 h; 600 mg PO at 3 h before ERCP	243	10.20	17.80	3.20	< 0.001
	Mosler[122]	Allopurinol 600 mg PO at 4 h; 300 mg PO at 1 h before ERCP	346	12.55	12.14	12.96	0.520
	Budzynska[123]	Allopurinol 200 mg PO at 15 h; 200 mg PO at 3 h before ERCP	300	10.70	7.90	12.10	0.320
N-acetylcystine							
	Milewski[134]	NAC 600 mg IV BID × 2 d after ERCP	106	9.43	11.76	7.27	NS
	Katsinelos[135]	NAC 70 mg/kg 2 h before and 35 mg/kg 4 h intervals for 24 h after procedure	249	10.80	9.60	12.10	> 0.500
ANTIBIOTICS							
Cephtazidime							
	Räty[129]	Cephtazidime 2g IV 30 min before ERCP	321	NR	9.38	2.58	0.009
INTERLEUKIN-10							
Interlukin-10							
	Sherman[54]MC	IL-10 8 μg/kg IV 15-30 min before ERCP	305	17.38	14.30	15.40	0.830
		IL-10 20 μg/kg IV 15-30 min before ERCP				22.00	0.140
	Devière[52]	IL-10 4 μg/kg IV 30 min before ERCP	144	29.90	24.40	10.41	0.046
		IL-10 20 μg/kg IV 30 min before ERCP				6.81	0.017
	Dumot[53]	IL-10 8 μg/kg IV 15 min before ERCP	200	10.00	9.10	10.90	0.650

PEP: Post-ERCP pancreatitis; ERCP: Endoscopic retrograde cholangiopancreatography; IL-10: Ingerlukin-10; NAC: N-acetyl cystine; NS: Not significant;
NR: Not reported/unable to acquire primary data from publication; MC: Multi-centered.

Table 2. Randomized controlled trails of drugs that decrease inflammation evaluated for reduction or prevention of post-ERCP pancreatitis.

			Rate of post-ERCP pancreatitis (%)				
Agent	Author	Factor studied	*n*	Overall	Control	Intervention	*P*value
Heparin							
	Barkay[37]	Unfractionated heparin 5000 IU SC 20-30 min before ERCP	106	NR	7.40	7.80	NS
	Rabenstein[133]	Low molecular weight heparin Certoparin 3000 IU SC the day before ERCP	448	8.50	8.81	8.14	0.870
Gabexate							
	Ueki[159]	Gabexate 600 mg IV 60-90 min before and 22 h after ERCP	68	2.90	NR	2.90	NS
	Manes[160]MC	Gabexate mesylate 500 mg within 1 h before ERCP	608	5.60	9.40	3.90	< 0.01
		Gabexate mesylate 500 mg within 1h after ERCP				3.40	< 0.01
	Xiong[161]	Gabexate 300 mg IV 30 min before gtt until 4 h after ERCP	200	6.70	10.50	3.10	0.04
	Fujishiro[162]	Gabexate 900 mg/1500 mL gtt for 13 h beginning 1 h before ERCP	139	NR	NR[a]	4.30	NS
	Andriulli[163]MC	Gabexate 500 mg 30 min before gtt until 6 h after ERCP	1127	5.60	4.80	5.80	NS
	Masci[87]MC	Gabexate 500 mg IV 30 min before gtt until 6.5 h after ERCP and 1 g IV for 13 h after ERCP	434	1.80	2.20	1.40	NS
	Andriulli[163]MC	Gabexate 500 mg IV 30 min before and 2 h after ERCP	579	8.60	6.50	8.10	NS
	Cavallini[164]MC	Gabexate 1 g IV 30-90 min before gtt until 12 h after ERCP	418	5.00	8.00	2.00	0.03
Ulinastatin							
	Yoo[166]	Ulinastatin 100 000 U gtt after ERCP for 5.5 h	227	6.20	5.60	6.70	0.715
	Ueki[159]	Ulinastatin 150 000 units 60-90 min before & for 22 h after ERCP	68	2.90	2.90	2.90	NS
	Fujishiro[162]MC	Ulinastatin 150 000 units 1 h before, during; 11 h after ERCP				6.50	NS
		Ulinastatin 50 000 units				8.50	NS
	Tsujino[167]MC	Ulinastatin 150 000 U gtt 10 min before ERCP	406	5.17	7.40	2.90	0.041

PEP: Post-ERCP pancreatitis; ERCP: Endoscopic retrograde cholangiopancreatography; NS: Not significant;NR: Not reported/unable to acquire primary data from publication; MC: Multi-centered.

Table 3. Randomized controlled trails of drugs that interrupt the activity of proteases evaluated for reduction or prevention of post-ERCP pancreatitis.

Agent	Author	Factor studied	Rate of post-ERCP pancreatitis (%)				
			n	Overall	Control	Intervention	*P*value
Beta-carotene							
	Lavy[127]	Natural beta-carotene 2 g at 12 h before ERCP	321	9.60	9.60	10.00	NR
Octreotide							
	Kisli[149]	Octreotide 0.1 mg gtt 60 min before ERCP and continued during and after ERCP	120	NR	11.49	15.15	NS
	Li[150]	Octreotide 0.3 mg gtt 1 h before -6 h after ERCP; then 0.1 mg SC; 12 h later 0.1 mg SC	832	3.85	5.26	2.42	0.046
	Thomopoulos[151]	Octreotide 500 µg TID starting 24 h before ERCP	201	10.89	8.90	2.00	0.03
	Testoni[152]	Octreotide 200 µg TID × 24 h before ERCP	114	NR	14.30	12.00	NS
	Hardt[153]	Octreotide 200 µg SC the night before ERCP	94	NR	NR	NR	NS
	Duvnjak[154]	Octreotide 0.5 mg SC 60 min before ERCP	209	NR	9.52	3.85	NS
	Arvanitidis[155]	Octreotide 0.1 mg SC 30 min before; 8 h and 16 h after ERCP	73	10.95	11.11	10.81	NS
	Tulassay[40]	Octreotide 0.1 mg SC 45 min after ERCP	1199	7.84	6.00	5.90	NS
	Arcidiacono[156]	Octreotide 0.1 mg SC 120 and 30 min before; 4 h after ERCP	151	6.62	NR	NR	NS
	Baldazzi[157]	Octreotide 0.1 mg SC 45 min before; 6 h after ERCP	100	NR	NR	NR	NR
	Testoni[158]	Octreotide 0.2 mg SC before ERCP	60	NR	NR	NR	NS
	Testoni[29]	Octreotide 200 µg TID × 3 d before ERCP	60	NR	NR	NR	NS
Somatostatin							
	Lee[171]MC	Somatostatin 3 mg in 500 mL NS gtt 12 h starting 30min before ERCP	391	6.65	9.60	3.60	0.02
	Andriulli[58]MC	Somatostatin 750 µg IV 30 min before and continued for 6 h after ERCP				6.30	NS
	Arvanitidis[172]	Somatostatin 4 µg/kg gtt 12 h on identification of the papilla and before introduction of the catheter	372	NR	9.80	1.70	< 0.05
		Somatostatin 3 mg gtt 12 h on identification of the papilla and before introduction of the catheter				1.70	< 0.05
	Poon[173]	Somatostatin 250 mg IV bolus immediately after ERCP	270	NR	13.30	4.40	0.01
	Andriulli[163]MC	Somatostatin 750 µg IV 30 min before and 2 h after ERCP				11.50	NS
	Poon[174]	Somatostatin 3 mg in 500 mL NS gtt for 12 h starting 30 min before ERCP	220	5.91	10.00	3.00	0.03
	Bordas[175]	Natural somatostatin 4 mg/kg IV on identification of the papilla and before introduction of the catheter	160	NR	10.00	2.50	< 0.05

PEP: Post-ERCP pancreatitis; ERCP: Endoscopic retrograde cholangiopancreatography; NS: Not significant; NR: Not reported/unable to acquire primary data from publication; MC: Multi-centered.

Table 4. Randomized controlled trails of inhibitors of pancreatic secretion evaluated for reduction or prevention of post-ERCP pancreatitis.

Agent	Author	Factor studied	Rate of post-ERCP pancreatitis (%) *n*	Overall	Control	Intervention	*P*value
Injected Botulinum toxin							
	Gorelick[128]	Botulinum toxin injection after biliary sphincterotomy	26	NR	43.00	25.00	0.340
Nifedipine							
	Prat[136]	Nifedipine 20 mg PO 3-6 h before ERCP	155	15.50	17.70	13.20	NS
	Sand[137]	Nifedipine 20 mg PO q 8 h the day of ERCP	166	3.61	4.00	4.00	NR
Nitroglycerin							
	Hao[138]	Glyceryl trinitrate 5 mg IV and 100 mg vitamin C 5 min before ERCP maneuvers	74	16.20	25.00	7.90	0.012
	Beauchant[139]MC	Nitroglycerin bolus of 0.1 mg, then 35 g/kg/min IV for 6 h after ERCP	208	12.00	15.00	10.00	0.260
	Kaffes[140]	Transdermal glyceryl trinitrate patch (15 mg) precordial area 30-40 min before ERCP	318	NR	7.40	7.70	NS
	Moretó[141]	Transdermal glyceryl trinitrate patch (15 mg) precordial area 30-40 min before ERCP	144	9.00	15.00	4.00	0.030
	Sudhindran[142]	Glyceryl trinitrate 2 mg SL 5 min before ERCP	186	13.00	18.00	8.00	< 0.050
Nafamostat mesylate							
	Choi[165]	Nafamostat mesylate 20 mg gtt 1 h before and for 24 h after ERCP	704	5.40	7.40	3.30	0.018
Pentoxifylline							
	Kapetanos[168]	Pentoxifylline 400 mg PO TID before ERCP	320	4.38	3.00	5.60	0.28
Recombinant PAF acetylhydrolase							
	Sherman[169]MC	Recombinant PAF acetylhydrolase (rPAF-AH) 1 mg/kg gtt< 1 h before ERCP	600	17.60	19.60	17.50	0.59
		Recombinant PAF acetylhydrolase (rPAF-AH) 5 mg/kg gtt< 1 h before ERCP				15.90	0.34
Semapimod							
	van Westerloo[170]	Semapimod IV 50 mg/100 mL glucose gtt 1 h before ERCP	242	11.98	14.88	9.09	0.117
SpryedEpineprine							
	Matsushita[117]	Epinephrine (10 mL of 0.02%) sprayed on papilla before cannulation	370	1.10	2.16	0.00	0.00 0.123
SprayedLidocaine							
	Schwartz[176]	Lidocaine (10 mL of 1%) sprayed on the major papilla before cannulation	294	4.08	3.04	4.32	0.73

ERCP: Endoscopic retrograde cholangiopancreatography; NS: Not significant;NR: Not reported/unable to acquire primary data from publication; MC: Multi-centered.

Table 5. Randomized controlled trails of drugs that decrease Sphincter of Oddi Pressure and miscellaneous drugs evaluated for reduction or prevention of post-ERCP pancreatitis.

mg by mouth given 30–90 min before ERCP and up to 4–6 h after ERCP showed no decrease in the incidence of PEP [146]. A small clinical trial by Senol and colleagues found no significant difference in the incidence of PEP in patients given ERCP with the use of 75 mg of diclofenac by the intramuscular route plus intravenous (IV) hydration versus those given placebo and IV solutions [147]. According to the European Society of Gastrointestinal Endoscopy, no other drug prophylaxis has been proven to be effective against PEP as rectal NSAIDs [148].

Glyceryl trinitrate [141], hydrocortisone [130], and IL-10 [52] were shown to be beneficial in one RCT. However, studies with larger numbers of patients [26,54,140] found no significant effects of these treatments. Gabexate [160,161,163], octreotide [150,151], somatostatin [171,174], and ulinastatin [167] have all been reported to reduce the incidence of PEP. However, studies evaluating each of these agents using similar designs have reported no significant reduction in the incidence of PEP. These differences might be explained by differences in the selection and number of patients, clinical presentation, and timing of administration or dosage of the agents under investigation.

7. Management of PEP

Not all patients with pain and hyperamylasemia following ERCP have acute pancreatitis, and clinicians may have difficulty establishing the diagnosis. As a result, some patients with severe post-ERCP pancreatitis may not be identified in the early stages of their illness when aggressive hydration is most important. Some endoscopists may have difficulty acknowledging that post-ERCP pancreatitis has occurred, as this requires accepting that there has been a complication. A sense of guilt on the part of the clinician performing the procedure is understandable. However, delay in either the diagnosis or treatment of post-ERCP pancreatitis may lead to adverse consequences.

Post-ERCP pancreatitis should be managed as for other causes of acute pancreatitis. This is sometimes complicated by the difficulty distinguishing mild from severe disease in the early stages. The elevations in serum amylase and lipase levels do not always correlate with disease severity.

Mild and moderate PEP usually resolve quickly with conservative therapy. Although there are no specific guidelines for the treatment of PEP, a recent study found that a protocol-based management strategy was associated with less severe pancreatitis, shorter length of hospital stay, the need for fewer imaging studies, and less use of antibiotics [109,177].

Practice guidelines for acute pancreatitis treatment are available and may be applicable to PEP as well [47]. In patients with persistent or severe PEP, two important markers of severity are multisystem organ failure and pancreatic necrosis, both of which require aggressive management [18]. Early identification of organ failure, pancreatic necrosis, perforation (especially in the setting of endoscopic sphincterotomy), biliary damage/leak and pancreatic fluid collections are important clinical branch points that may require more intensive intervention. Checking the levels of serum transaminases, amylase, and lipase is not routinely recommended after ERCP, but if assessed, postprocedure elevations occur often. These elevations are likely to be secondary to intermittent biliary, pancreatic, or papillary obstruction. In a recent study, 46% of patients had elevated liver test results after ERCP, but only 5.4% had PEP [110]. Asymptomatic elevation of liver markers is not an indication for a change in management and a repeat ERCP should be performed only with a clear indication. Although the use of enteral feeding during treatment of acute pancreatitis is controversial, patients who are unlikely to resume oral nutrition within 5 days require nutritional support, which can be provided via total parenteral nutrition or enteral routes [177]. There appear to be some advantages to enteral feeding. A recent study found that initiating oral nutrition after mild acute pancreatitis with a low-fat soft diet appeared to be safe but did not shorten the length of hospitalization [111].

8. Conclusion

Acute pancreatitis is a well-recognized and frequent complication that can occur in 1%–15% of patients undergoing ERCP. Clinical research to prevent PEP using depurate endoscopic techniques and pharmacological prophylaxis is intense and so far indicates that the use of NSAIDs and pancreatic stenting, coupled with appropriate selection of eligible patients and performed by an experienced endoscopist are the most effective preventive measures to reduce the incidence and severity this complication.

9. References

[1] Freeman ML, DiSario JA, Nelson DB, Fennerty MB, Lee JG, Bjorkman DJ, et al. Risk factors for post-ERCP pancreatitis: a prospective, multicenter study. Gastrointest Endosc 2001;54(4):425-34.
[2] Rabenstein T, Hahn EG. Post-ERCP pancreatitis: New momentum. Endoscopy 2002; 34: 325-9.
[3] Frank CD, Adler DG. Post-ERCP Pancreatitis and its prevention. Nat Clin Pract Gastroenterol Hepatol 2006;3:680-8.
[4] LaFerla G, Gordon S , Archibald M, Murray WR. Hyperamylasaemia and acute pancreatitis following endoscopic retrograde cholangiopancreatography. Pancreas. 1986;1(2):160-63.
[5] Badalov N, Tenner S, Baillie J. The Prevention, recognition and treatment of post-ERCP pancreatitis. JOP. 2009;10(2):88-97.
[6] Vandervoort J, Soetikno RM, Tham TC, Wong RC, Ferrari AP Jr, Montes H, et al. Risk factors for complications after performance of ERCP. Gastrointest Endosc. 2002;56(5):652-6.
[7] García-Cano Lizcano J, González Martín JA, Morillas Ariño J, Pérez Sola A. Complications of endoscopic retrograde cholangiopancreatography. A study in a small ERCP unit. Rev Esp Enferm Dig. 2004;96(3):163-73.
[8] Cheng CL, Sherman S, Watkins JL, Barnett J, Freeman M, Geenen J, et al. Risk factors for post-ERCP pancreatitis: a prospective multicenter study. Am J Gastroenterol. 2006;101(1):139-47.
[9] Williams EJ, Taylor S, Fairclough P, Hamlyn A, Logan RF, Martin D, et al. Risk factors for complication following ERCP; results of a large-scale, prospective multicenter study. Endoscopy. 2007;39(9):793-801.
[10] Freeman ML, Guda NM. Prevent ion of post - ERCP pancreatitis: a comprehensive review. Gastrointest Endosc. 2004;59(7):845-64
[11] Ito K, Fujita N, Noda Y, Kobayashi G, Horaguchi J, Takasawa O, Obana T.Relationship between post-ERCP pancreatitis and the change of serum amylase level after the procedure. World J Gastroenterol 2007; 13:3855-60.

[12] Bilbao MK, Dotter CT, Lee TG, Katon RM. Complications of endoscopic retrograde cholangiopancreatography (ERCP). A study of 10,000 cases. Gastroenterology. 1976;70(3):314-20.
[13] Skude G, Wehlin L, Maruyama T, Ariyama J. Hyperamylasaemia after duodenoscopy and retrograde cholangiopancreatography. Gut. 1976;17(2):127-32.
[14] Silviera ML, Seamon MJ, Porshinsky B, Prosciak MP, Doraiswamy VA, Wang CF, et al. Complications related to endoscopic retrograde cholangiopancreatography: a comprehensive clinical review. J Gastrointestin Liver Dis. 2009;18(1):73-82.
[15] Wang P, Li ZS, Liu F, Ren X, Lu NH, Fan ZN, et al. Risk factors for ERCP-related complications: a prospective multicenter study. Am J Gastroenterol. 2009;104(1):31-40.
[16] Cohen S, Bacon BR, Berlin JA, Fleischer D, Hecht GA, Loehrer PJ Sr, et al. National Institutes of Health State-of-the-Science Conference Statement: ERCP for diagnosis and therapy, January 14-16, 2002. Gastrointest Endosc. 2002;56(6):803-9.
[17] Brugge WR, Van Dam J. Pancreatic and biliary endoscopy. N Engl J Med. 1999;341(24):1808-16.
[18] Cotton PB, Lehman G, Vennes J, Geenen JE, Russell RC, Meyers WC, et al. Endoscopic sphincterotomy complications and their management: an attempt at consensus. Gastrointest Endosc. 1991;37(3):383-93.
[19] Testoni PA, Bagnolo F, Caporuscio S, Lella F. Serum amylase measured four hours after endoscopic sphincterotomy is a reliable predictor of postprocedure pancreatitis. Am J Gastroenterol. 1999;94(5):1235-41.
[20] Testoni PA, Cicardi M, Bergamaschini L, Guzzoni S, Cugno M, Buizza M, et al. Infusion of C1-inhibitor plasma concentrate prevents hyperamylasemia induced by endoscopic sphincterotomy. Gastrointest Endosc. 1995;42(4):301-5.
[21] Testoni PA, Bagnolo F. Pain at 24 hours associated with amylase levels greater than 5 times the upper normal limit as the most reliable indicator of post-ERCP pancreatitis. Gastrointest Endosc. 2001;53(1):33-9.
[22] Testoni PA, Bagnolo F, Natale C, Primignani M. Incidence of post-endoscopic retrograde-cholangiopancreatography/sphincterotomy pancreatitis depends upon definition criteria. Dig Liver Dis. 2000;32(5):412-8.
[23] Weiner GR, Geenen JE, Hogan WJ, Catalano MF. Use of corticosteroids in the prevention of post-ERCP pancreatitis. Gastrointest Endosc. 1995;42(6):579-83.
[24] Freeman ML, Nelson DB, Sherman S, Haber GB, Herman ME, Dorsher PJ, et al. Complications of endoscopic biliary sphincterotomy. N Engl J Med. 1996;335(13):909-18.
[25] Johnson GK, Geenen JE, Johanson JF, Sherman S, Hogan WJ, Cass O. Evaluation of post-ERCP pancreatitis: potential causes noted during controlled study of differing contrast media. Midwest Pancreaticobiliary Study Group. Gastrointest Endosc. 1997;46(3):217-22.
[26] De Palma GD, Catanzano C. Use of corticosteriods in the prevention of post-ERCP pancreatitis: results of a controlled prospective study. Am J Gastroenterol. 1999;94(4):982-5.
[27] Sherman S, Ruffolo TA, Hawes RH, Lehman GA. Complications of endoscopic sphincterotomy. A prospective series with emphasis on the increased risk

associated with sphincter of Oddi dysfunction and nondilated bile ducts. Gastroenterology. 1991;101(4):1068-75.
[28] Sherman S, Hawes RH, Rathgaber SW, Uzer MF, Smith MT, Khusro QE, et al. Post-ERCP pancreatitis: randomized, prospective study comparing a low- and high-osmolality contrast agent. Gastrointest Endosc. 1994;40(4):422-427.
[29] Testoni PA, Lella F, Bagnolo F, Caporuscio S, Cattani L, Colombo E, et al. Long-term prophylactic administration of octreotide reduces the rise in serum amylase after endoscopic procedures on Vater's papilla. Pancreas. 1996;13(1):61-5.
[30] Masci E, Toti G, Mariani A, Curioni S, Lomazzi A, Dinelli M, et al. Complications of diagnostic and therapeutic ERCP: a prospective multicenter study Am J Gastroenterol. 2001;96(2):417-23.
[31] Abid GH, Siriwardana HP, Holt A, Ammori BJ. Mild ERCP induced and non-ERCP-related acute pancreatitis: two distinct clinical entities? J Gastroenterol. 2007;42(2):146-51.
[32] Chen CC, Wang SS, Lu RH, Lu CC, Chang FY, Lee SD. Early changes of serum proinflammatory and anti-inflammatory cytokines after endoscopic retrograde cholangiopancreatography. Pancreas. 2003;26(4):375-80.
[33] Bradley EL 3rd. A clinically based classification system for acute pancreatitis. Summary of the International Symposium on Acute Pancreatitis, Atlanta, Ga, September 11 through 13, 1992. Arch Surg. 1993;128(5):586-90.
[34] Knaus WA, Zimmerman JE, Wagner DP, Draper EA, Lawrence DE. APACHE-acute physiology and chronic health evaluation: a physiologically based classification system. Crit Care Med. 1981;9(8):591-7.
[35] Ranson JH, Rifkind KM, Roses DF, Fink SD, Eng K, Spencer FC. Prognostic signs and the role of operative management in acute pancreatitis. Surg Gynecol Obstet. 1974;139(1):69-81.
[36] Bhatia V, Garg PK, Tandon RK, Madan K. Endoscopic retrograde cholangiopancreatography-induced acute pancreatitis often has a benign outcome. J Clin Gastroenterol. 2006;40(8):726-31.
[37] Barkay O, Niv E, Santo E, Bruck R, Hallak A, Konikoff FM. Low-dose heparin for the prevention of post-ERCP pancreatitis: a randomized placebo-controlled trial. Surg Endosc. 2008;22(9):1971-76.
[38] Conwell DL, O'Connor JB, Ferguson DR, Vargo JJ, Barnes DS, et al. Pretreatment with methylprednisolone to prevent ERCP-induced pancreatitis: a randomized, multicenter, placebo-controlled clinical trial. Am J Gastroenterol. 1998;93(1):61-5.
[39] Murray B, Carter R, Imrie C, Evans S, O'Suilleabhain C. Diclofenac reduces the incidence of acute pancreatitis after endoscopic retrograde cholangiopancreatography. Gastroenterology. 2003;124(7):1786-91.
[40] Tulassay Z, Döbrönte Z, Prónai L, Zágoni T, Juhász L. Octreotide in the prevention of pancreatic injury associated with endoscopic cholangiopancreatography. Aliment Pharmacol Ther. 1998;12(11):1109-12.
[41] Sherman S, Lehman GA. ERCP and endoscopic sphincterotomy-induced pancreatitis. Pancreas. 1991;6(3):350-67.
[42] Pezzilli R, Romboli E, Campana D, Corinaldesi R. Mechanisms involved in the onset of post-ERCP pancreatitis. JOP. 2002;3(6):162-8.

[43] Messmann H, Vogt W, Holstege A, Lock G, Heinisch A, von Fürstenberg A, et al. Post-ERP pancreatitis as a model for cytokine induced acute phase response in acute pancreatitis. Gut. 1997;40(1):80-5.
[44] Oezcueruemez-Porsch M, Kunz D, Hardt PD, Fadgyas T, Kress O, Schulz HU, et al. Diagnostic relevance of interleukin pattern, acute-phase proteins, and procalcitonin in early phase of post-ERCP pancreatitis. Dig Dis Sci. 1998;43(8):1763-69.
[45] Cooper ST, Slivka A. Incidence, risk factors, and prevention of post-ERCP pancreatitis. Gastroenterol Clin North Am. 2007;36(2):259-76.
[46] Mohseni Salehi Monfared SS, Vahidi H, Abdolghaffari AH, Nikfar S, Abdollahi M. Antioxidant therapy in the management of acute, chronic and post-ERCP pancreatitis: a systematic review. World J Gastroenterol 2009;15:4481-90.
[47] Banks PA, Freeman ML; Practice Parameters Committee of the American College of Gastroenterology. Practice guidelines in acute pancreatitis. Am J Gastroenterol. 2006;101(10):2379-400.
[48] Kilciler G, Musabak U, Bagci S, Yesilova Z, Tuzun A, Uygun A, et al. Do the changes in the serum levels of IL-2, IL-4, TNFalpha, and IL-6 reflect the inflammatory activity in the patients with post-ERCP pancreatitis? Clin Dev Immunol. 2008;2008:481560.
[49] Sultan S, Baillie J. What are the predictors of post-ERCP pancreatitis, and how useful are they? JOP. 2002;3(6):188-94.
[50] Demols A, Deviere J. New frontiers in the pharmacology prevention of post-ERCP pancreatitis: the cytokines. JOP. 2003;4(1):49-57.
[51] Pande H, Thuluvath P. Pharmacological prevention of postendoscopic retrograde cholangiopancreatography pancreatitis. Drugs. 2003;63(17):1799-812.
[52] Devière J, Le Moine O, Van Laethem JL, Eisendrath P, Ghilain A, Severs N, et al. Interleukin 10 reduces the incidence of pancreatitis after therapeutic endoscopic retrograde cholangiopancreatography. Gastroenterology. 2001;120(2):498-505.
[53] Dumot JA, Conwell DL, Zuccaro G Jr, Vargo JJ, Shay SS, Easley KA, et al. A randomized, double blind study of interleukin 10 for the prevention of ERCP-induced pancreatitis. Am J Gastroenterol. 2001;96(7):2098-102.
[54] Sherman S, Cheng CL, Costamagna G, Binmoeller KF, Puespoek A, Aithal GP, et al. Efficacy of recombinant human interleukin-10 in prevention of post-endoscopic retrograde cholangiopancreatography pancreatitis in subjects with increased risk. Pancreas. 2009;38(3):267-74.
[55] Deschamps JP, Allemand H, Janin Magnificat R, Camelot G, Gillet M, Carayon P. Acute pancreatitis following gastrointestinal endoscopy without ampullary cannulation. Endoscopy. 1982;14(3):105-6.
[56] Williams EJ, Taylor S, Fairclough P, Hamlyn A, Logan RF, Martin D, et al. Risk factors for complication following ERCP; results of a large-scale, prospective multicenter study. Endoscopy. 2007;39(9):793-801.
[57] Freeman ML, DiSario JA, Nelson DB, Fennerty MB, Lee JG, Bjorkman DJ, et al. Risk factors for post-ERCP pancreatitis: a prospective, multicenter study. Gastrointest Endosc. 2001;54(4):425-34.
[58] Andriulli A, Solmi L, Loperfido S, Leo P, Festa V, Belmonte A, et al. Prophylaxis of ERCP-related pancreatitis: a randomized, controlled trial of somatostatin and gabexate mesylate. Clin Gastroenterol Hepatol. 2004;2(8):713-8.

[59] Cheon YK, Cho KB, Watkins JL, McHenry L, Fogel EL, Sherman S, et al. Frequency and severity of post-ERCP pancreatitis correlated with extent of pancreatic ductal opacification. Gastrointest Endosc. 2007;65(3):385-93.
[60] Jowell PS, Baillie J, Branch MS, Affronti J, Browning CL, Bute BP. Quantitative assessment of procedural competence. A prospective study of training in endoscopic retrograde cholangiopancreatography. Ann Intern Med. 1996;125(12):983-9.
[61] Baron Baron TH, Petersen BT, Mergener K, Chak A, Cohen J, Deal SE, et al. Quality indicators for endoscopic retrograde cholangiopancreatography. Am J Gastroenterol. 2006;101(4):892-7.
[62] Kapral C, Duller C, Wewalka F, Kerstan E, Vogel W, Schreiber F. Case volume and outcome of endoscopic retrograde cholangiopancreatography: results of a nationwide Austrian benchmarking project. Endoscopy. 2008;40(8):625-30.
[63] Cotton PB, Garrow DA, Gallagher J, Romagnuolo J. Risk factors for complications after ERCP: a multivariate analysisof 11,497 procedures over 12 years. Gastrointest Endosc. 2009;70(1):80-8.
[64] Williams EJ, Taylor S, Fairclough P, Hamlyn A, Logan RF, Martin D, et al. Are we meeting the standards set for endoscopy? Results of a large-scale prospective survey of endoscopic retrograde cholangio-pancreatograph practice. Gut. 2007;56(6):821-9.
[65] Vitte RL, Morfoisse JJ; Investigator Group of Association Nationale des Gastroentérologues des Hôpitaux Généraux. Evaluation of endoscopic retrograde cholangiopancreatography procedures performed in general hospitals in France. Gastroenterol Clin Biol. 2007;31(8-9 Pt 1):740-9.
[66] Freeman ML, Guda NM. ERCP cannulation: a review of reported techniques. Gastrointest Endosc. 2005;61(1):112-25.
[67] Cortas GA, Mehta SN, Abraham NS, Barkun AN. Selective cannulation of the common bile duct: a prospective randomized trial comparing standard catheters with sphincterotomes. Gastrointest Endosc. 1999;50(6):775-9.
[68] Lella F, Bagnolo F, Colombo E, Bonassi U. A simple way of avoiding post-ERCP pancreatitis. Gastrointest Endosc. 2004;59(7):830-834.
[69] Artifon EL, Sakai P, Cunha JE, Halwan B, Ishioka S, Kumar A. Guidewire cannulation reduces risk of post-ERCP pancreatitis and facilitates bile duct cannulation. Am J Gastroenterol. 2007;102(10):2147-53.
[70] Ito K, Fujita N, Noda Y, Kobayashi G, Obana T, Horaguchi J, et al. Pancreatic guidewire placement for achieving selective biliary cannulation during endoscopic retrograde cholangio-pancreatography. World J Gastroenterol. 2008;14(36):5595-6000.
[71] Lee TH, Park do H, Park JY, Kim EO, Lee YS, Park JH, et al. Can wire-guided cannulation prevent post-ERCP pancreatitis? A prospective randomized trial. Gastrointest Endosc. 2009;69(3 Pt 1):444-9.
[72] Bailey AA, Bourke MJ, Williams SJ, Walsh PR, Murray MA, Lee EY, et al. A prospective randomized trial of cannulation technique in ERCP: effects on technical success and post-ERCP pancreatitis. Endoscopy. 2008;40(4):296-301.
[73] Barkin JS, Casal GL, Reiner DK, Goldberg RI, Phillips RS, Kaplan S. A comparative study of contrast agents for endoscopic retrograde pancreatography. Am J Gastroenterol. 1991;86(10):1437-41.

[74] Johnson GK, Geenen JE, Bedford RA, Johanson J, Cass O, Sherman S, et al. A comparison of nonionic versus ionic contrast media: results of a prospective, multicenter study. Midwest Pancreaticobiliary Study Group. Gastrointest Endosc. 1995;42(4):312-6.

[75] George S, Kulkarni AA, Stevens G, Forsmark CE, Draganov P. Role of osmolality of contrast media in the development of post-ERCP pancreatitis: a metanalysis. Dig Dis Sci. 2004;49(3):503-8.

[76] Tarnasky PR, Palesch YY, Cunningham JT, Mauldin PD, Cotton PB, Hawes RH. Pancreatic stenting prevents pancreatitis after biliary sphincterotomy in patients with sphincter of Oddi dysfunction. Gastroenterology. 1998;115(6):1518-24.

[77] Harewood GC, Pochron NL, Gostout CJ. Prospective, randomized, controlled trial of prophylactic pancreatic stent placement for endoscopic snare excision of the duodenal ampulla. Gastrointest Endosc. 2005;62(3):367-370.

[78] Sofuni A, Maguchi H, Itoi T, Katanuma A, Hisai H, Niido T, et al. Prophylaxis of postendoscopic retrograde cholangiopancreatography pancreatitis by an endoscopic pancreatic spontaneous dislodgement stent. Clin Gastroenterol Hepatol. 2007;5(11):1339-46.

[79] Freeman ML. Pancreatic stents for prevention of postendoscopic retrograde cholangiopancreatography pancreatitis. Clin Gastroenterol Hepatol. 2007;5(11):1354-65.

[80] Tarnasky PR. Mechanical prevention of post-ERCP pancreatitis by pancreatic stents: results, techniques, and indications. JOP. 2003;4(1):58-67.

[81] Fazel A, Quadri A, Catalano MF, Meyerson SM, Geenen JE. Does a pancreatic duct stent prevent post-ERCP pancreatitis?. A prospective randomized study. Gastrointest Endosc. 2003;57(3):291-4.

[82] Simmons DT, Petersen BT, Gostout CJ, Levy MJ, Topazian MD, Baron TH. Risk of pancreatitis following endoscopically placed large-bore plastic biliary stents with and without biliary sphincterotomy for management of postoperative bile leaks. Surg Endosc. 2008;22(6):1459-63.

[83] Smithline A, Silverman W, Rogers D, Nisi R, Wiersema M, Jamidar P, et al. Effect of prophylactic main pancreatic duct stenting on the incidence of biliary endoscopic sphincterotomy-induced pancreatitis in high-risk patients. Gastrointest Endosc 1993; 39: 652-7

[84] Tsuchiya T, Itoi T, Sofuni A, Itokawa F, Kurihara T, Ishii K et al. Temporary pancreatic stent to prevent post endoscopic retrograde cholangiopancreatography pancreatitis: a preliminary, single-center, randomized controlled trial. J Hepatobiliary Pancreat Surg. 2007;14(3):302-307.

[85] Fogel EL, Eversman D, Jamidar P, Sherman S, Lehman GA. Sphincter of Oddi dysfunction: pancreaticobiliary sphincterotomy with pancreatic stent placement has a lower rate of pancreatitis than biliary sphincterotomy alone. Endoscopy. 2002;34(4):280-5.

[86] Andriulli A, Forlano R, Napolitano G, Conoscitore P, Caruso N, Pilotto A, et al. Pancreatic duct stents in the prophylaxis of pancreatic damage after endoscopic retrograde cholangiopancreatography: a systemic analysis of benefits and associated risks. Digestion. 2007;75(2-3):156-163.

[87] Masci E, Mariani A, Curioni S, Testoni PA. Risk factors for pancreatitis following endoscopic retrograde cholangiopancreatography: a meta-analysis. Endoscopy. 2003;35(10):830-4.
[88] Singh P, Das A, Isenberg G, Wong RC, Sivak MV Jr, Agrawal D, et al. Does prophylactic pancreatic stent placement reduce the risk of post-ERCP acute pancreatitis? A meta-analysis of controlled studies. Gastrointest Endosc. 2004;60(4):544-50.
[89] Mazaki T, Masuda H, Takayama T. Prophylactic pancreatic stent placement and post-ERCP pancreatitis: a systematic review and meta-analysis. Endoscopy. 2010;42(10):842-53.
[90] Choudhary A, Bechtold ML, Arif, M, Szary NM, Puli SR, Othman MO, Pais WP, Antillon MR, et al. Pancreatic stents for prophylaxis against post-ERCP pancreatitis: a meta-analysis and systematic review. Gastrointest Endosc. 2011;73(2):275-82.
[91] Deviere J. Pancreatic Stents. Gastrointest Endosc Clin N Am. 2011;21(3):499-510.
[92] Arnold JC, Benz C, Martin WR, Adamek HE, Riemann JF. Endoscopic papillary balloon dilation vs. sphincterotomy for removal of common bile duct stones: a prospective randomized pilot study. Endoscopy. 2001;33(7):563-7.
[93] Disario JA. Endoscopic balloon dilation for extraction of bile duct stones: the devil is in the details. Gastrointest Endosc. 2003;57(2):282-5.
[94] Fujita N, Maguchi H, Komatsu Y, Yasuda I, Hasebe O, Igarashi Y, et al. Endoscopic sphincterotomy and endoscopic papillary balloon dilatation for bile duct stones: A prospective randomized controlled multicenter trial. Gastrointest Endosc 2003; 57: 151-5.
[95] Vlavianos P, Chopra K, Mandalia S, Anderson M, Thompson J, Westaby D. Endoscopic balloon dilatation versus endoscopic sphincterotomy for the removal of bile duct stones: a prospective randomised trial. Gut. 2003;52(8):1165-9.
[96] Song SY, Lee KS, Na KJ, Ahn BH. Tension pneumothorax after endoscopic retrograde pancreatocholangiogram. J Korean Med Sci. 2009;24(1):173-5.
[97] García-Cano J. Fatal pancreatitis after endoscopic balloon dilation for extraction of common bile duct stones in an 80-year-old woman. Endoscopy. 2007;39 Suppl 1:E132.
[98] Mao Z, Zhu Q, Wu W, Wang M, Li J, Lu A, et al. Duodenal perforations after endoscopic retrograde cholangiopancreatography: experience and management. J Laparoendosc Adv Surg Tech A. 2008;18(5):691-5.
[99] Margantinis G, Sakorafas GH, Kostopoulos P, Kontou S, Tsiakos S, Arvanitidis D. Post-ERCP/endoscopic sphincterotomy duodenal perforation is not always a surgical emergency. Dig Liver Dis. 2006;38(6):434-6.
[100] Park DH, Kim MH, Lee SK, Lee SS, Choi JS, Song MH, et al. Endoscopic sphincterotomy vs. endoscopic papillary balloon dilation for choledocholithiasis in patients with liver cirrhosis and coagulopathy. Gastrointest Endosc. 2004;60(2):180-5.
[101] Cotton PB. ERCP is most dangerous for people who need it least. Gastrointest Endosc. 2001;54(4):535-6.
[102] Woods KE, Willingham FF. Endoscopic retrograde cholangiography associated pancreatitis: A 15-year review. World J Gastrointest Endosc 2010;2: 165-78.

[103] Loperfido S, Angelini G, Benedetti G, Chilovi F, Costan F, De Berardinis F, et al. Major early complications from diagnostic and therapeutic ERCP: a prospective multicenter study. Gastrointest Endosc. 1998;48(1):1-10.

[104] Christoforidis E, Goulimaris I, Kanellos I, Tsalis K, Demetriades C, Betsis D. Post-ERCP pancreatitis and hyperamylasemia: patient-related and operative risk factors. Endoscopy. 2002;34(4):286-92.

[105] Tarnasky P, Cunningham J, Cotton P, Hoffman B, Palesch Y, Freeman J, et al. Pancreatic sphincter hypertension increases the risk of post-ERCP pancreatitis. Endoscopy. 1997;29(4):252-7.

[106] Deenadayalu VP, Blaut U, Watkins JL, Barnett J, Freeman M, Geenen J, et al. Does obesity confer an increased risk and/or more severe course of post-ERCP pancreatitis?: a retrospective, multicenter study. J Clin Gastroenterol. 2008;42(10):1103-9.

[107] Lukens FJ, Howell DA, Upender S, Sheth SG, Jafri SM. ERCP in the very elderly: outcomes among patients older than eighty. Dig Dis Sci. 2010;55(3):847-51.

[108] Debenedet AT, Raghunathan TE, Wing JJ, Wamsteker EJ, DiMagno MJ. Alcohol use and cigarette smoking as risk factors for post-endoscopic retrograde cholangiopancreatography pancreatitis. Clin Gastroenterol Hepatol. 2009;7(3):353-8e4.

[109] Reddy N, Wilcox CM, Tamhane A, Eloubeidi MA, Varadarajulu S. Protocol-based medical management of post-ERCP pancreatitis. J Gastroenterol Hepatol. 2008;23(3):385-92.

[110] Silverman WB, Thompson RA. Management of asymptomatically/minimally symptomatic post-ERCP serum liver test elevations: first do no harm. Dig Dis Sci. 2002;47(7):1498-501.

[111] Jacobson BC, Vander Vliet MB, Hughes MD, Maurer R, McManus K, Banks PA. A prospective, randomized trial of clear liquids versus low-fat solid diet as the initial meal in mild acute pancreatitis. Clin Gastroenterol Hepatol. 2007;5(8):946-51.

[112] Dundee PE, Chin-Lenn L, Syme DB, Thomas PR. Outcomes of ERCP: prospective series from a rural centre. ANZ J Surg. 2007;77(11):1013-7.

[113] Barthet M, Lesavre N, Desjeux A, Gasmi M, Berthezene P, Berdah S, et al. Complications of endoscopic sphincterotomy: results from a single tertiary referral center. Endoscopy. 2002;34(12):991-7.

[114] Andriulli A, Loperfido S, Napolitano G, Niro G, Valvano MR, Spirito F, et al. Incidence rates of post- ERCP complications: a systematic survey of prospective studies. Am J Gastroenterol. 2007;102(8):1781-8.

[115] Disario JA, Freeman ML, Bjorkman DJ, Macmathuna P, Petersen BT, Jaffe PE, et al. Endoscopic balloon dilation compared with sphincterotomy for extraction of bile duct stones. Gastroenterology. 2004;127(5):1291-9.

[116] Bergman JJ, Rauws EA, Fockens P, van Berkel AM, Bossuyt PM, Tijssen JG, et al. Randomised trial of endoscopic balloon dilation versus endoscopic sphincterotomy for removal of bileduct stones. Lancet. 1997;349(9059):1124-9.

[117] Matsushita M, Takakuwa H, Shimeno N, Uchida K, Nishio A, Okazaki K. Epinephrine sprayed on the papilla for prevention of post-ERCP pancreatitis. J Gastroenterol 2009; 44: 71-5

[118] Dumot JA, Conwell DL, O'Connor JB, Ferguson DR, Vargo JJ, Barnes DS, et al. Pretreatment with methylprednisolone to prevent ERCP-induced pancreatitis: a randomized, multicenter, placebo-controlled clinical trial. Am J Gastroenterol 1998; 93: 61-5.

[119] Martinez-Torres H, Rodriguez-Lomeli X, Davalos-Cobian C, Garcia-Correa J, Maldonado-Martinez JM, Medrano-Muñoz F, et al. Oral allopurinol to prevent hyperamylasemia and acute pancreatitis after endoscopic retrograde cholangiopancreatography. World J Gastroenterol. 2009;15(13):1600-6.

[120] Katsinelos P, Kountouras J, Chatzis J, Christodoulou K, Paroutoglou G, Mimidis K, et al. Highdose allopurinol for prevention of post-ERCP pancreatitis: a prospective randomized double-blind controlled trial. Gastrointest Endosc. 2005;61(3):407-15.

[121] Romagnuolo J, Hilsden R, Sandha GS, Cole M, Bass S, May G, et al. Allopurinol to prevent pancreatitis after endoscopic retrograde cholangiopancreatography: a randomized placebo-controlled trial. Clin Gastroenterol Hepatol. 2008;6(4):465-71.

[122] Mosler P, Sherman S, Marks J, Watkins JL, Geenen JE, Jamidar P, et al. Oral allopurinol does not prevent the frequency or the severity of post-ERCP pancreatitis. Gastrointest Endosc. 2005;62(2):245-50.

[123] Budzyńska A, Marek T, Nowak A, Kaczor R, Nowakowska-Dulawa E. A prospective, randomized, placebo-controlled trial of prednisone and allopurinol in the prevention of ERCP-induced pancreatitis. Endoscopy. 2001;33(9):766-72.

[124] Dai H-F, Wang X-W, Zhao K. Role of nonsteroidal anti-inflammatory drugs in the prevention of post-ERCP pancreatitis: a meta-analysis. Hepatobiliary Pancreat Dis Int 2009; 8: 11 - 6.

[125] Elmunzer B, Waljee A, Elta G, Taylor JR, Fehmi SM, Higgins PD. A meta-analysis of rectal NSAIDs in the prevention of post-ERCP pancreatitis. Gut 2008; 57: 1262-7.

[126] Zheng M-H, Xia H, Chen Y-P. Rectal administration of NSAIDs in the prevention of post-ERCP pancreatitis: a complementary meta-analysis. Gut 2008; 57: 1632-3.

[127] Lavy A, Karban A, Suissa A, Yassin K, Hermesh I, Ben-Amotz A. Natural beta-carotene for the prevention of post-ERCP pancreatitis. Pancreas 2004; 29(2): e45-e50.

[128] Gorelick A, Barnett J, Chey W, Anderson M, Elta G. Botulinum toxin injection after biliary sphincterotomy. Endoscopy 2004; 36(2): 170-3.

[129] Räty S, Sand J, Pulkkinen M, Matikainen M, Nordback I. Post-ERCP pancreatitis: reduction by routine antibiotics. J Gastrointest Surg 2001; 5(4): 339-45.

[130] Kwanngern K, Tiyapattanaputi P, Wanitpukdeedecha M, Navicharern P. Can a single dose corticosteroid reduce the incidence of post-ERCP pancreatitis? A randomized, prospective control study. J Med Assoc Thai 2005; 88 Suppl 4:S42-5.

[131] Manolakopoulos S, Avgerinos A, Vlachogiannakos J, Armonis A, Viazis N, Papadimitriou N, et al. Octreotide versus hydrocortisone versus placebo in the prevention of post-ERCP pancreatitis: a multicenter randomized controlled trial. Gastrointest Endosc 2002; 55(4):470-5.

[132] Sherman S, Blaut U, Watkins JL, Barnett J, Freeman M, Geenen J, et al. Does prophylactic administration of corticosteroid reduce the risk and severity of post-ERCP pancreatitis: a randomized, prospective, multicenter study. Gastrointest Endosc 2003; 58(1):23-9.

[133] Rabenstein T, Fischer B, Wiessner V, Schmidt H, Radespiel-Tröger M, Hochberger J, et al. Low-molecular-weight heparin does not prevent acute post-ERCP pancreatitis. Gastrointest Endosc. 2004;59(6):606-13.

[134] Milewski J, Rydzewska G, Degowska M, Kierzkiewicz M, Rydzewski A. N-acetylcysteine does not prevent postendoscopic retrograde cholangiopancreatography hyperamylasemia and acute pancreatitis. World J Gastroenterol. 2006;12(23):3751-5.

[135] Katsinelos P, Kountouras J, Paroutoglou G, Beltsis A, Mimidis K, Zavos C. Intravenous N-acetylcysteine does not prevent post-ERCP pancreatitis. Gastrointest Endosc. 2005;62(1):105-11.

[136] Prat F, Amaris J, Ducot B, Bocquentin M, Fritsch J, Choury AD, et al. Nifedipine for prevention of post-ERCP pancreatitis: a prospective, double-blind randomized study. Gastrointest Endosc. 2002;56(2):202-8.

[137] Sand J, Nordback I. Prospective randomized trial of the effect of nifedipine on pancreatic irritation after endoscopic retrograde cholangiopancreatography Digestion. 1993;54(2):105-11.

[138] Hao JY, Wu DF, Wang YZ, Gao YX, Lang HP, Zhou WZ. Prophylactic effect of glyceryl trinitrate on post-endoscopic retrograde cholangiopancreatography pancreatitis: a randomized placebo-controlled trial. World J Gastroenterol. 2009;15(3):366-8.

[139] Beauchant M, Ingrand P, Favriel JM, Dupuychaffray JP, Capony P, Moindrot H, et al.. Intravenous nitroglycerin for prevention of pancreatitis after therapeutic endoscopic retrograde cholangiography: a randomized, double-blind, placebo-controlled multicenter trial. Endoscopy. 2008;40(8):631-6.

[140] Kaffes AJ, Bourke MJ, Ding S, Alrubaie A, Kwan V, Williams SJ. A prospective, randomized, placebo-controlled trial of transdermal glyceryl trinitrate in ERCP: effects on technical success and post-ERCP pancreatitis. Gastrointest Endosc. 2006;64(3):351-7

[141] Moretó M, Zaballa M, Casado I, Merino O, Rueda M, Ramírez K, et al. Transdermal glyceryl trinitrate for prevention of post-ERCP pancreatitis: A randomized double-blind trial. Gastrointest Endosc. 2003;57(1):1-7.

[142] Sudhindran S, Bromwich E, Edwards PR. Prospective randomized double-blind placebo-controlled trial of glyceryl trinitrate in endoscopic retrograde cholangiopancreatography-induced pancreatitis. Br J Surg. 2001;88(9):1178-82.

[143] Khoshbaten M, Khorram H, Madad L, Ehsani Ardakani MJ, Farzin H, Zali MR. Role of diclofenac in reducing post-endoscopic retrograde cholangiopancreatography pancreatitis. J Gastroenterol Hepatol. 2008;23(7 Pt 2):e11-6.

[144] Montaño-Loza A, Rodriguez-Lomeli X, Garcia-Correa J, Fuentes Orozco C, González Ojeda A, Medrano Munoz F, et al. Effect of rectal administration of indomethacin on amylase serum levels after endoscopic retrograde cholangiopancreatography, and its impact on the development of secondary pancreatitis episodes. Rev Esp Enferm Dig 2007;99(6):330–6.

[145] Sotoudehmanesh R, Khatibian M, Kolahdoozan S, Ainechi S, Malboosbaf R, Nouraie M. Indomethacin may reduce the incidence and severity of acute pancreatitis after ERCP. Am J Gastroenterol. 2007;102(5):978-83.

[146] Cheon YK, Cho KB, Watkins JL, McHenry L, Fogel EL, Sherman S, et al. Efficacy of diclofenac in the prevention of post-ERCP pancreatitis in predominantly high-risk

patients: a randomized double blind prospective trial. Gastrointest Endosc. 2007;66(6):1126 - 32.
[147] Senol A, Saritas U, Demirkan H. Efficacy of intramuscular diclofenaco and fluid replacement in prevention of post-ERCP pancreatitis. World J Gastroenterol 2009;15(32):3999-4004.
[148] Dumonceau JM , Andriulli A, Deviere J, Mariani A, Rigaux J , Baron TH, et al. European Society of Gastrointestinal Endoscopy (ESGE) Guideline: Prophylaxis of post-ERCP pancreatitis. Prophylaxis. Endoscopy 2010; 42: 503 – 15
[149] Kisli E, Baser M, Aydin M, Guler O. The role of octreotide versus placebo in the prevention of post-ERCP pancreatitis. Hepatogastroenterology. 2007;54(73):250-3.
[150] Li ZS, Pan X, Zhang WJ, Gong B, Zhi FC, Guo XG, et al. Effect of octreotide administration in the prophylaxis of post-ERCP pancreatitis and hyperamylasemia: A multicenter, placebo-controlled, randomized clinical trial. Am J Gastroenterol. 2007;102(1):46-51.
[151] Thomopoulos KC, Pagoni NA, Vagenas KA, Margaritis VG, Theocharis GI, Nikolopoulou VN. Twenty-four hour prophylaxis with increased dosage of octreotide reduces the incidence of post-ERCP pancreatitis. Gastrointest Endosc. 2006;64(5):726-31.
[152] Testoni PA, Bagnolo F, Andriulli A, Bernasconi G, Crotta S, Lella F, et al. Octreotide 24-h prophylaxis in patients at high risk for post-ERCP pancreatitis: results of a multicenter, randomized, controlled trial. Aliment Pharmacol Ther. 2001;15(7):965-72.
[153] Hardt PD, Kress O, Fadgyas T, Doppl W, Schnell-Kretschmer H, Wüsten O, et al. Octreotide in the prevention of pancreatic damage induced by endoscopic sphincterotomy. Eur J Med Res. 2000;5(4):165-70.
[154] Duvnjak M, Supanc V, Simicević VN, Hrabar D, Troskot B, Smircić-Duvnjak L, et al. Use of octreotideacetate in preventing pancreatitis-like changes following therapeutic endoscopic retrograde cholangiopancreatography. Acta Med Croatica. 1999;53(3):115-8.
[155] Arvanitidis D, Hatzipanayiotis J, Koutsounopoulos G, Frangou E. The effect of octreotide on the prevention of acute pancreatitis and hyperamylasemia after diagnostic and therapeutic ERCP. Hepatogastroenterology. 1998 ;45(19):248-52.
[156] Arcidiacono R, Gambitta P, Rossi A, Grosso C, Bini M, Zanasi G. The use of a long-acting somatostatin analogue (octreotide) for prophylaxis of acute pancreatitis after endoscopic sphincterotomy. Endoscopy. 1994;26(9):715-8.
[157] Baldazzi G, Conti C, Spotti EG, Arisi GP, Scevola M, Gobetti F, et al. Prevention of post-ERCP acute pancreatitis with octreotide. G Chir. 1994;15(8-9):359-62.
[158] Testoni PA, Lella F, Bagnolo F, Buizza M, Colombo E. Controlled trial of different dosages of octreotide in the prevention of hyperamylasemia induced by endoscopic papillosphincterotomy. Ital J Gastroenterol. 1994;26(9):431-6.
[159] Ueki T, Otani K, Kawamoto K, Shimizu A, Fujimura N, Sakaguchi S, et al. Comparison between ulinastatin and gabexate mesylate for the prevention of post-endoscopic retrograde cholangiopancreatography pancreatitis: a prospective, randomized trial. J Gastroenterol. 2007;42(2):161-7.
[160] Manes G, Ardizzone S, Lombardi G, Uomo G, Pieramico O, Porro GB. Efficacy of postprocedure administration of gabexate mesylate in the prevention of post-ERCP

pancreatitis: a randomized, controlled, multicenter study Gastrointest Endosc. 2007;65(7):982-7.

[161] Xiong GS, Wu SM, Zhang XW, Ge ZZ. Clinical trial of gabexate in the prophylaxis of post-endoscopic retrograde cholangiopancreatography pancreatitis. Braz J Med Biol Res. 2006;39(1):85-90

[162] Fujishiro H, Adachi K, Imaoka T, Hashimoto T, Kohge N, Moriyama N, et al. Ulinastatin shows preventive effect on post-endoscopic retrograde cholangiopancreatography pancreatitis in a multicenter prospective randomized study. J Gastroenterol Hepatol. 2006;21(6):1065-9.

[163] Andriulli A, Clemente R, Solmi L, Terruzzi V, Suriani R, Sigillito A, et al. Gabexate or somatostatin administration before ERCP in patients athigh risk for post-ERCP pancreatitis: a multicenter, placebo controlled, randomized clinical trial. Gastrointest Endosc. 2002;56(4):488-95.

[164] Cavallini G, Tittobello A, Frulloni L, Masci E, Mariana A, Di Francesco V. Gabexate for the prevention of pancreatic damage related to endoscopic retrograde cholangiopancreatography. Gabexate in digestive endoscopy--Italian Group. N Engl J Med. 1996;335(13):919-23.

[165] Choi CW, Kang DH, Kim GH, Eum JS, Lee SM, Song GA, et al. Nafamostat mesylate in the prevention of post-ERCP pancreatitis and risk factors for post-ERCP pancreatitis. Gastrointest Endosc. 2009 Apr;69(4):e11-8.

[166] Yoo JW, Ryu JK, Lee SH, Woo SM, Park JK, Yoon WJ, et al. Preventive effects of ulinastatin on post-endoscopic retrograde cholangiopancreatography pancreatitis in high-risk patients: a prospective, randomized, placebo-controlled trial. Pancreas. 2008;37(4):366-70.

[167] Tsujino T, Komatsu Y, Isayama H, Hirano K, Sasahira N, Yamamoto N, et al. Ulinastatin for pancreatitis after endoscopic retrograde cholangiopancreatography: a randomized, controlled trial. Clin Gastroenterol Hepatol. 2005;3(4):376-83.

[168] Kapetanos D, Kokozidis G, Christodoulou D, Mistakidis K, Sigounas D, Dimakopoulos K, et al.. A randomized controlled trial of pentoxifylline for the prevention of post-ERCP pancreatitis. Gastrointest Endosc. 2007;66(3):513-8.

[169] Sherman S, Alazmi WM, Lehman GA, Geenen JE, Chuttani R, Kozarek RA, et al. Evaluation of recombinant platelet-activating factor acetylhydrolase for reducing the incidence and severity of post-ERCP acute pancreatitis. Gastrointest Endosc. 2009;69(3 Pt 1):462-72.

[170] van Westerloo DJ, Rauws EA, Hommes D, de Vos AF, van der Poll T, Powers BL, et al. Pre-ERCP infusion of semapimod, a mitogen-activated protein kinases inhibitor, lowers post-ERCP hyperamylasemia but not pancreatitis incidence. Gastrointest Endosc. 2008;68(2):246-54.

[171] Lee KT, Lee DH, Yoo BM. The prophylactic effect of somatostatin on post-therapeutic endoscopic retrograde cholangiopancreatography pancreatitis: a randomized, multicenter controlled trial. Pancreas. 2008;37(4):445-8.

[172] Arvanitidis D, Anagnostopoulos GK, Giannopoulos D, Pantes A, Agaritsi R, Margantinis G, et al. Can somatostatin prevent post-ERCP pancreatitis? Results of a randomized controlled trial. J Gastroenterol Hepatol. 2004;19(3):278-82.

[173] Poon RT, Yeung C, Liu CL, Lam CM, Yuen WK, Lo CM, et al. Intravenous bolus somatostatin after diagnostic cholangiopancreatography reduces the incidence of

pancreatitis associated with therapeutic endoscopic retrograde cholangiopancreatography procedures: a randomized controlled trial. Gut. 2003;52(12):1768-73.
[174] Poon RT, Yeung C, Lo CM, Yuen WK, Liu CL, Fan ST. Prophylactic effect of somatostatin on post-ERCP pancreatitis: a randomized controlled trial. Gastrointest Endosc. 1999;49(5):593-8.
[175] Bordas JM, Toledo-Pimentel V, Llach J, Elena M, Mondelo F, Ginès A, et al. Effects of bolus somatostatin in preventing pancreatitis after endoscopic pancreatography: results of a randomized study. Gastrointest Endosc. 1998;47(3):230-4.
[176] Schwartz JJ, Lew RJ, Ahmad NA, Shah JN, Ginsberg GG, Kochman ML, et al. The effect of lidocaine sprayed on the major duodenal papilla on the frequency of post-ERCP pancreatitis. Gastrointest Endosc. 2004;59(2):179-84.
[177] Talukdar R, Vege SS. Early Management of Severe Acute Pancreatitis. Curr Gastroenterol Rep 2011;13(2):123–30.

13

Endoscopic Retrograde Cholangiopancreatography (ERCP) Related Acute Pancreatitis

Zoltán Döbrönte
University of Pécs, Faculty of Health Sciences and Markusovszky Teaching Hospital, Department of Gastroenterology and Internal Medicine, Szombathely, Hungary

1. Introduction

Despite the significant development in endoscope technology and in availability of endoscopic accessories and the spreading of well structured ERCP training the incidence of ERCP-related acute pancreatitis has been little changed in the last three decades. One of the explanations of this contradiction may be that post-ERCP pancreatitis occurs nowadays more often in case of therapeutic intervention compared to the diagnostic ERCP and the need for solely diagnostic ERCP is rapidly declining due to the development of less invasive imaging methods such as magnetic resonance cholangiopancreatography (MRCP) and endoscopic ultrasonography (EUS). ERCP has become an almost exclusive therapeutic procedure.

2. Incidence of post-ERCP pancreatitis

Endoscopic retrograde cholangiopancreatography (ERCP) has the greatest potential for complications among the gastrointestinal endoscopic procedures. The most common complication is acute pancreatitis with an overall incidence of 2-10 %, which can reach even 30 % in the presence of certain risk factors. The post-ERCP pancreatitis is most often mild, or less commonly moderate, but in about 10% of cases (about 0.4-0.6 % of the procedures performed) it is severe and potentially fatal. The mortality rate is about 0.1-0.5 %. Furthermore asymptomatic hyperamylasemia occurs in 35-70 % in patients undergoing ERCP. The wide interval of the published incidence of pancreatitis can be explained by and, depends on the criteria used for diagnosis, the type and duration of follow-up of patients involved in the studies, the levels of endoscopic expertise and, the frequency of patients- and procedure-related risk factors in the patient population (Cotton et al. 2009).

3. Definition of post-ERCP pancreatitis

A transient elevation in the serum amylase concentration without clinical signs of pancreatitis is common following ERCP and abdominal pain is also a frequent complaint due to distension caused by intestinal retention of air insufflated during the procedure. Therefore clear definition is mandatory for exact evaluation of clinical trials, for comparing the results of different publications and for the standardised management in the prevention and treatment of ERCP related pancreatitis.

The current definition is based on an attempt at consensus in 1991 (Cotton et al.). According to this proposal post-ERCP pancreatitis was originally defined as „clinical pancreatitis with serum amylase at least three times normal at more than 24 hours after the procedure, requiring hospital admission or a prolongation of planned admission". On the basis of this definition the widely excepted criteria for the diagnosis of post-ERCP pancreatitis are the followings: pancreatic-type abdominal pain and symptoms with onset after ERCP and severe enough to require hospital stay or to extend the length of stay of already hospitalised patients, serum amylase and/or lipase at least 3 times higher than the upper limit of normal values in 24 hours after the procedure, and/or CT/MRI consistent with the diagnosis of acute pancreatitis.

The *severity* of attack was graded by the above consensus report as mild, moderate and severe. A mild post-ERCP pancreatitis was defined as a need for hospital stay up to 3 days, a moderate pancreatitis was defined as a need for hospital stay for 4-10 days, and a severe pancreatitis as more than 10 days with a significant complication. The European Society of Gastrointestinal Endoscopy (ESGE) guideline recommends a more specific grading system of the severity of pancreatitis for the future (Dumonceau et al. 2010). The Atlanta classification can also be used for the estimation of severity of the post-ERCP pancreatitis, on the basis of the absence or presence of local (documented by CT) or systemic complications, independently of the duration of the hospital stay.

4. Pathophysiology of post-ERCP hyperamylasemia and pancreatitis

Pathomechanism of post-ERCP pancreatitis is of multifactorial nature, but it has not been fully understood yet. It seems to be an inflammatory response to mechanical, hydrostatic, thermal, bacterial and chemical insults that results from canulation and other instrumentation of the papilla and injection of contrast medium into the pancreatic duct. These initiating factors may act independently or in combination.

Mechanical trauma: repeated cannulation attempts or prolonged manipulation around the papillary orifice may cause injury of the pancreatic sphincter or proximal pancreatic duct and may lead to mechanical obstruction due to oedema of the pancreatic sphincter or to prolonged spasm in patients with sphincter of Oddi hypertension.

Hydrostatic factor: pressure increase in the pancreatic duct may be related to overinjection of contrast medium (parenchymography) or to pancreatic manometry without distal aspiration. The consecutive capillary endothelial injury leads to an increase in capillary permeability. It has been suggested that this capillary injury might be mediated by oxygen-derived free radicals.

Thermal injury: electrocautery current may produce edema of the pancreatic orifice and thermal damage of the periampullary acinar cells. Coagulation or blended current causes more tissue injury than cutting current.

Infection: bacterial injury from contaminated endoscope channel or accessories may occur.

Chemical factor: injection of contrast medium into the pancreatic duct may result in chemical injury. High osmolarity contrast agents are thought to play a role in the induction of hyperamylasemia, although a meta-analysis (George et al. 2004) could not confirm it.

Enzymatic factor: intestinal content may activate intrapancreatic proteolytic enzymes.

The above initiating factors lead to autodigestion due to premature intracellular activation of pancreatic proteolytic enzymes, and to release of inflammatory cytokines producing both local and systemic effects (Demols & Deviere 2003, Karne & Gorelick 1999). The severity of pancreatitis is determined by the intensity of the inflammatory cascade and systemic response. The process itself is believed the same as for other forms of acute pancreatitis.

5. Risk factors of ERCP related pancreatitis

Stratification of patients into low or high risk categories is important pre-investigational information to take the potential benefit and risk of procedure into account, to consider patient referral to a tertiary centre, and for selection of prophylactic measures. A number of risk factors acting independently or in combination have been identified. They can be categorised as patient related, procedure related, and investigator related risk factors.

5.1 Patient related risk factors

A multivariate analysis of prospective studies found as significant patient-related risk factors the followings: young age, female gender, suspected sphincter of Oddi dysfunction, previous post-ERCP pancreatitis, recurrent acute pancreatitis, and lack of evidence of chronic pancreatitis (Freeman & Guda, 2004). The European Society of Gastrointestinal Endoscopy (ESGE) guideline further differentiates between definite and likely risk factors based on the strength of evidence from prospective studies (Dumonceau et al., 2010) (Table 1.). These risk factors can act synergistically, putting patients at high risk for post-ERCP pancreatitis.

Definite risk factors
Suspected sphincter of Oddi dysfunction
Female gender
Previous pancreatitis
Likely risk factors
Younger age
Non-dilated extrahepatic bile ducts
Absence of chronic pancreatitis
Normal serum bilirubin

Table 1. Patient-related risk factors of post-ERCP pancreatitis (Adapted from ref. Dumonceau et al., 2010)

The association of these predictors to post-ERCP pancreatitis proved to be the strongest in patients with *known or suspected sphincter of Oddi dysfunction* with a complication rate of 10-30 %. All of the risk factors are independently important, but they may have a *cumulative effect*. In a prospective multicentre study (Freeman et al. 2001) the highest risk (42%) was found in the following combination of the predictors for post-ERCP pancreatitis: female patients, normal serum bilirubin level, suspected sphincter of Oddi dysfunction, and difficult bile duct cannulation. It can be postulated that a prolonged pancreatic sphincter spasm may be an important common factor in the induction of pancreatitis in the group of patients with increased risk for post-ERCP pancreatitis, and that this group of patients have a lower threshold for developing pancreatitis after ERCP.

The higher risk in *younger age* might depend on the lack of age-related atrophy of the pancreatic glands and on the higher prevalence of sphincter of Oddi dysfunction in young people, predominantly in *females*. Similarly to the aging, the *protective role of chronic pancreatitis* can be explained by atrophy and decreased enzymatic activity. Patients with *normal serum bilirubin* and *non-dilated stonefree bile ducts* reported as predictors for developing post-ERCP pancreatitis may also have sphincter of Oddi dysfunction not having been taken into consideration in the diagnosis, especially regarding patients complaining also biliary pain. A *history of acute pancreatitis* independently of the etiology is the second most important risk factor after sphincter of Oddi dysfunction, and it should be taken into consideration before planning an ERCP.

5.2 Procedure related risk factors

Procedure-related risk factors are similarly important as patient-related factors in determining the incidence and severity of post-ERCP pancreatitis (Fig 1.). Various procedures are associated with higher risk of post-ERCP pancreatitis (Table 2.), most of them documented by multivariate analyses. For example role of papillectomy has not been analysed, but it can be considered as a definitive risk factor on the basis of prospective studies.

Definite risk factors
Pancreatic duct cannulation and contrast injection
Multiple attempts of cannulation
Precut sphincterotomy
Endoscopic papillectomy
Other risk factors
Balloon dilation of the sphincter
Sphincter of Oddi manometry
Pancreatic sphincterotomy
Pancreatic brush cytology
Failure to clear bile duct stones
Difficult or failed cannulation

Table 2. Procedure-related risk factors of post-ERCP pancreatitis

Repeated attempts at cannulating, also without pancreatic duct contrast injection is associated with high incidence of pancreatitis. This fact supports that papillary edema and sphincter spasm, rather than hydrostatic ductal and contrast agent injury are the major factors in the induction of post-ERCP pancreatitis. The risk rate seems to progressively increase with the number of attempts. More than 10 cannulation attempts can increase the risk of pancreatitis about 15-fold (Testoni et al. 2010).

The *contrast injection* itself can induce pancreatitis due to hydrostatic injury from pancreatic duct overfilling, which is the most pronounced in cases of parenchymography. The use of lower ionic contrast agents does not result in lower frequency of pancreatitis than that of the conventional ones.

Pre-cut sphincterotomy is associated with a threefold increase of post-procedure pancreatitis, however the risk is likely mainly investigator dependent and seems to be lower in experts hands. Moreover, early pre-cut may be safer than delayed pre-cut performed after multiple cannulation attempts. The overall risk of pancreatitis after pre-cut sphincterotomy is less than after repeated attempts at standard cannulation. Out of the two techniques of needle knife precut, fistulotomy where the precut is separate from the papillary orifice, seems to be accompanied with less pancreatitis than precut starting at the papillary orifice

(Mavrodiannis et al. 1999), although high level evidence fails to support the preference of fistulotomy.

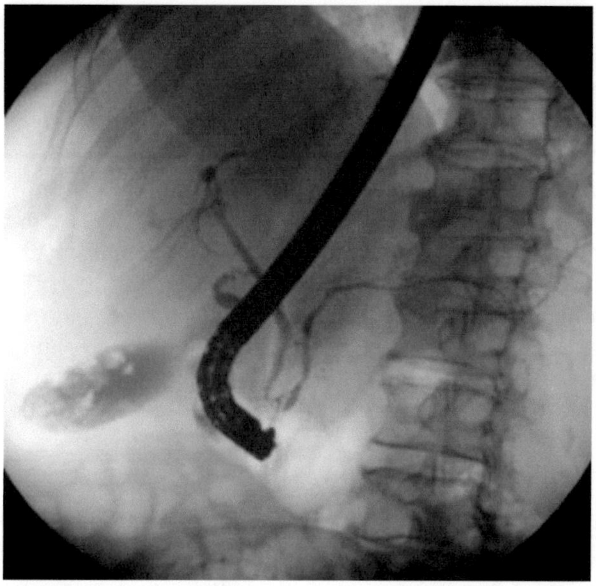

Fig. 1. Endoscopic retrograde cholangiopancreatogram of a young woman with gallbladder stones. Non-dilated bile ducts, young age, and female gender represent patient related risk factors, and contrast injection into the pancreatic duct a procedure related risk factor for post-ERCP pancreatitis

Pancreatitis occurs after *endoscopic papillectomy* performed like a snare polypectomy using a side-viewing duodenoscope in 15-20 %. Therefore papillectomy (ampullectomy) should perform only by well-trained and experienced endoscopists. The incidence and severity of this complication can be significantly reduced by prophylactic pancreatic duct stenting (Wong, 2004). Pancreatitis caused by stenosis of the pancreatic duct orifice can also be a late complication after papillectomy (Norton et al., 2002).

Biliary sphincterotomy itself is not associated with an increased risk of pancreatitis. Currently the use of pure cut current is advisable, because it causes less tissue injury and edema than coagulation current. On the contrary to biliary sphincterotomy *balloon dilatation* of the intact biliary sphincter has been associated with a high incidence of pancreatitis, therefore its use is not advisable in the presence of patient-related risk factors, especially in patients with sphincter of Oddi hypertension. Large diameter *biliary stent without sphincterotomy* can also induce pancreatitis due to compression of the pancreatic sphincter (Tarnasky et al., 1997). On the contrary, biliary-stent exchange in sphincterotomised patients causes less-frequent pancreatitis compared to other ERCP procedures (Cotton et al. 2008).

Sphincter of Oddi manometry using standard perfusion catheter is associated with a substantial incidence of pancreatitis. The risk can be significantly reduced by using modified triple lumen catheter with simultaneous aspiration or by using a microtransducer catheter. In two randomised controlled studies the incidence of post-ERCP pancreatitis was found using the alternative catheters in comparison with the standard perfusion catheter 3.0% vs. 23.5 % and 3.1% vs. 13.8 % (Sherman et al. 1990, Wehrmann et al. 2003).

Pancreatic sphincterotomy was associated with high risk of pancreatitis in a recent prospective multicentre study only in univariate analysis (Testoni et al., 2010), in agreement with some earlier reports (Freeman et al., 2001, Cheng et al. 2006). As independent risk factor proved have to been only *minor papilla sphincterotomy.*
What other procedure risk factors concerns, *pancreatic brush cytology* can cause pancreatitis due to edema in consequence of mechanical trauma of the pancreatic duct. In case of failure to clear the bile duct during ERCP *residual stones* can induce biliary pancreatitis.

5.3 Investigator related risk factors

Data about a potential relationship between post-ERCP pancreatitis incidence and endoscopist's experience in the technique defined as annual case volume (the median number of ERCPs per endoscopists/year) are conflicting. Endoscopist's inexperience and trainee participation may be associated with a higher incidence as it was shown in some of the studies, while others could not confirm it. This might be explained by the fact that in high-volume centres there are more patients with high risk for potential post-ERCP pancreatitis and larger number of procedures at higher degree of difficulty.

6. Prophylaxis of ERCP related pancreatitis

6.1. Mechanical techniques

6.1.1 Pancreatic stent placement

The purpose of placing a temporary pancreatic duct stent is to sustain the pancreatic outflow in the face of relative obstruction due to edema and sphincter of Oddi spasm caused by manipulations of the papilla. A meta-analysis of eight randomized controlled trials demonstrated that short term pancreatic stent placement reduces the incidence of post-ERCP pancreatitis (Mazaki et al 2010) (Fig. 2.). Sofuni et al (2007) found significant benefit of stent placement only in patients at high risk for pancreatitis, and it seems to be not cost-effective in patients at average risk (Das A et al. 2007). Therefore, the use of prophylactic pancreatic stenting is generally proposed only for patients who are at high risk for developing pancreatitis after ERCP. Similar standpoint is represented also in the recommendation of the ESGE guideline (Dumonceau et al. 2010).

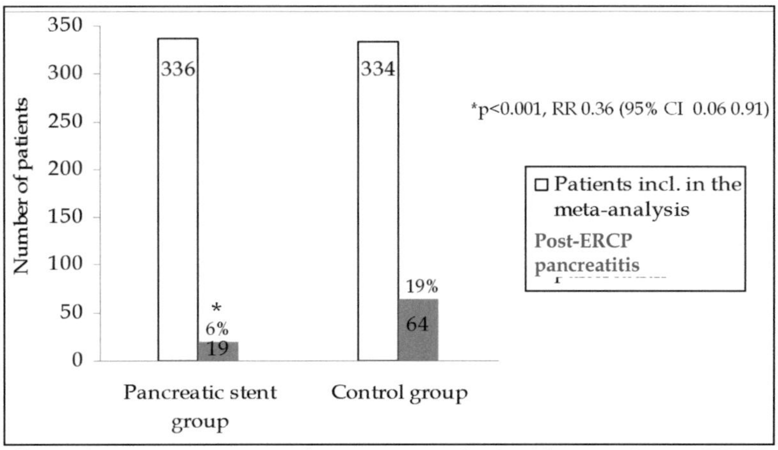

Fig. 2. The effect of pancreatic stent placement on the incidence of post-ERCP pancreatitis according to meta-analysis (Mazaki et al. 2010)

What kind of plastic stent should be used? 3 mm long 3 -5 Fr straight polyethylene plastic stents without internal flanges (for promoting of spontaneous elimination in few days following the insertion) and with one or two external flanges (for preventing proximal migration) are recommended for prophylactic purpose (Fig.3). Stents of 3-Fr and 5-Fr in diameter proved to be similarly effective, but the insertion of 5-Fr stents seems to be easier and faster (Zolotarevsky et al. 2011).

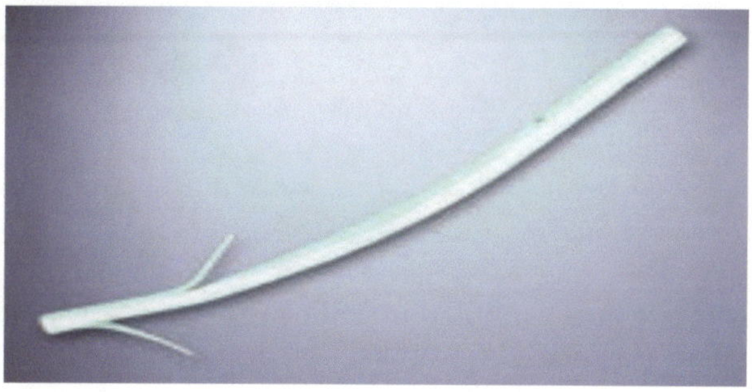

Fig. 3. Pancreatic stent without internal flanges

The stent migrates spontaneously into the duodenum within two weeks in most of the cases. Within 5 to 10 days after the stent insertion an X-ray control and, when the stent is in place yet, endoscopic stent removal is recommended because of the risk of stent-induced damage to the pancreatic duct. Adverse events including pancreatitis following stenting of the main pancreatic duct occur in 4.2-4.6 %, but the incidence of pancreatitis after failed cannulation attempts may reach even 65 % (Freeman et al. 2004). Therefore this is a technique for experienced endoscopist.

6.1.2 Pancreatic guide wire placement for facilitation of bile duct cannulation

Data about the effectiveness of pancreatic guide wire placement in the prevention of post-ERCP pancreatitis are still controversial. In patients with difficult bile duct cannulation successful biliary cannulation can be achieved by pancreatic guide wire-assisted technique in more than 70% of the cases (Dumonceau et al. 2010). If this method is used, a pancreatic stent should be placed for prophylaxis of pancreatitis (Fig 4.). For the same reason pancreatic stenting can be useful also in cases in which biliary cannulation remains unsuccessful.

6.1.3 Guide wire-assisted deep biliary cannulation

Insertion of 0.035-inch diameter guide-wire into the papilla directly or advancing the guide-wire through the sphincterotome inserted into the papilla for deep biliary cannulation reduces the risk of post-ERCP pancreatitis due to promotion of selective primary cannulation. This method may namely diminish traumatic injury to the pancreatic duct and hydrostatic pressure increase associated with injection of contrast material. Therefore, the guide wire-assisted technique is advised for deep biliary cannulation by the ESGE guideline (Dumonceau et al. 2010). However, in a prospective randomised trial this technique was associated with a lower rate of post-ERCP pancreatitis only with the exception of cases where the technique was performed in patients with sphincter of Oddi dysfunction or where unintentional pancreas guide wire cannulation occurred (Lee et al 2009).

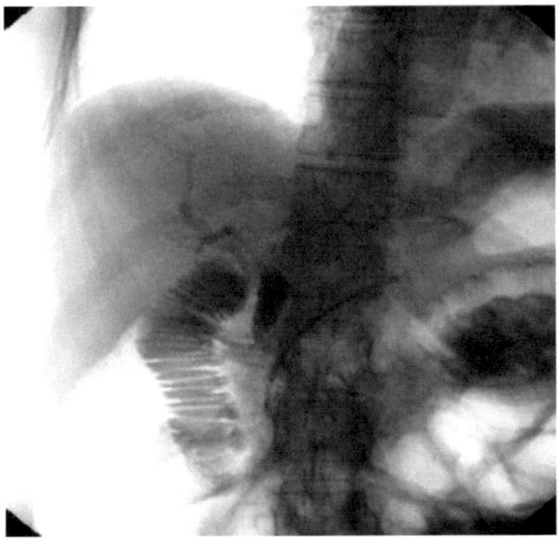

Fig. 4. A case of difficult bile duct cannulation. Following pancreatic guide wire-assisted technique pancreatic stent was placed for prevention of post-ERCP pancreatitis

6.2 Pharmacological agents

Several agents have been tested experimentally and in clinical trials for potential efficacy in the prevention of ERCP induced pancreatitis. Chemoprevention studies have targeted the following mechanism of action: reduction of pancreatic secretion, prevention of intra-acinar trypsinogen activation, interruption of inflammatory cascade, relaxation of sphincter of Oddi, and prevention of infection. The majority of the investigated pharmacological agents appeared promising in initial randomised single-centre clinical studies however, conflicting results were obtained from larger multi-centre trials (Table 3.).

Drug	Efficacy
Somatostatin	Conflicting data
Octreotide	Conflicting data
Gabexate mesilate	Conflicting data
Ulanistatin	Conflicting data
Nitroglycerin	Conflicting data
Nifedipin	No
Lidocain spray	No
Epinephrine spray	No
Botulinum toxin intrapapillary	No
Ceftazidime	Need for more trials
N-acethylcysteine	No
Beta-carotene	No
Allopurinol	Conflicting data
Glucocorticoids	No
Pentoxifylline	No
Semapimod	No
Acethylhydrolase	No
Indomethacin	Yes, but need for more trials
Diclofenac	Yes, but need for more trials

Table 3. Medications tested for prophylaxis of post-ERCP pancreatitis

6.2.1 Reduction of pancreatic enzyme secretion

Somatostatin and its long-acting analogue ocreotide affect the exocrine function of the pancreas directly by reducing the secretion of digestive enzymes and indirectly by inhibiting the production of secretin and cholecystokinin. According to a meta-analysis pooling the data from ten high-quality randomised controlled trials it can be concluded, that *somatostatin* did not influence the overall incidence of post-ERCP pancreatitis (Dumonceau et al. 2010). Although a significant risk reduction of post-ERCP pancreatitis was found in four randomised controlled trial, when somatostatin was administered in continuous infusion for longer than 12 hours, and in two studies, when somatostatin was given as a single bolus, the question is yet open, weather using specific dose-schedules somatostatin might be more efficacious (Arvanatidis et al. 2004).

Concerning the long-acting somatostatin analogue *ocreotide* the same conclusion can be drawn based on an ad hoc meta-analysis of eight randomised controlled trials (Dumonceau et al. 2010). Octreotide can reduce the ERCP-induced hyperamylasemia, but this effect can only be shown, if endoscopic sphincterotomy is simultaneously performed (Tulassay et al. 1997). Octreotide increases namely the tone of the sphincter of Oddi, and therefore this partial beneficial effect of the reduced enzyme secretion may be effective only with sphincterotomy together. Some data suggest that the effect of octreotide may be dose-dependent and more than 0.5 mg of octreotide may be beneficial (Zhang Y et al. 2009), but it should yet be clarified in future studies.

6.2.2 Protease inhibitors

Antiprotease agents were tested for prophylaxis of post-ERCP pancreatitis with the purpose of prevention of intra-acinar trypsinogen activation to trypsin and that of the subsequent inflammatory cascade. *Gabexate mesilate* in six randomised controlled trials, while *ulanistatin* in four randomised controlled trials have been evaluated. Furthermore, the prophylactic effect of gabexate with ulanistatin was compared in two clinical trials. The results can be summarised by stating that, although there is a small risk reduction, particularly in the ulanistatin subgroup, there is no solid evidence that antiprotease drugs significantly influence the incidence of post-ERCP pancreatitis. The same conclusion can be drawn from a recently published meta-analysis (Seta & Noguchi 2011) on the basis of which it can be stated that the primary studies were not of high quality enough to come to the proper consequences. Nevertheless, protease inhibitors are costly.

6.2.3 Sphincter relaxants

Nitroglycerin (glycerine trinitrate) proved to be effective in some reports, but ineffective in others. Based on two meta-analyses (Bang et al. 2009, Shao et al. 2010) of pooled data from five randomised controlled trials it can be concluded that nitroglycerin administered orally or sublingual may reduce the incidence of post-ERCP pancreatitis, but transdermal nitroglycerin is ineffective. The use of nitroglycerin is often associated with transient hypotension and headache, therefore the ESGE guideline does not recommend its routine use in the prophylaxis of post-ERCP pancreatitis (Dumonceau et al. 2010).

Nifedipin was also tested, because calcium channel blockers have proved to be effective in the prevention of experimental pancreatitis. In clinical trials, however, nifedipin failed to show a significant effect in the prevention of post-ERCP pancreatitis (Prat et al. 2002).

Other drugs (lidocaine spray, epinephrine spray, Botulinum toxin injected intrapapillary) tested with the intention of reducing the sphincter of Oddi pressure failed to show any efficacy (Gorelick et al. 2004, Matsushita et al. 2009, Schwartz et al. 2004).

6.2.4 Antibiotics

There is only a single study evaluating the *ceftazidime* for prophylaxis of post-ERCP pancreatitis. This antibiotic was given in a dose of 2 g intravenously 30 min prior to the investigation and a significant reduction in the incidence of post-ERCP pancreatitis was observed (Raty et al. 2001). Further data are necessary to establish the real place of antibiotics in the prevention of ERCP-related pancreatitis.

6.2.5 Antioxidants

The following antioxidant agents were investigated for prevention of ERCP related pancreatitis: *N-acetylcysteine* (Katsinelos P. et al. 2005), *beta-carotene* (Lavy et al. 2004) *and allopurinol*. The free radical scavenger *N-acetylcysteine* and *beta-carotene* failed to show any beneficial effect. *Allopurinol* is a xanthine oxidase inhibitor and an antioxidant with antiapoptotic property. Four randomised clinical trials dealing with its effect in the prevention of post-ERCP hyperamylasemia and pancreatitis were published. Three of them reported negative outcomes but in two studies allopurinol proved to be effective in the reduction of the incidence of hyperamylasemia, and in one of them also in that of acute pancreatitis, particularly in patients submitted to high risk procedures (Martinez-Torres et al. 2009). Allopurinol was administered orally in a dose of 300 mg at 15 and 3 hours before ERCP.

6.2.6 Antiinflammatory drugs

Several agents acting by interruption of the inflammatory cascade were tested. *Glucocorticoids* do not reduce the incidence of post-ERCP pancreatitis according to a meta-analysis based on six randomised controlled trials (Bay et al. 2008). Similarly to glucocorticoids *pentoxifylline, semapimod,* and *acethylhydrolase* (a recombinant platelet-activating factor) all proved to be ineffective. *Interleukin-10* reduced the incidence and severity of post-ERCP pancreatitis in an initial study (Deviere et al. 2001), but further trials could not confirm its effectiveness. As suggested by observational and animal studies, *heparin* has also an anti-inflammatory effect, inhibit the activity of pancreatic proteases and improves pancreatic circulation, but in clinical randomised controlled trials neither unfractionated heparin (Barkay et al. 2008), nor low molecular-weight heparin (Rabenstein T et al 2004) proved to be effective in the prophylaxis of post-ERCP pancreatitis.

Nonsteroidal anti-inflammatory drugs (NSAIDs) inhibit phospholipase A2 which has an early role in the inflammatory cascade in acute pancreatitis. Inhibition of phospholipase A2 results in suppression of several important classes of proinflammatory lipids (prostaglandins, leukotriens, platelet-activating factor). Furthermore, NSAIDs inhibit neutrophyl-endothelial cell attachment. Indomethacin followed by diclofenac is the most potent NSAID with regard to phospholipase A2 inhibition. Indomethacin has shown to decrease the mortality of experimental pancreatitis in animals (Wildenhain et al 1989). Four prospective randomised controlled clinical studies have been published until now that compared rectally administered indomethacin or diclofenac vs. placebo (Murray et al. 2003, Sotoudehmanesh R et al. 2007, Montano Loza et al. 2007, Koshbaten M et al. 2008) (Fig. 5.).

On the basis of three meta-analyses using the data of these studies rectally administered indomethacin and diclofenac in a dose of 100 mg proved to be effective in the decrease of incidence of post-ERCP pancreatitis (Elmunser et al. 2008, Zheng et al. 2008, Dai et al. 2009).

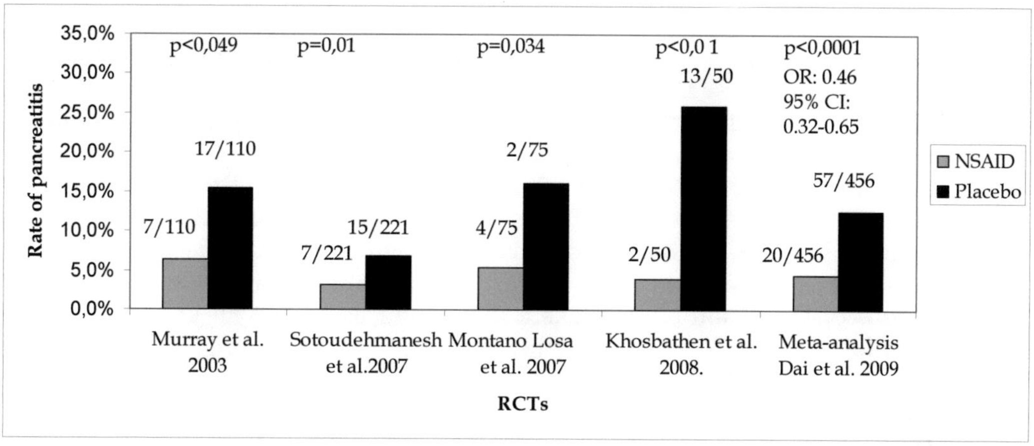

(RCT: randomised controlled trial)

Fig. 5. Incidence of post-ERCP pancreatitis: rectally administered NSAIDs versus placebo.

The reduction seems to be similar regardless of the degree of the risk (Zheng et al. 2008). Limitation of the original studies is the small number of the trials performed only in three countries. Therefore some scepticism related to the clinical efficacy of NSAIDs in the prophylaxis of post-ERCP pancreatitis exists, all the more because several agents tested before have shown promise in early single-centre studies, but the results were disappointing in larger multicentre randomised controlled trials. Furthermore it has to be mentioned that diclofenac administered intramuscularly or orally did not proved to be effective in lowering the rate of post-ERCP pancreatitis significantly (Cheon et al. 2007, Senol et al 2009). Further multicentre controlled studies are awaited for confirmation of the promising results of the foregoing trials. Nevertheless NSAIDs in a single dose are relatively safe, cheap, and easy to use. Therefore 100 mg of indomethacine or diclofenac administered rectally immediately before or after ERCP is routinely recommended. This standpoint is reflected also in the ESGE guidelines (Dumonceau et al. 2010).

6.3 Post-procedure management (Follow-up after ERCP)

Post-ERCP pancreatitis is an unforeseen complication but it can be predicted by measuring the serum amylase concentration at 2-4 hours after the procedure. It should be taken into account, however, that hyperamylasemia without pancreatitis following ERCP is well recognised and abdominal discomfort for some hours after ERCP due to intestinal distension by air insufflated during the investigation is a commonly occurring symptom, in particular in patients with functional gastrointestinal dysfunction. It is advisable to restrict oral intake of water for four hours and until serum amylase value is available. Serum amylase concentration less than 1.5 times the upper limit of normal value almost excludes post-ERCP pancreatitis and the patient can be discharged on the day of ERCP. For patients with four hours serum amylase levels more than twice the upper limit, with ongoing abdominal pain / tenderness or fever, fasting and parenteral fluid replacement is recommended. The same policy is advised in the presence of any risk factor of post-procedural pancreatitis at least for 24 hour after ERCP. Further management is depending on the 24 hour serum amylase level and clinical signs of pancreatitis.

6.4 Principles of prevention and reduction of severity of ERCP-induced pancreatitis

Following factors listed below should be considered when indicating and performing ERCP.

1. Because post-ERCP pancreatitis can be severe, life-threatening or even fatal, careful and adequate patient selection is one of the most important and the most effective preventive measures. ERCP should not be performed when the indication is not clear or the procedure is unlikely to benefit the patient. In borderline indications and when the aim of ERCP is solely diagnostic, non-invasive imaging methods, magnetic resonance cholangiopancreatography (MRCP) and endoscopic ultrasound should be performed first. Endoscopists should always take a risk-benefit analysis with knowledge of the identified patient related risk factors, when deciding whether to perform an ERCP.
2. Referral of patients at high risk for post-ERCP pancreatitis to a great volume specialist centre should be considered.
3. Minimal use of contrast material, avoidance of repeated attempts of pancreatic cannulation and use of guide wire to gain access or use of dual wire technique can be effective measures for prophylaxis in certain cases.
4. Risk related ERCP techniques should be avoided when possible.
5. Pharmacological prophylaxis with periprocedural rectal administration of NSAIDs (indomethacine or diclofenac) as a cheap, practical and safe method is routinely recommended.
6. Prophylactic placement of short 5 Fr pancreatic stent without inner flanges should be strongly considered for patients at high risk for development of post-ERCP pancreatitis.
7. Early screening for post-ERCP pancreatitis following the procedure and appropriate management is also important for the prevention or for reduction of the severity of ERCP-related pancreatitis.

The recommendations above are in concordance with the European Society of Gastrointestinal Endoscopy guideline (Dumonceau et al., 2010).

7. Therapy of post-ERCP pancreatitis

The treatment of ERCP related pancreatitis is the same as that of the acute pancreatitis of other etiologies and it depends considerably on the severity of the pancreatitis. The therapy is mainly supportive including fasting, adequate correction of hypovolemia, and maintenance of optimal fluid balance, close monitoring for signs of local and systemic complications, and adequate pain control. Patients with mild pancreatitis can generally begin oral food intake in few days. The outflow of the pancreatic juice can be tried to improve with spasmolytics, nitroglycerin or theophyllin. Morphine should be avoided because this drug may produce high outflow resistance due to sphincter of Oddi spasm, but pethidine / meperidine are allowed if the patient requires it for pain relief. If the efficacy of pethidine / meperidine is insufficient, epidural anesthesia is the best choice or fentanyl can be given. In cases of severe pancreatitis early nasojejunal feeding can be crucial for the maintenance of integrity of the gut mucosal barrier, hereby preventing bacterial translocation into the systemic circulation. Translocated pathogen intestinal flora is namely one of the main sources of septic complications. Enteral feeding with appropriate energy intake has also a role in the correction of the nutritional imbalance due to the prolonged hypermetabolic state in severe acute pancreatitis. Adequate intravenous substitution is also very important, likewise early antibiotic prophylaxis in necrotizing pancreatitis - although still controversial, and effective antimicrobial treatment of the inflammatory complications. Infected pancreatic necrosis and infected pancreatic and peripancreatic fluid collections should be treated by surgery or by endoscopic or CT guided intervention. Treatment of the systemic complications has to be managed in an intensive care unit with close monitoring of the vital functions.

8. Conclusion

Acute pancreatitis is the most common and feared complication of ERCP. Post-ERCP pancreatitis is severe and potentially fatal in a significant proportion. The incidence rate has been little changed over the last decades despite important advances in endoscope and in accessory technology.

The widely accepted criteria for the diagnosis of post-ERCP pancreatitis are serum amylase and/or lipase at least 3 times higher than the upper limit of normal values in 24 hours after the procedure accompanied by new pancreatic-type abdominal pain and symptoms and severe enough to require hospital stay or to extend the length of stay of already hospitalised patients, and/or CT/MRI consistent with the diagnosis of acute pancreatitis.

The pathomechanism is not fully understood. It seems to be an inflammatory response to mechanical, hydrostatic, enzymatic, thermal, microbiological, and probably chemical insults that results from cannulation attempts and contrast material injection into the pancreatic duct.

A number of risk factors for developing pancreatitis after ERCP are known, they can categorised as patient related, procedure related, and investigator related risk factors. It is essential to identify patients at high risk to avoid unnecessary procedures or adopt protective technical or pharmacological measures. If patient related risk factors are present, first of all it is advised to consider patient's referral to a specialist centre, or for selection of prophylactic measures. In borderline indications non-invasive imaging methods should be preferred. Out of procedure related risk factors papillary edema and sphincter spasm are the major factors in the induction of post-ERCP pancreatitis. For minimizing the risk of pancreatitis during the procedure the following measures should be kept in mind: atraumatic manipulation of the papilla, avoidance of repeated pancreatic duct cannulation and contrast injection, avoidance of balloon catheter dilatation of the intact sphincter, limited use of precut sphincterotomy and pancreatic sphincterotomy, avoiding placement of biliary stent through intact papilla, using soft-tipped guide wire to access bile duct, and using pure cut electrosurgical current.

Despite selecting patients and using protective technical measures post-ERCP pancreatitis can occur unexpectedly. Therefore prophylactic pharmacological intervention is routinely advised by means of rectal indomethacine or diclofenac immediately before or after the procedure. The administration of indomethacine and diclofenac in a single dose is safe, cheap, and easy and based on the few randomised controlled trials it seems to be effective in the decrease of the incidence of post-ERCP pancreatitis. Further randomised controlled trials are needed to prove the real efficacy of NSAIDs in the reduction of *severe* ERCP related pancreatitis. For high-risk ERCPs prophylactic placement of short pancreatic stent proved to be beneficial in experienced hands, therefore its use is recommended for few days in these cases.

Careful follow up, early screening for pancreatitis and appropriate management of the complication are crucial for the outcome. The treatment of post-ERCP pancreatitis itself does not differ from that of the acute pancreatitis of whatever etiology.

9. References

Andriulli A, Caruso N, Quitadamo M, Forlano R, Leandro G, Spirito F & De Maio G (2003): Antisecretory vs. antiproteasic drugs in the prevention of post-ERCP pancreatitis: the evidence-based medicine derived from a meta-analysis study. JOP Vol. 4, No. 1, pp. 41-48. ISSN 1590-8577

Andriulli A, Forlano R, Napolitano G, Conoscitore P, Caruso N, Pilotto A, Di Sebastiano PL & Leandro G (2007): Pancreatic duct stent in the prophylaxis of pancreatic damage after endoscopic retrograde cholangiopancreatography: a systematic analysis of benefits and associated risks. Digestion Vol. 75, No. 2-3, pp. 156-163. ISSN 0012-2823

Bai Y, Gao J, Shi X, Zou D & Li Z (2008): Prophylactic corticosteroids do not prevent post-ERCP pancreatitis: a meta-analysis of randomized controlled trials. Pancreatology Vol. 8, No. 4-5, pp. 504-509. ISSN 1424-3903

Bang UC, Nojgaard C, Andersen PK & Matzen P (2009): Meta-analysis: nitroglycerin for prevention of post-ERCP pancreatitis. Aliment. Pharmacol. Ther. Vol. 29, No. 10, pp. 1078-1085. ISSN 0269-2813

Barkay O, Niv E, Santo E, Bruck R, Hallak A & Konikoff FM (2008): Low-dose heparin for the prevention of post-ERCP pancreatitis: a randomised placebo-controlled trial. Surg. Endosc. Vol. 22, No. 9, pp. 1971-1976. ISSN 1432-2218

Cheng CL, Sherman S, Watkins IL, Barnett J, Freeman M, Geenen J, Ryan M, Parker H, Frakes JT, Fogel EL, Silvermn WB, Dua KS, Aliperti G, Yakhse P, Uzer M, Jones W, Goff J, Lazzell-Pannell L, Rashdan A, Temkit M & Lehman GA (2006): Risk factors for post-ERCP pancreatitis : a prospective, multicenter study. Am. J. Gastroenterol. Vol. 101, No. 1, pp.139-147. ISSN 0002-9270

Cheon YK, Cho KB, Watkins JL, McHenry L, Fogel EL, Sherman S, Schnidt S, Lazzell-Pannell L, Lehman GA (2007): Efficacy of diclofenac in the prevention of post-ERCP pancreatitis in predominantly high-risk patients : a randomized double-blind prospective trial. Gastrointest. Endosc. Vol. 66, No. 6, pp.1126-1132. ISSN 0016-5107

Cotton PB, Lehman G, Vennes J, Geenen JE, Russell RC, Meyers WC, Liguory C & Nickl N (1991): Endoscopic sphincterotomy complications and their management: An attempt at consensus. Gastrointest. Endosc. Vol. 37, No. 3, pp. 383-93. ISSN 0016-5107

Cotton PB, Garrow DA, Gallagher J & Romagnuolo J (2009): Risk factors for complications after ERCP: a multivariate analysis of 11,497 procedures over 12 years. Gastrointest. Endosc. Vol. 70, No. 1, pp. 80-88. ISSN 0016-5107

Dai XF, Wang XW & Zhao K (2009): Role of nonsteroidal anti-inflammatory drugs in the prevention of post-ERCP pancreatitis : a meta-analysis. Hepatobiliary Pancreat. Dis. Int. Vol 8, No. 1, pp 11-16. ISSN 1499-3872

Das A, Singh P, Sivak MV, Chak A (2007): Pancreatic stent-placement for prevention of post-ERCP pancreatitis: a cost-effectiveness analysis. Gastrointest. Endosc. Vol. 65, No. 7, pp. 960-968. ISSN 0016-5107

Demols A & Deviere J. (2003): New frontiers in the pharmacological prevention of post-ERCP pancreatitis: the cytokines. JOP Vol. 4, No. 1, pp. 49-57. ISSN 1590-8577

Deviere J, Le Moine O, Van Leathem J-L, Eisendrath P, Ghilain A, Sevsrs N & Cohard M (2001): Interleukin-10 reduces the incidence of pancreatitis after therapeutic retrograde cholangiopancreatography. Gastroenterology Vol. 120, No. 2, pp. 498-505. ISSN 0016-5085

Dumonceau J-M, Andriulli A, Deviere J, Mariani A, Rigaux J, Baron TH & Testoni PA (2010): European Society of Gastrointestinal Endoscopy (ESGE) guideline: prophylaxis of post-ERCP pancreatitis. Endoscopy Vol. 42, No. 6. pp. 503-515. ISSN 0013-726X

Elmunser BJ, Waljee AK, Elta GH, Taylor JR, Fehmi SMA & Higgins PDR (2008): A meta-analysis of rectal NSAIDs in the prevention of post-ERCP pancreatitis. Gut Vol. 57 No. 9, pp. 1262-1267. ISSN 0017-5749

Freeman ML, DiSario JA, Nelson DB, Fennerty MB, Lee JG, Bjorkman DJ, Overby CS, Aas J, Ryan ME, Bochna GS, Shaw MJ, Snady HW, Erickson RV, Moore JP & Roel JP (2001): Risk factors for post-ERCP pancreatitis : a prospective, multicenter study. Gastrointest. Endosc. Vol. 54, No. 4, pp. 425-434. ISSN 0016-5107

Freeman ML & Guda MN (2004): Prevention of post-ERCP pancreatitis : a comprehensive review. Gastrointest. Endosc. Vol. 59, No. 7, pp. 845-864. ISSN 0016-5107

Freeman ML, Overby C & Qi D (2004): Pancreatic stent insertion : consequences of failure and results of a modified technique to maximize success. Gastrointest. Endosc. Vol. 59, No. 1, pp. 8-14. ISSN 0016-5107

George S, Kulkarni A, Stevens G Forsmark CE & Draganov P (2004): Role of osmolarity of contrast media in the development of post-ERCP pancreatitis: a meta-analysis. Dig. Dis. Sci. Vol. 49, No. 3, pp. 503-508. ISSN 0002-9211

Gorelick A, Barnett J, Chey W, Anderson M & Elta G (2004): Botulinum toxin injection after endoscopic sphincterotomy. Endoscopy Vol. 36, No. 2, pp.170-173. ISSN 0013-726X

Karne S & Gorelick ES (1999): Etiopathogenesis of acute pancreatitis. Surg. Clin. North Am. Vol. 79, No. 4, pp. 699-710. ISSN 1061-3315

Katsinelos P, Kountouras J, Paroutoglou G, Beltsis A, Mimidis K & Zavos C (2005): Intravenous N-acetylcysteine does not prevent post-ERCP pancreatitis. Gastrointest. Endosc. Vol. 62, No. 1, pp. 105-111. ISSN 0016-5107

Khoshbaten M, Khorram H, Madad L, Ehsani Ardakani MJ, Farzin H & Zali MR (2008): Role of diclofenac in reducing post-endoscopic retrograde cholangiopancreatography pancreatitis. J. Gastroenterol. Hepatol. Vol. 23, No. 7, Pt 2, e 11-16. ISSN 1687-223X

Lavy A, Karban A, Suissa A, Yassin K, Hermesh I & Ben-Amotz A (2004): Natural beta-carotene for the prevention of post-ERCP pancreatitis. Pancreas, Vol. 29, No. 2, pp. e45-e50. ISSN 1536-4828

Lee TH, Park DH, Park J-Y, Kim EO, Lee YS, Park JH, Lee S-H, Chung I-K, Kim HS, Park S-H & Kim S-J (2009): Can wire-guided cannulation prevent post-ERCP pancreatitis ? Gastrointest. Endosc. Vol. 69, No. 3, pp. 444-452. ISSN 0016-5107

Matsushita M, Takakuwa H, Shimeno N Uchida K, Nishio A & Okazaki K (2009): Epinephrine sprayed on the papilla for prevention of post-ERCP pancreatitis. J Gastroenterol Vol. 44, No. 1, pp. 71-75. ISSN 0944-1174

Mavrogiannis C, Liatsos C, Romanos A, Petoumenos C, Nakos A & Karvountzis G (1999): Needle-knife fistulotomy versus needle-knife precut papillotomy for the treatment of common bile duct stones. Gastrointest Endosc Vol. 50, No. 3, pp. 334-339. ISSN 0016-5107

Mazaki T, Masuda H & Takayama T (2010): Prophylactic pancreatic stent placement and post-ERCP pancreatitis : a systematic review and meta-analysis. Endoscopy Vol. 42, No. 10, pp. 842-852. ISSN 0013-726X

Martenez-Torres H, Rodrigez-Lomeli X, Davalos-Cobian C , Garcia-Correa J, Maldonado-Martinez JM, Medrano-Munoz F, Fuentes-Orosco C & Gonzalez-Ojeda A (2009): Oral allopurinol to prevent hyperamylasemia and acute pancreatitis after endoscopic retrograde cholangiopancreatography. World J Gastroenterology Vol. 15, No. 13, pp. 1600-1606. ISSN 1007-9327

Murray B, Carter R, Imrie C Evans S & O'Suilleabhain C (2003): Diclofenac reduces the incidence of acute pancreatitis after endoscopic retrograde cholangiopancreatography. Gastroenterology, Vol. 124, No. 7, pp. 1786-91. ISSN 0016-5085

Murray WR (2005): Reducing the incidence and severity of post ERCP pancreatitis. Scand. J. Surg. Vol. 94, No. 2, pp. 112-116. ISSN 0036-5521

Montano Loza A, Lomeli XR, Garcia Correa J, Cobian CD, Guevara GC, Munoz FM, Orozco CF & Ojeda AG (2007): Effect of the rectal administration of indomethacin on amylase serum levels after endoscopic retrograde cholangiopancreatography, and its impact on the development of secundary pancreatitis episodes. Rev. Esp. Enferm. Dig. Vol. 99, No. 6, pp. 330-336. ISSN 1130-0108

Norton ID, Gostout CJ, Baron TH, Geller A, Petersen BT & Wiersema MJ (2002): Safety and outcome of endoscopic snare excision of the major duodenal papilla. Gastrointest. Endosc. Vol. 56, No. 2, pp. 239-243. ISSN 0016-5107

Prat F, Amaris J, Ducot B, Bocquentin M, Fritsch J, Choury AD, Pelletier G, Buffet C (2002): Nifedipin for prevention of post-ERCP pancreatitis : a prospective double-blind randomized study. Gastrointest. Endosc. Vol. 56, No. 2, pp. 202-208. ISSN 0016-5107

Rabenstein T, Fischer B, Wiessner W Schmidt H, Radespiel-Tröger M & Hochberger J (2004): Low-molecular-weight heparin does not prevent acute post-ERCP pancreatitis. Gastrointest. Endosc. Vol. 59, No. 6, pp. 606 -613. ISSN 0016-5107

Raty S, Sand J, Pulkkinen M, Matikainen N & Nordback I (2001): Post-ERCP pancreatitis : reduction by routine antibiotics. J. Gastrointest. Surgery Vol. 5, No. 4, pp. 339-345. ISSN 1091-255X

Senol A, Saritas U, Demirkan H (2009): Efficacy of intramuscular diclofenac and fluid replacement in prevention of post-ERCP pancreatitis. World J. Gastroenterol. Vol. 15, No. 32, pp. 3999-4004. ISSN 1007-9327

Seta T & Noguchi J (2011): Protease inhibitors for preventing complications associated with ERCP : an updated meta-analysis. Gastrointest. Endosc. Vol. 73, No. 4, pp. 700-706. ISSN 0016-5107

Shao LM, Chen QY, Chen MY, Cai JT (2010): Nitroglycerin in the prevention of post-ERCP pancreatitis : a meta-analysis. Dig. Dis. Sci. Vol 55, No. 1, pp. 1-7. ISSN 0002-9211

Sherman S, Troiano FP, Hawes RH & Lehman GA (1990): Sphincter of Oddi manometry : decreased risk of clinical pancreatitis with use of a modified aspirating catheter. Gastrointest. Endosc. Vol.36, No. 5, pp. 462-466. ISSN 0016-5107

Schwatrz JJ, Lew RJ, Ahmad NA Shah JN, Ginsberg GG, Kochman ML, Brensinger CM & Long WB (2004): The effect of lidocaine sprayed on the major duodenal papilla on the frequency of post-ERCP pancreatitis. Gastrointest. Endosc. Vol. 59, No. 2, pp. 179-184. ISSN 0016-5107

Sotoudehmanesh R, Khatibian M, Kolahdoozan S Ainechi S, Malboosbaf R & Nouraie M (2007): Indomethacin may reduce the incidence and severity of acute pancreatitis after ERCP. Am. J. Gastroenterol. Vol. 102, No. 5 pp. 978-83. ISSN 0002-9270

Tarnasky PR, Cunningham JT, Hawes RH Hoffman BJ, Uflacker R, Vujic I & Cotton PB (1997): Transpapillary stenting of proximal biliary strictures: does biliary sphincterotomy reduce the risk of postprocedure pancreatitis? Gastrointest. Endosc. Vol. 45, No. 1, pp. 46-51. ISSN 0016-5107

Testoni PA, Marani A, Giussani A, VailatiC, Masci E, Macarri G, Ghezzo L, Familiari L, Giardullo N, Mutignani M, Lornbardi G, Talarnini G, Spadaccini A, Briglia R, Piazzi L & SEIFRED Group (2010): Risk factors for post-ERCP pancreatitis in high and low volume centers and among expert and non-expert operators: a prospective, multicenter study. Am. J. Gastroenterol. Vol. 105, No. 4, pp.1753-1761. ISSN 0002-9270

Tulassay Z, Döbrönte Z, Prónai L, Zágoni T & Juhász L (1998) : Octreotide in the prevention of pancreatic injury associated with endoscopic cholangiopancreatography. Aliment. Pharmacol. Ther. Vol.12, No. 11, pp. 1109-1112 ISSN 0269-2813

Wehrmann T, Stergiou N, Schmitt T, Dietrich CE & Seifert H (2003): Reduced risk for pancreatitis after endoscopic microtransducer manometry of the sphincter of Oddi : a randomised comparison with the perfusion manometry technique. Endoscopy Vol. 35, No. 6, pp. 472-477. ISSN 0013-726X

Wildenhain PM, Melhem MF, Birsic WI Sell HW & Rao KN (1989): Acute hemorrhagic pancreatitis in mice: improved survival after indomethacin administration. Digestion, Vol. 44, No. 1, pp. 41-51. ISSN 0012-2823

Wong RF & DiSario JA (2004): Approaches to endoscopic ampullectomy. Curr. Opin. Gastroenterol. Vol. 20, No. 5, pp. 360-467. ISSN 0267-1379

Zheng M-H, Xia H H-X & Chen Y-P (2008): Rectal administration of NSAIDs in the prevention of post-ERCP pancreatitis : a complementary meta-analysis. Gut Vol. 57 No. 11, pp. 1632-1633. ISSN 0017-5749

Zhang Y, Chen QB, Gao ZY, Xie WF (2009): Meta-analysis : octreotide prevents post-ERCP pancreatitis, but only at sufficient doses. Aliment. Pharmacol. Ther. Vol. 29, No. 11, pp. 1155-1164. ISSN 0269-2813

Zolotarevsky E, Fehmi SM, Anderson MA, Schoenfeld PS, Elmunzer BJ, Kwon RS, Piraka CR, Wamsteker EJ, Scheiman JM, Korsnes SJ, Normolle DP, Myra Kim H, Elta GH (2011): Prophylactic 5-Fr pancreatic duct stents are superior to 3-Fr stents : a randomized controlled trial. Endoscopy Vol. 43, No. 4, pp. 325-330. ISSN 0013-726X

14

Nutrition Assessment and Therapy in Acute Pancreatitis

Vanessa Fuchs-Tarlovsky[1] and Krishnan Sriram[2]
[1]*Servicio de Oncología, Hospital General de México, Mexico City,*
[2]*Stroger Cook County Hospital, Rush University, Chicago Illinois,*
[1]*Mexico*
[2]*USA*

1. Introduction

The impact of nutritional status in acute pancreatitis (AP) has not been fully elucidated, but it is probable that severe malnutrition will adversely affect outcomes, as occurs in other critical diseases. Malnutrition is known to occur in 50-80% of chronic alcoholics and alcohol is a major etiological factor in AP. Morbid obesity is also associated with poorer prognosis (Gianotti L et al, 2009). Assessment of the severity of AP, together with the patient´s nutritional status is crucial in the decision-making process that determines the need or otherwise for nutrition support. Both should be done on admission and at frequent intervals thereafter.

Substrate metabolism in AP is similar to that in response to severe sepsis or trauma. There is an increase in protein catabolism, characterized by an inability of exogenous glucose to inhibit gluconeogenesis, increased energy expenditure, increased insulin resistance and increase dependence of fatty acid oxidation to provide energy substrates. Energy needs may differ and change substantially according to the severity and stage of AP, comorbidities, and specific complications occurring during the clinical course of AP.

Assessment criteria that can serve as early predictors of AP severity are often complex and not sufficiently accurate. However, several recently described criteria that rely on criteria such as the body mass index, physical findings, and simple laboratory measurements could prove useful if validated in large prospective studies (Talukdar R et al, 2009).

The factors that influence mortality in different degrees of severity of AP are various. Etiology, age, sex, race, ethnicity, genetic makeup, severity on admission, and the extent and nature of pancreatic necrosis (sterile vs. infected) influence the mortality. Other factors include treatment modalities such as administration of prophylactic antibiotics, parenteral nutrition (PN) vs. enteral (EN), endoscopic retrograde cholangio pancreatography with sphincterotomy, and surgery in selected cases. Epidemiological studies indicate that the incidence of AP is increasing along with an increase in obesity, a bad prognostic factor. Since Ranson reported early prognostic criteria, a number of attempts have been made to simplify or add new clinical or laboratory studies in the early assessment of severity. Obesity, hemoconcentration on admission, presence of pleural effusion, increased fasting blood sugar, as well as creatinine, elevated C-Reactive Protein in serum, and urinary trypsinogen levels are some of the well-documented factors (Pitchumoni CS et al, 2005).

We found evidence that some indicators of nutritional status could be of help in trying to predict mortality in AP, since nutritional status may be associated with final prognosis. Specifically in the case of severe AP, excess body fat, lack of lean body mass, muscle wasting and poor immune status seems to be related with poor prognosis (Fuchs-Tarlovsky V et al, 2010; Fuchs-Tarlovsky V et al, 1997).

PN in the past has always appeared ideally suited as the preferred route for nutrition support over EN in patients with AP. The pathophysiology of the disease process involves a catabolic stress state, elevated caloric requirements; reduction in pancreatic stimulation or "pancreatic rest" appeared to be needed to allow resolution of inflammation within the gland. However, evidence has emerged that other pathophysiologic processes outside the pancreas itself may contribute to the stress state seen in these patients. Failure to use the gut may actually exacerbate the stress response, prolong the duration and severity of the disease, and increase the likelihood of complications (McClave SA et al, 2006; Lugli AK et al, 2007).

More recent clinical trials have suggested that EN in comparison to PN may maintain gut integrity, reduce intestinal permeability, and down regulate the systemic immune response syndrome (SIRS), thereby favorably affecting clinical outcome (Jabbar A et al, 2003). Further evidence suggests that not only is the route of feeding a factor in outcome, but specific agents in EN or PN (immune-modulating agents) such as probiotics or ω-3 fish oil may influence hospital length of stay (LOS) and rate of complications (Olah A et al, 2002; Lasztity N, 2005).

2. Nutrition assessment in AP

Severe AP is associated with high mortality. Adequate nutrition support improves clinical outcome. Nevertheless, several recent trials have focused primarily on the route of nutrition support and neglected the role of nutrition status assessment in tailoring nutrition support to individual needs (Lugli AK et al, 2007).

Definition of an optimal nutritional regimen requires knowledge of energy requirements. Because pancreatitis is a serious disease, it is presumed to be associated with marked increases in energy expenditure. However, data for measured resting energy expenditure (REE) in patients with pancreatitis are limited. In a study aimed to assess the REE of patients with pancreatitis, Dickerson et al found a significantly higher value in those patients complicated by sepsis than those with pancreatitis alone. Septic patients had the largest percentage of hypermetabolic REE, >110% of predicted energy expenditure. They measured REE ranged from 77% to 139% of predicted energy expenditure according to Harris-Benedict equation. The authors concluded that REE is variable in patients with pancreatitis; and the Harris-Benedict equation is an unreliable estimate of caloric expenditure. Septic complications are associated with hypermetabolism and may be the most important factor influencing REE (Dickerson R et al, 1991).

AP increases the catabolism and proteolysis of skeletal muscle by as much as 80% in comparison with normal controls. Further, nitrogen losses have been shown to increase to as much as 20 to 40 g/d (Dickerson R, et al 1991). Decreased levels of total plasma proteins and rapid turnover proteins and marked decrease of the ratio of branched-chain to aromatic amino acid further characterize the hypermetabolic state (Havala T et al 1989; Shaw JHF, 1986). Significant decrease in plasma essential aminoacids, with marked reductions of

almost all amino acids by skeletal muscle mass, have been reported clinically and experimentally (Bouffard YH et al. 1989).
Another study reported the changes in body composition, plasma proteins, and REE during 14 days of PN in patients with AP. Total body protein (TBP), total body water (TBW), and total body fat (TBF) were measured by neutron activation analysis and tritium dilution before and after PN. They studied 15 patients with AP, most of them with severe disease. The gains in body weight, TBW, TBP, Fat Free Mass, TBF and resting energy expenditure after 14 days were not significant. The authors concluded that body composition is preserved in AP during 14 days of PN. In patients without sepsis or recent surgery, PN was able to significantly increase body protein stores (Chandrasegaram MD et al, 2005).
We have found that there are some nutritional parameters associated with mortality in AP. From the nutritional indicators measured, body fat reserves, renal function, muscle mass and immune function were the parameters that associated better with mortality in AP (Fuchs-Tarlovsky et al 1997). In another study aimed to validate these findings, we found that the group with higher mortality was associated with higher fat reserves, lower immune function or lymphocyte count and lower muscle reserves (Fuchs-Tarlovsky et al., 2010).

3. Pancreatic rest and secretions

Today, the validity of this concept of "pancreatic rest" is no longer accepted (Petrov MS et al, 2008; Ioannidis O et al, 2008; Talukdar R et al, 2009). Efforts to keep up with the increased energy demands in the case of AP are thwarted by the adage to put the pancreas at rest and the avoidance of pancreatic stimulation via gut luminal nutrition. The "pancreatic rest concept" assumes that the pancreatic rest promotes healing, decreases pain, and reduces secretion and leakage of the pancreatic juices in pancreas parenchyma and pancreas tissue (McClave SA et al, 1997). This concept disregards the presence of basal pancreatic exocrine secretion. Protein enzyme output is the responsible component for autodigestion of the gland and perpetuation of inflammatory process. Suppression of protein enzymes output alone with continued bicarbonate and fluid volume output may therefore be adequate in putting the pancreas to rest.

3.1 Pancreatic secretion

Pancreatic secretion and gut motility are tightly interwoven. Basal enzyme secretion is 20% of maximal enzyme secretion and it is regulated by cholinergic and cholecystokinin (CCK)-mediated mechanisms. Feeding by mouth increases pancreatic secretion by involving 3 stimulation levels: cephalic, gastric and intestinal level or phase (Spanier BM et al, 2011). The mere sight of food begins the process of pancreatic secretion and prepares the gut for digestion. Once the food enters the mouth and is chewed and swallowed there is a strong vagal stimulation which fortifies this response. The passage of food into the stomach produces mechanical effects, which further amplify the vagal response and, in addition, lead to gastric acid secretion. Finally, the movement of food and secretions through the pylorus into the duodenum culminates in the maximal stimulatory effect mediated by humoral CCK and secretin and also cholinergic excitation. For many years it was considered that CCK was the chief stimulus for pancreatic enzyme secretion but now it is known that the response id complex and possibly mediated through cholinergic activation (O'Kaffe SJ et al, 2006).

Further studies have demonstrated that as food progresses through the gastrointestinal (GI) tract, there are a series of feedback loops all the way down from the stomach to the colon. Passage of food into the jejunum also inhibits gastric emptying and intestinal transit. The presence of food in the ileum inhibits jejunal motility, presence of nutrients in the ileum inhibits not only pancreatic secretion but also gastric emptying and intestinal transit, and finally the transit of digested food into the colon augments the activation of the ileal brake (Van Citters GW, 1999).

The duration of pancreatic enzyme response increases with greater caloric load. The pancreatic response is also influenced by the physical properties of the meal: mixed solid-liquid meals induce a higher response than liquid or homogenized meals with similar energy content. In both instances, the rate of gastric emptying and thus duodenal delivery of nutrients are the key factors which determine the duration of the pancreatic secretion. The proportion of fat, carbohydrate, and protein contents within a meal also influence the duration and enzyme composition of the pancreatic response (Spanier BM et al, 2011).

3.2 Pancreatic secretion with Enteral Nutrition (EN)

The degree to which the pancreas is stimulated by EN is determined by the site in the GI tract at which feeding is infused. Feeding infused into the jejunum beyond the ligament of Treitz may bypass the cephalic, gastric, and intestinal phase of stimulation of pancreatic secretion, is less likely to stimulate CCK and secretin, and may stimulate inhibiting polypeptides (Abou S et al 2002, Russell MK at al, 2004, Scolapio JS et al, 1999). It has been demonstrated in human studies during jejunal feeding that the pancreatic enzyme output increased significantly over basal levels when it was delivered at the ligament of Treitz, whereas there was no significant increase during more distal jejunal feeding, 60 cm beyond the ligament of Treitz (Vu MK et al, 1999).

Also, the composition of the infused feeds is important. There is some evidence to support an added benefit of elemental formulae for putting the pancreas to rest compared to standard formulae with intact protein or blenderized diets. Elemental diets cause less stimulation than standard formulas, because of their low fat content, the presence of free amino acids instead of intact proteins which bind to free trypsin in the gut, causing trypsin levels to fall, and less acid production from the stomach (Spanier MS et al, 2011).

4. Nutrition therapy

Nutrition therapy in the past has been governed by the principle that the gut should be put at rest with avoidance of any stimulation of pancreatic exocrine secretion. These concepts should now be replaced by the principle that pancreatic stimulation should be reduced to basal rates, but that the gut integrity should be maintained and that the stress response should be contained the likelihood of multiorgan failure (MOF), nosocomial infections, and mortality (McClave SA et al, 1998).

Usually, the initial treatment of AP consists of a nil per os (NPO) regimen and administration of analgesics and ample intravenous fluids (Pandol SJ et al, 2007; Forsmark CE et al, 2007). However, within 24-48 hours EN should be initiated. The rationale for a period without food intake is the assumption that pancreatic stimulation by enteral feeding may aggravate pancreatic inflammation. Moreover, many patients are anorectic and may suffer increasing pain sensation when eating and ileus-related nausea and vomiting, and delayed return of appetite (Banks PA et al, 2006; Forsmark CE et al, 2007; Meier R et al, 2005; Gianotti L et al, 2009).

There have been studies regarding PN and PN supplemented with special nutrients. A Chinese study by Xian-Li et al evaluated the effects of supplemental parenteral glutamine. Forty one patients with severe AP were randomized to receive either PN or PN with glutamine. Use of PN with parenteral glutamine was associated with significantly less pancreatic infection (0.0% vs 23.8%, $p<0.05$) and fewer overall complications (20% vs 52%, $p<0.05$) compared to the use of PN alone without supplemental glutamine (Xian-Li H et al, 2004).

However today's data trends more to the use of EN rather than PN as will be discussed below.

4.1 Enteral vs Parenteral Nutrition

Traditionally, patients with AP were either treated with strict rest or given PN to allow the pancreas to "rest" until the serum enzyme levels returned to normal. Unfortunately, some disadvantages are associated with the use of PN; one of the most serious is catheter related sepsis. Currently, EN is preferred for patients with AP because it is more cost effective than PN and results in fewer complications (Siow E, 2008).

Despite fears that EN may exacerbate AP because of the stimulatory effect of luminal nutrients on trypsinogen synthesis, several randomized clinical trials have shown that outcome is better and the cost is lower if EN is used instead of PN (McClave SA et al, 1997; Abou-Assi S et al, 2002; Kalfarentzos F et al, 1997). EN can improve survival and reduce the complications accompanying severe AP. The explanations are: EN avoids PN related complications; luminal nutrition maintains intestinal health; enteral aminoacids are more effective in supporting splanchnic protein synthesis; EN may prevent the progression of MOF (Ionnidis O et al, 2008).

In addition to its mucosal protective and immunomodulatory effects, EN is the most effective way of supporting intestinal metabolism. By down-regulating splachnic cytokine production and modulating the acute phase response, EN reduces catabolism and preserves protein (Winsdor AC et al, 1998). In addition, EN with a diet enriched with glutamine has beneficial effect on recovery of IgG and IgM-proteins with a trend to shorter disease duration (Grant J et al, 1984).

There are some clinical studies that compared the use of PN versus EN in AP; the end points analyzed were mortality and complications. From 1996 to 2006 there were 5 studies which studied these outcomes; none of the studies yielded evidence of a difference in the mortality rates between patients given EN and patients given PN. Louie at al reported no deaths among patients given EN and 3 deaths among patients given PN. Those deaths however were attributed to complications of pancreatitis rather than to the mode of nutrition (Louie BE et al, 2005).

Most of the randomized clinical studies reviewed reported higher complication rates among patients given PN than among the EN groups. Kalfatenzos at al reported significantly lower total number of complications for patients given EN compared with the PN group. Complications such as sepsis, nosocomial infection, catheter-related infection, and hyperglycemia are common findings in all studies, especially in patients who were given PN (Kalfarenzos FE et al, 1991). Abou-Assi et al showed a significant difference in rates of catheter–related infections between patients given EN and those with PN. The patients with

infections eventually required removal of the venous catheter and antibiotic treatment (Abou-Assi S et al, 2002). McClave at al. on the other hand, observed equal increases in the risk of infectious complications and the incidences of fluid and electrolyte imbalances (McClave SA et al, 1997).
Louie at al found that the mean number of days of elevated blood glucose levels was 2.7 in the enteral group and 3.6 in the parenteral group (Louie BE, 2005). In all the above mentioned studies, the patients who received EN required fewer days to the start of oral diet than did the PN groups. Abou-Assi et al showed significant evidence that the patients given EN received 4.1 fewer days of nutritional support than the PN group. After disease resolution, 80% of the patients in EN progressed to oral diet without problem, compared with 63% in the PN group (Abou-Assi S et al, 2002).
In addition, all of these clinical trials demonstrated that EN is cheaper than PN. Gupta et al provided significant evidence that patients given EN require a shorter length of hospitalization than patients given PN (Gupta R et al, 2003).
In a recent systematic review about EN vs PN in pancreatitis the authors compared the effect of PN vs EN in patients with AP. The searches or randomized clinical trials were from 2000 to 2008. Eight trials with a total of 348 participants were included. Comparing EN to PN in AP, the relative risk (RR) for deaths was 0.5 (95% CI 0.28 to 0.91), for MOF was 0.55 (95% CI 0.37 to 0.81), for systemic infection was 0-39 (95% CI 0.23 to 0.65), for operative interventions was 0.44 (95% CI 0.29 to 0.67), for local septic complications was 0.74 (95% CI 0.40 to 1.35), and for other local complications was 0.70 (95% CI 0.43 to 1.13). Mean LOS was reduced by 2.37 days in EN vs PN groups (95% CI - 7.18 to 2.44). Furthermore, a subgroup analysis for EN vs PN in patients with severe AP showed a RR for death of 0.18 (95% CI 0.06 to 0.58) and RR for MOF of 0.46 (95% CI 0.16 to 1.29) (Al-Omran M et al, 2010).
McClave et al concluded after performing a systematic review of literature comparing EN vs PN in AP that EN reduces oxidative stress, hastens resolution of the disease process, and costs less. Insufficient data exists to determine whether EN improves outcome over standard therapy. However, in those patients requiring surgery for complications of AP, meta-analysis of 2 trials indicates that provision of EN postoperatively may reduce mortality (RR_0.26; 95% CI 0.0-1.09; p=0.06) compared with standard therapy (McClave SA et al, 2006).
In patients with AP, EN significantly reduced mortality, MOF, systemic infections, and the need for operative interventions compared with those who received PN. In addition, there was a trend towards a reduction in LOS. These data suggest that EN should be considered the standard of care for patients with AP requiring nutritional support. This recommendation is supported by the 2009 American Society for Parenteral and Enteral Nutrition (ASPEN) and Society for Critical Care Medicine (SCCM) Guidelines (McClave SA et al, 2009). Although hypertriglyceridemia may occasionally be the cause of AP, several years of clinical use has shown that PN containing lipid emulsions are safe in this condition (Leibowitz AB, 1992). Serum triglyceride levels should be monitored. Addition of heparin to PN infusate may decrease triglyceride levels in some patients (Benderly A et al, 1983). Table 1 summarizes the available information on the special nutrients in enteral feedings.

4.2 Nasojejunal (NJ) vs Nasogastric feeding (NG)

NJ feeding tubes are placed blindly at the bedside, expecting spontaneous transpyloric migration or by using endoscopic or radiologic control.

Reference Author, year	Study design	Type of nutrition	Results	Conclusion
Abou -Assi et al, 2002	Randomized controlled comparative clinical trial	EN(NJ) vs. PN	Duration of feeding was shorter in the EN (6.7 vs. 10.8 days, $p<0.05$) and nutrition costs were lower in the EN group. Metabolic ($p<0.003$) and septic ($p=0.01$) complications were lower in the EN group.	EN seems to be safer and less expensive than PN in AP.
Kalfarentzos F et al, 1997	Randomized controlled comparative clinical trial	EN vs. PN	Patients who received EN experienced fewer complications ($P<0.05$) , specially septic complications ($P<0.01$) than those receiving PN. PN costs were three times higher than EN.	EN should be used preferentially in patients with severe AP.
Winsdor AC et al, 1998	Randomized controlled comparative clinical trial	EN vs. PN	The acute phase response and disease severity scores were significantly improved following EN (CRP: 156(117-222) to 84(50-141), $p<0.005$; APACHE II scores 8(6-10) to 6(4- 8), $P<0.0001$) without change in the CT scan scores. In the PN group, these parameters did not change but there was an increment in the EndoCAb antibody levels and reduction in the CT scan scores. EN did not show changes in the level EndoCAb level but there was an increase in the CT scan scores.	EN moderates the acute phase response, and improves disease severity and clinical outcome despite unchanged pancreatic injury on CT scan. EN reduced systemic exposure to endotoxin and reduced oxidative stress; it also modulates the inflammatory and sepsis response in PA.
Luie BE et al, 2005	Randomized controlled comparative clinical trial	PN vs. EN	Reduction of CRP levels by 50% was 5 days faster with EN than with PN. Nutrition support costs were lower in the EN group.	EN shows a trend toward faster attenuation of inflammation, with fewer septic complications and is the preferred therapy in terms of cost - effectiveness.
Gupta R et al, 2003	Randomized controlled comparative clinical trial	EN vs. PN	Fatigue improved in groups but faster with EN. Oxidative stress was similar in both groups. There were no significant differences in complication rate and LOS was shorter in EN group (7(4-14)vs10(7-26)days; $p=0.05$) The cost in the EN group was considerably less than PN.	EN is safe in severe AP. It is as effective as PN and may be beneficial in the clinical course of disease.

Abbreviations: AP= Acute Pancreatitis / EN = Enteral Nutrition / PN = Parenteral Nutrition / LOS = Length of Hospital Stay

Table 1. Comparative studies between EN and PN

Eatock at al. performed a randomized controlled study on early NG versus NJ feeding in severe AP (Eatock FC et al , 2000; Eatock FC et al, 2005). They found that NG feedings were very well tolerated and recommended that NG feedings should be considered a therapeutic option because of its simplicity, obviating the need for endoscopic or radiologic procedures. This study had several limitations, one of them being the failure to fluoroscopically confirm that the NJ tubes were appropriately positioned in the jejunum. There is no indication whether the NJ tubes were placed distal enough (at least 60 cms from the ligament of Treitz) to avoid gastric and pancreatic stimulation. The failure to find difference may have been related to continued gastric and duodenal stimulation occurring in both groups of patients. Similar findings from randomized studies were reported by Eckerwall et al who performed a randomized clinical trial to compare the efficacy and safety of early EN via NG tubes with PN. The authors reported that early NG EN in patients with severe AP was feasible, and resulted in better glucose control. No beneficial effects on the intestinal permeability or on the inflammatory response were seen by EN treatment (Eckerwall GE et al, 2006).

Kumar et al performed a randomized clinical trial to compare early NJ with NG feeding in severe AP, and showed that that EN at a slow infusion is well tolerated by both NJ and NG routes in patients with severe AP. Neither feedings leads to recurrence or worsening of pain in patients with severe AP. They also reported that nutritional parameters remained unaffected because of inadequate caloric intake during the first week of feeding (Kumar A et al, 2006).

Vu et al studied the activation of pancreatic secretion in 8 healthy volunteers in response to proximal or more distal jejunal delivery of nutrients into the small intestine. The authors concluded that continuous feeding into the distal jejunum does not stimulate exocrine pancreatic secretion (Vu MK et al, 1999).

Piciucchi M et al assessed the rate of spontaneous tube migration and to compare the effects of naso-intestinal (NI) tube feeding in AP. They defined NI location as those tubes placed beyond the ligament of Treitz. The authors showed that spontaneous tube migration to an NI site occurred in 10 of 25 or 25% of the patients, while in 15 (60%) EN was started with an NG tube. EN through NG or NI were similar in terms of tolerability, safety, clinical goals, complications and hospital stay. As a conclusion, EN by NG tubes seem to provide a pragmatic alternative opportunity with similar outcomes in AP (Piciucchi M et al, 2010).

McClave SA et al also commented in their meta-analysis that a wide range of tolerance to EN exists, irrespective of known influences such as mode (continuous versus bolus) and level of infusion within the GI tract (gastric versus postpyloric) (McClave SA et al, 2006).

Patients with severe necrotizing pancreatitis may have gastric outlet obstruction or severe gastroparesis and many may have to be approached differently. Feeding into the stomach may be ineffective and possibly hazardous. Further multicenter randomized trials studies are needed to confirm whether NG feeding is a practical and effective form of management for patients with severe AP (Ioannidis O et al, 2008). Table 2 summarizes the available information on the special nutrients in enteral feedings.

4.3 When to start nutrition support

Per oral ingestion of nutrients is often hampered by abdominal pain with food aversion, nausea, vomiting, gastric atony, and paralytic ileus or by partial duodenal obstruction from pancreatic gland enlargement. The application of early EN may be limited by the severity of the pancreatitis attack and the occurrence of ileus (Spanier BWM, et al. 2011).

Reference	**Study design**	**Via or Enteral Feeds**	**Results**	**Conclusion**
Eatock FC et al, 2005	Randomized controlled comparative clinical trial	NG vs. NJ	Clinical differences between the two groups were not significant. Overall mortality was 24.5% with five deaths in the NG group and seven in the NJ group.	The simpler, cheaper, and easier to use NG feeding is as good as NJ feeding in patients with objectively graded severe AP.
Kumar A et al, 2006	Randomized controlled comparative clinical trial	NJ vs. NG	Group1 (NG): Diarrhea occurred in 4 patients and there were 5 deaths, 1 patient underwent surgery. Group 2(NJ): Diarrhea occurred in 3 patients, there were 4 deaths, and 2 patients underwent surgery.	EN at a slow infusion is well tolerated by both NJ and NG routes in patients with AP. Neither NJ nor NG feeding leads to recurrence or worsening of pain in AP. Nutritional parameters remained unaffected because of inadequate calorie intake during the first week of feeding.
Piciucchi M et al, 2010	Randomized controlled comparative clinical trial	NG vs. NJ	Spontaneous tube migration to NJ site occurred in 10/25(40%) prospectively enrolled severe AP patients; while in 15 (60%) nutrition was started with a NG tube. CT severity index was higher in NG tube patients than in NI (mean 6.2 vs. 4.7, P = 0.04).	Spontaneous distal tube migration is successful in 40% of severe AP patients, with higher CT severity index predicting IG retention; in such cases EN by NG tubes seems to provide a pragmatic alternative opportunity with similar outcomes.

Abbreviations: AP= Acute Pancreatitis / NJ = Nasojejunal feeding / NG = Nasogastric feeding /IG = Intragastric/NI=Nasointestinal

Table 2. Comparative studies between NJ and NG

The precise timing for initiating enteral support has not been specifically addressed in the pancreatitis population but has been studied to a large extent in the critically ill population. EN has been described as a rational and acceptable option of supporting critically ill patients after major abdominal surgery, as well as in patients with AP (Windsor AC et al, 1998). Early EN starting prior to 48 hours from admission in critically ill patients is associated with a significant 24% reduction in infectious complications and 32% reduction in mortality compared with delay feedings started after that point time (McClave SA et al, 2009; Heyland DK et al, 2003)

Olah et al demonstrated that early jejunal feeding with an elemental diet within 48 hours after the onset of symptoms when possible, and was more useful and cheaper than PN. They concluded that early jejunal feeding reduced septic complications in necrotizing AP in combination with adequate antibiotic prophylaxis (Olah A et al, 2002).

Pupelis G et al performed a randomized clinical trial measuring the feasibility and effectiveness of jejunal feeding after surgery due to peritonitis in severe AP. They concluded that early jejunal feeding resulted in 3.3% mortality as opposed to 23.3% in the control group (p=0.05) and that jejunal feeding is feasible and effective in postoperative treatment of patients due to secondary peritonitis because of AP (Pupelis G et al, 2001). Table 3 summarizes the available information on the special nutrients in enteral feedings.

Author, reference, year	**Study design**	**Time to start nutrition therapy**	**Results**	**Conclusion**
Pupelis G et al, 2001	Randomized controlled comparative clinical trial	Patients in EN group received the daily mean of 1294.6 (362.6) kcal including 830.6 (372.7) kcal enterally, versus 472.8 (155.8) kcal daily in the control group (P < 0.0001).	The first surgical intervention resulted in 3.3% of re-laparotomies in EN patients, caused by unresolved peritonitis, versus 26.7% in the control subjects (P = 0.03). Recovery of bowel transit took significantly less time in the EN patients (mean: 54.6 h versus 76.8 h in control subjects, P = 0.01). EN resulted in 3.3% mortality as opposed to 23.3% in the control group (P = 0.05).	EN is feasible and effective in postoperative treatment of patients due to secondary peritonitis or severe pancreatitis. Improved bowel and peritoneal function could be the main impact of EN.
Oláh et al, 2002	Randomized controlled comparative clinical trial	1st phase: PN was compared with early (within 24-72 h after the onset symptoms) EN.	Septic complications were lower in the EN group (P = 0.08, chi(2) test)	The combination of early EN and selective, adequate antibiotic prophylaxis may prevent multiple organ failure in patients with AP.
Kalfarentzos, 1991	Randomized controlled comparative clinical trial	Group1:EN in the first 72 hours an EN later in the course of the disease	Group 1: 23% complications and 13% mortality Group 2: 95.6% complications rate and 38% mortality P<0.01	Early EN reduced complications rate and mortality in AP

Abbreviations: Se=Selenium / AP= Acute Pancreatitis / EN = Enteral Nutrition

Table 3. Comparative studies between early and late EN

4.4 Types of enteral formula recommended

A few studies to date compare the results of feeding elemental, semielemental, and polymeric diets to patients with AP (Marik PE, 2009 and Talukdar R et al, 2009). Elemental formulas are completely predigested and consist of aminoacids, simple sugars, and enough fat to prevent essential fatty acid deficiency. Semielemental formulas required less digestion than polymeric foods and contain peptides of varying chain length, simple sugars, glucose polymer, or starch and fat primarily as medium chain triglycerides. Polymeric feeds contain non-hydrolyzed proteins, complex carbohydrates, and longchain triglycerides. Based on the assumption that elemental and semielemental formulas cause less pancreatic stimulation than standard formulas, most EN studies have used an elemental or semielemental formula. Although there is a variety of data on the use of standard enteral formula in such patients (Spanier BWM et al, 2011), both Windsor et al and Pupelis et al have shown that polymeric formula can be safely fed through jejunal tubes in AP patients (Windsor ACJ, 1998; Pupelis G et al., 2001).

A few studies have defined the benefits of semielemental versus polymeric formulas in severe AP. Cravo et al found a similar tolerance in 102 patients with AP given semielemental versus polymeric formulas (Cravo M et al, 1989). In a randomized trial using semielemental and polymeric formulas in 30 AP patients, Tiegou et al showed that both formulas were well tolerated and well absorbed, but the semielemental group had less weight loss and shorter LOS compared with the polymeric group (Tiegou IE, 2006). Petrov et al performed an adjusted meta-analysis using 20 randomized controlled trials, including 1070 patients. None of the studies was associated with a significant difference in feeding tolerance when comparing the tolerance and safety of EN formulations in patients with AP. The use of a semielemental diet versus polymeric formulation did not show significant differences (RR= 0.62). The authors concluded that the use of polymeric compared with semielemental formulation, does not lead to a significant higher risk of feeding intolerance, infectious complications, or death in AP patients (Petrov MS et al, 2008; Petrov MS et al, 2009). Table 4 summarizes the available information on the special nutrients in enteral feedings.

It should be remembered that semielemental or elemental diets are sevenfold as expensive as polymeric feeds, and in some countries perhaps even more expensive. In summary, the evidence base to use just semielemental or elemental formulas becomes less clear (Spanier BWM et al, 2011).

4.5 Use of supplements or special nutrients in Enteral Nutrition

The routine use of glutamine, immunonutrition, prebiotics and probiotics in AP is not supported by large scale clinical studies. Two studies evaluated immune-enhancing formulas that contain glutamine, arginine and fibers or glutamine, arginine and ω-3 fatty acids, vitamins, and micronutrients (Hallay J et al, 2001; Pearce CB et al, 2006). Hallay et al compared a standard formula with a glutamine-enriched formula on immunologic parameters in 16 patients with AP; they found that the recovery of the immunological parameters was better and the time of disease recovery was shorter in the glutamine treated group. Other authors also reported the beneficial effect of a glutamine-rich multifiber diet as compared to a standard fiber diet; the trend of IgG and IgM, as well as visceral proteins (prealbumin and Retinol Binding Protein) with shorter disease duration was seen in the treatment group (Hallay J et al, 2001).

Author, reference, year	Study design	Types of formula	Results	Conclusion
Tiegou IE, 2006	Randomized comparative prospective controlled clinical trial	Semi-elemental vs polymeric formula.	Tolerance was good in both groups (semi-elemental vs. polymeric: VAS, 7.4 +/- 0.6 vs. 7.1 +/- 0.6 NS; number of stools per 24 hours, 1.7 +/- 0.4 vs. 1.8 +/- 0.4, NS). Steatorrhea was lower than normal in both groups. In the semi-elemental formula group, the hospital LOS was shorter (23 +/- 2 vs. 27 +/- 1, p = .006) and weight loss was less marked (1 +/- 1 vs. 2 +/- 0, p = .01). One patient in semi-elemental group and 3 patients in polymeric group developed an infection (NS).	Semi-elemental and polymeric nutrition are very well tolerated in patients with AP. Nutrition with a semi-elemental formula supports the hypothesis of a more favorable clinical course than nutrition with a polymeric formula.
Windsor ACJ, 1998	Randomized Clinical trial	Polymeric formula "Osmolite"®,"Fresubin"®	Following seven days of enteral nutritional support there was a significant reduction in serum CRP from 156 (117–222) mg/l to 84 (50–141) mg/l ($p<0.005$) and APACHE II scores fell from 8 (6–10) to 6 (4–8) ($p<0.0001$) in the enterally fed group.	Polymeric formula can be safely fed through NJ tubes in AP patients. Enteral feeding in acute pancreatitis is practical. Furthermore is both feasible and desirable in the management of patients with acute pancreatitis.
Cravo M et al, 1989	Prospective	Elemental (group 1/ n=47) vs polymeric formula (group 2 / n=44)	Mean nutrient intake was higher in group II ($p<0.001$): Kcal: 1447+228 vs 1161+182; protein: 45+9 vs 30+8g; fat: 31+10 vs 4+3g. Local complications rate was similar (17% in group I vs 7% in group II) and LOS was: In group I -6.6±3 .2 vs Group II-6.3±2.2d.	Elemental diets offer no advantage upon polymeric balanced diets.

Abbreviations: NS=Non significant / AP= Acute Pancreatitis / EN=Enteral Nutrition /NJ=Nasojejunal/ LOS=Length of hospital stay

Table 4. Comparative studies between the efficacies of the different types of EN

Pearce at al supplemented arginine, glutamine, ω-3 fatty acids and antioxidants in 31 patients with severe AP in a randomized control trial; their findings suggest that an increase in C-Reactive Protein was found in the supplemented group compared with the control group. No significant differences were found in the length of hospital stay. Although a lower incidence of pneumonia and MOF, and shorter length of ICU and hospital stay was observed in the immunonutrition group, none of these differences reached statistical significance (Pearce CB et al, 2006).

De Beaux et al randomized 14 patients with severe AP to receive standard PN of isocaloric, isonitrogenous, glutamine-enriched PN; only 13 patients completed the study. There was a trend for the glutamine supplemented group to show improved lymphocyte proliferation, increased T-cell DNA synthesis and decrease release of the pro-inflammatory cytokine IL-8 (De Beaux AC et al, 1998).

A double blind randomized clinical trial by Olah et al evaluated the effects of probiotics added to EN. They proposed that the rapid disappearance of commensal flora in AP, combined with overgrowth of potentially pathogenic organisms, provided the rationale for probiotic therapy. The authors divided patients into 2 groups; the treatment group, who received a preparation containing *Lactobacillus plantarum* together with a substrate of oat fiber for one week by NJ tube; and the control group who received heat inactivated *Lactobacillus* strain preparation. Infected pancreatic necrosis and abscesses occurred in 4% of the patients in the treatment group as compared to 30% in the control group ($p=0.023$). The mean hospital LOS was shorter in the treatment group as well ($p<0.05$) (Olah A et al, 2002).

Lasztity evaluated whether provision of ω-3 polyunsaturated fatty acids (ω-3 PUFA) or fish oil could alter the course of disease in AP through modulation of eicosanoid synthesis. Supplementation of EN with 3.3 g/d of ω-3 PUFA for 7 days in the treatment group resulted in a significant decrease in hospital LOS ($p<0.05$) and duration of nutrition therapy (Lasztity N, 2005).

Author, reference, year	Study design	Special nutrient in formula	Results	Conclusion
Hallay J et al, 2001	Randomized clinical trial	"Stresson " ® Multi Fibre vs "Nutrison" ® Fibre	The treatment with glutamine-rich "Stresson" ® resulted in significant elevations in the serum levels of IgG, retinol binding protein, compared to the effects of Nutrison Fibre. In addition, the recovery of treated patients was significantly shorter in the "Stresson" ® Multi Fibre group than in the "Nutrison " ® Fibre group.	The "Stresson" ® Multi Fibre nutrient treatment of patients treated for AP seems to have clinical benefit based upon the fast recovery of IgG, IgM proteins and the immunological defense mechanisms.
Pearce CB et al, 2006	Double-blind Randomized controlled trial	Glutamine, arginine, tributyrin and antioxidants vs an isocaloric isonitrogenous	After 3 days of feeding, in the study group 2/15 (13%) of patients had reduced their CRP by 40 mg/L or more. In the control group 6/16 (38%) of patients had reduced their CRP by this	The cause of the unexpectedly higher CRP values in the study group is unclear.

Author, reference, year	Study design	Special nutrient in formula	Results	Conclusion
			amount. This difference was found to be near the statistical significant limit (P=0.220).	
Oláh A et al, 2002	Randomized clinical trial	Group 1: Received Lactobacillus plantarum together with a substrate of oat fibre. Group 2(control): Received a isonitrogenous formula but the Lactobacillus was inactivated by heat.	Infected pancreatic necrosis and abscesses occurred in 1 of 22 patients in the treatment group, compared with 7 of 23 in the control group (P = 0.023). The mean length of stay was 13.7 days in the treatment group versus 21.4 days in the control group (p=NS).	Supplementary L. plantarum was effective in reducing pancreatic sepsis and the number of surgical interventions.
Lasztity, 2005	Randomized clinical trial	N-3 PUFAs (fish oil) enterally (3.3g/day for 5-7 days).	The n-3 to n-6 LCPUFA ratios increased significantly in serum lipids of the patients receiving supplementation. The SOD activity was significantly higher at day 3 in the supplemented group (P<0.05).	The use of enteral formula enriched with n-3 PUFAs in the treatment of AP seems to have clinical benefits based upon the shortened time of jejunal feeding and hospital stay
Kuklinski B et al, 1995	Randomized clinical trial	Antioxidant treatment sodium selenite as a water soluble redox substance represented an alternative	With a well-timed selenium therapy the rates of lethality complications and operation dropped drastically. Complications occurred if the therapy began too late (if patients were administered too late) and in biliary forms.	An improvement in the prognosis of acute pancreatitis can be achieved if antioxidant selenium therapy with sodium Se is introduced in time. In rare cases total necroses and complications in organs only occurred in those patients who were admitted to this therapy too late.

Abbreviations: Se=Selenium / AP= Acute Pancreatitis / PUFA = Polyunsaturated fatty acids / SOD= Superoxide dismutase

Table 5. Special Nutrients in Enteral Feeding

In a study by Kuklinski et al. reduction of plasma selenium levels was noted in patients with AP; positive results after the addition of selenium into the intestinal diet of these patients was reported (Kuklinski B et al, 1995). Despite the limited number of reports on this subject, the European Society of Parenteral and Enteral Nutrition (ESPEN) Guidelines recommend the use of PN with selenium in patients with AP (Meier R et al, 2006).

In summary, the beneficial effect of EN on patient outcome in AP may be enhanced by providing certain supplements. Although adding arginine, glutamine, ω-3 fatty acids, or specific probiotic preparation to the EN in patients with AP may result in reduction of hospital LOS, duration of nutrition therapy, or certain complications (when compared with the use of EN alone without the supplements), not enough information is available to make firm and specific recommendations. The addition of parenteral glutamine to PN should be considered in order to shorten hospital LOS and duration of nutrition therapy (when compared with PN alone without the supplement (McClave SA et al, 2006). Table 5 summarizes the available information on the special nutrients in enteral feedings.

5. Conclusions

Most patients with AP have mild disease and do not need additional nutrition support during admission. According to guidelines, nutritional support is generally indicated if patients cannot consume normal food after 5-7 days when it becomes evident that the patients will not be able to tolerate oral intake for prolonged period of time (7 days or more) (Spanier BM et al, 2011). However, in a malnourished patient, especially if critically ill, nutrition therapy in some form must be provided earlier, to avoid caloric deficits.

Nutrition therapy by enteral route is now the modality of choice for patients with severe AP. Recent guidelines have summarized the levels 1 and 2 evidence in support of the preferred role of EN according to safety, cost, and ease of administration. Patients with AP should be provided EN early because such therapy modulates the stress response, promotes more rapid resolution of the disease process, and results in better outcome. EN has beneficial influence on the disease course and should be initiated as early as possible (within 48 hours of admission). Large multicenter studies are still needed to confirm the safety and effectiveness of NG feeding when compared with NJ feeding and to investigate the role of early (within 48 hours) versus late nutrition support. When distal jejunal access is not possible to attain or maintain, intragastric feeding can be cautiously initiated, following safe practice standards. The clinical evidence to use semielemental diets is still weak. Routine use of supplementation formulas with glutamine and probiotics or immune-enhancing diets in AP cannot be recommended at this time.

6. References

Abou-Assi S, Craig K, O'Kaffe JD. Acute pancreatitis: results of a randomized comparative study. Am J Gastroenterol. 2002; 97(9):2255-2262.

Al-Omran M, Albawi ZH, Tashkandi MF et al. Enteral versus parenteral nutrition for acute pancreatitis. Cochrane Database systematic reviews. (1):CD002837, 2010.

Banks PA, Freeman ML, Fass R. Practice guidelines in acute pancreatitis. Am J Gastroenterol, 2006;101(10): 2379-2400.

Benderly A, Rosenthal E, Levi J, Brook G. Effect of heparin on lipoprotein profile during parenteral nutrition. J Parenter Enteral Nutr JPEN. 7:37-39, 1983.

Bouffard YH, Delafosse BX, Annat GJ et al. Energy expenditure during severe acute pancreatitis. JPEN J Parenter Enteral Nutr 1989; 13: 26.

Chandrasegaram MD, Plank LD, Windsor JA. The impact of Parenteral nutrition on body Composition of patients with acute pancreatitis. JPEN J Parenter Enteral Nutr. 2005;29(2):65-73.

Cravo M, Camilo ME. Marques A at al. Early tube feeding in acute pancreatitis: a prospective study. Clin Nutr. 1989:A8-A14.

Dickerson R, Vehe K, Mullen J el al. Resting energy expenditure in patients with pancreatitis. Critical Care Medicine. 1991; 19(4):484-490.

De Beaux AC, O'Riordan MG, Ross JA et al. Glutamine-supplemented total parenteral nutrition reduced blood mononuclear cell interleukin-8 release in severe acute pancreatitis. Nutrition 1998; 14:261-5.

Eatock FC, Brombacher GD, Steven A et al. Nasogastric feeding in severe acute pancreatitis may be practical and safe. Int J Pancreatol. 2000; 28(1): 23-29.

Eatock FC, Chong O, Menezes N et al. A randomized study of early nasogastric versus nasojejunal feeding in severe acute pancreatitis. Am J Gastroenterol. 2005; 244(6): 432-439.

Eckerwall GE, Axelsson JB, Andersson RG. Early nasogastric feeding in predicted severe acute pancreatitis: a clinical, randomized study. Ann Surg. 2006; 244(6):959-965.

Forsmark CE, Baillie J. AGA Institute technical review on acute pancreatitis. Gastroenterology. 2007; 132(5):2022-2044.

Fuchs-Tarlovsky V, Ize L, Tapia J, Avila H. Estado nutricio y Pancreatitis aguda grave. Propuesta de un modelo analítico pronóstico. Cirujano General. 19(2);1997:109-115

Fuchs-Tarlovsky V, Espinoza Z, Quintana C, Gutiérrez Salmeán G. Validation of a prognostic index through nutritional status indicators in patients with severe acute pancreatitis. Nutr Hosp. 2010; 25(3):378-381.

Gianotti L, Meier R, Lobo DN et al. ESPEN guidelines on Parenteral Nutrition: Pancreas. Clin Nutr 28, 2009:429-435.

Grant J, James S, Grabowski V et al. Total Parenteral nutrition in pancreatic disease. Ann Surg. 1984; 200:627-31.

Gupta R, Patel K, Calder PC, Yaqoob P, Primrose JN, Johnson CD. A randomized clinical trial to assess the effect of total enteral and total parenteral nutritional support on metabolic, inflammatory and oxidative markers in patients with predicted severe acute pancreatitis (APACHE II ≥ 6). Pancreatology. 2003; 3(5):406-413.

Hallay J, Kovacs G, Szatmari et al. Early jejunal nutrition and changes in the immunological parameters of patients with acute pancreatitis. Hepatogastroenterology. 2001; 48(41): 1488-1492.

Havala T, Shronts E, Cerra F. Nutritional support in acute pancreatitis. Gastroenterol Clin N Am. 1989;18:525

Heyland DK, Dhaliwal R, Drover JW et al. Canadian clinical practice guidelines for nutrition support in mechanically ventilated, critically ill adult patients. JPEN J Parenter Enteral Nutr. 2003; 27(5) : 355-373.

Ioannidis O, Lavrentieva A, Botsios D. Nutrition support in acute pancreatitis. J pancr. 2008; 9(4):375-390.

Jabbar A, Chang WK, Dryden GW et al . Gut immunology and the different response to feeding and starvation. Nutr Clin Pract. 2003; 18:461-482.

Kalfarentzos FE, Karavias DD, Karatzas TM, Alevizatos BA, Androulakis JA. Total parenteral nutrition in severe acute pancreatitis. J Am Coll Nutr. 1991;10:156-162.

Kalfarenzos F, Kehagias J, Mead N et al. Enteral nutrition is superior to Parenteral nutrition in severe acute pancreatitis: results of a randomized prospective trial. Br J Surg. 1997;84:1665-9.

Kulinski B, Zimmermann T, Schweder R. Decreasing mortality in acute pancreatitis with sodium selenite. Clinical results of 4 years antioxidany therapy. Med Klin (Munich) 1995; 90 suppl 1:36-41.

Kumar A, Singh N, Prakash S et al. Early enteral nutrition in severe acute pancreatitis: a prospective randomized controlled trial comparing nasojejunal and nasogastric routes. J Clin Gastroenterol. 2006; 40(5): 431-434.

Lasztity N. Effect of enterally administered n-3 polyunsaturated fatty acids in acute pancreatitis: a prospective randomized clinical trial. Clin Nutr. 2005; 24:198-205.

Leibowitz AB, O'Sullivan P, Iberti TJ. Intravenous fat emulsion and the pancreas: a review. Mt Sinai J Med. 1992; 51(1): 38-42.

Louie BE, Noseworthy T, Hailey D, Gramlich, LM, Jacobs P, Warnock GL. Enteral or parenteral nutrition for severe pancreatitis: a randomized controlled trial and health technology assessment. Can J Surg. 2005; 48(4):298-306.

Lugli AK, Carli F, Wykes L. The importance of nutrition status assessment: the case of severe acute pancreatitis. Nutr Rev. 2007; 65(7):329-34.

Marik PE. What is the best way to feed patients with pancreatitis?. Curr Opin Crit Care. 2009; 15(2):131-138.

McClave SA, Spain DA, Snider HL. Nutritional management in acute and chronic pancreatitis. Gastroenterol Clin N Am. 1998; 27(2):421-434.

McClave SA, Chang WK, Rupinder D et al. Nutrition support in Acute pancreatitis: A systematic Review of the literature. JPEN J Parenter Enteral Nutr. 2006; 30(2): 143-156.

McClave SA, Snider H, Owens, et al. Clinical Nutrition in pancreatitis. Digest Dis Sci 1997; 42(10):2035-2044.

McClave SA, Greene LM, Snider HL, et al. Comparison of the safety of early enteral vs parenteral nutrition in mild acute pancreatitis. JPEN J Parenter Enteral Nutr. 1997;21(1):14-20.

McClave SA and Heyland DK. The physiologic response and associated clinical benefits from provision of early enteral nutrition. Nutr Clin Pract. 2009; 24(3):305-315.

McClave SA, Martinadle RG, Venek VW at al. Guidelines for the provision and assessment of nutrition support therapy in the adult critically ill patients: Society of Critical Care Medicine, and American Society for Parenteral and Enteral Nutrition. JPEN J Parenter Enteral Nutr 2009; 33:277-316.

Meier R, Ockenga J, Pertkiewicz M et al. ESPEN guidelines on parenteral nutrition: pancreas. Clin Nutr. 2006; 25(2):275-284.

O'Kaffe SJD, Steven JD. Physiological response of the human pancreas to enteral and Parenteral feeding. Curr Opin Clin Nutr Metab Care. 2006;9(5):622-628.

Olah A, Pardavi G, Belagyi T et al. Early feeding in acute pancreatitis is associated with lower complication rate. Nutrition. 2002; 18: 259-262.

Olah A, Belaguyi T, Issekutz A et al. Randomized clinical trial of specific lactobacillus and fiber supplemented to early enteral nutrition in patients with acute pancreatitis. Br J Surg 2002; 89: 1103-1107.

Osina VA, Kuzmina TN. Enteral nutrition in the therapy of gastrointestinal diseases (according to materials of the European Association of Parenteral and Enteral Nutrition)]. Eksp Klin Gastroenterol. 2007;(3):92-98,129.

Pandol SJ, Saluja AK, Imire CW et al. Acute pancreatitis: bench to the bedside. Gastroeneterology. 2007; 132(3):1127-1151.

Pearce CB, Sandek SA, Walters Am et al. A double- blind, randomized controlled trial to study the effect of enteral feed supplemented with glutamine, arginine, and omega-3 fatty acid in predicted acute severe pancreatitis. J Pancr. 2006; 7-84): 361-371

Petrov MS, Pylypchuk RD, Emelyanov NV. Systematic review: nutritional support in acute pancreatitis. Alim Pharmacol Ther 2008;28(6):704-12.

Petrov MS, Loveday BP, Pylypchuk RD et al. Systematic review and meta-analysis of enteral nutrition formulations in acute pancreatitis. Br J Surg. 2009; 96(11):1243-52.

Piciucci M, Merola E, Marigiani M et al. Nasogastric or nasointestinal feeding in acute pancreatitis. World J Surg. 2010; 16(29):3692-6

Pitchumoni CS, Patel NM, Shah P. Factors influencing mortality in acute pancreatitis: can we alter them?. J Clin Gastroenterol. 2005; 39(9):798-814.

Pupelis G, Selga G, Austrums E et al. Jejunal feeding, even when instituted late, improves outcome in patients with severe pancreatitis and peritonitis. Nutrition. 2001; 17(2):91-94.

Russell MK. Acute pancreatitis: a review of pathophysiology and nutrition management. Nutr Clin Pract.2004;19(1):16-24

Scolapio JS, Malhi-Chowla N, Ukleja A. Nutrition supplementation in patients with acute and chronic pancreatitis. Gastroenterol Clin N Am, 1999;28(3):695-707.

Siow E. Enteral vs parenteral nutrition for acute pancreatitis. Critical Care Nurse, 2008; 28(4):19-25.

Shaw JHF, Wolfe RR. Glucose, fatty acid, and urea kinetics in patients with severe acute pancreatitis. Ann Surg 1986;204:665

Spanier BM, Bruno MJ, Mathus-Vliegen EMH. Enteral nutrition in Acute Pancreatitis. A Review. Gastroenterology research and practice 201. Hindawi Publishing Corporation, 9 pages.

Taldukdar R, Vegue SS. Recent developments in acute pancreatitis. Clin Gatroenterol Hepatol. 2009; 7: S3-S9.

Tiegou LE, Gloro R, Pouzoulet J et al. Semielemental formula or polymeric formula: is there a better choice for enteral nutrition in acute pancreatitis? Randomized comparative study. . JPEN J Parenter Enteral Nutr. 2006; 30(1):1-5.

Van Citters GW, Lin HC. The ileal brake: A fifteen-year progress report. Curr Gastroenterol Reports 1999; 1:404-409.

Vu MK, Van Der Veek PJJ, Frölich M et al. Does jejunal feeding activate exocrine pancreatic secretion?. Europ J Clin Investigation 1999; 29(12):1053-1059.

Winsdor AC, Kanwar S, Li AG et al. Compared with Parenteral nutrition, enteral feeding attenuates the acute phase response and improves disease severity in acute pancreatitis. Gut. 1998; 42:431-435.

Xian-Li H, Quing-Jiu M, Jian-Guo L et al. Effect of TPN with or without glutamine dipeptide supplementation on outcome in severe acute pancreatitis. Clin Nutr (Suppl). 2004;1:43-47.

Part 4

Treatment

15

Changes in the Management of Treatment in Acute Pancreatitis Patients

Juraj Bober, Jana Kaťuchová and Jozef Radoňak
University of Pavol Jozef Šafarik/University Hospital, Slovakia

1. Introduction

Acute pancreatitis is an inflammatory condition with a variable clinical course from mild to the most severe with serious complications that attempt the life of a patient. According to the Atlanta classifications the severe acute pancreatitis occurs approximately at 25% of all patients with acute pancreatitis and it is associated with 10-20% of mortality. Death of the acute pancreatitis patients is often connected of at least one organ.

There are two phases of the severe acute pancreatitis relating to the mortality. The first phase, two weeks after onset of syndrome, is characterized by hypovolemia or even by the shock. It is accompanied by the systemic inflammatory responsive syndrome with production of inflammatory mediators and cytokines, which cause consecutive injury of lungs, livers and cardiovascular system. The multi organ failure is a very common appearance in the case of the severe acute pancreatitis and it happens very often even when the infection is absent. The second phase of this disease (third-forth week) is characterized by the complications caused by the infection of pancreatic necrosis. About 40-70% patients with necrotic acute pancreatitis is afflicted by the infection of the pancreatic necrosis, which causes the deaths of acute pancreatitis patients (Beger et al., 1997). The extent of the pancreatic necrosis and the duration of disease are the risk factors of the local pancreatic infection. Its incidence tends to culminate in third week of disease, though it may appear in whichever phase of the disease (Büchler et al., 2000). Severe acute pancreatitis requires treatment at the hospital, which is developed from personal, professional and technical point of view, where is a possibility to do the full diagnosis and therapy and the interdivisional cooperation, what is the basic presumption for treatment and diagnosis of acute pancreatitis.

Diagnosis is based upon clinical presentation, laboratory indicates and imaging studies, whilst illness severity can be assessed by clinical scoring systems, such as Ranson, Glasgow or Apache II criteria, or by radiological assessments such as the computer tomography severity index. Mild disease is often self-limiting and inflammation resolves with simple medical management. However, a minority of patients (up to 20%) will develop severe disease that carries substantial morbidity and mortality.

Over the past decades, management of severe acute pancreatitis changed from an early operative treatment to a more conservative approach. Nowadays there is clearly no more doubt that surgery is not the first choice of treatment for patients suffering from severe acute pancreatitis. Surgical debridement is the gold standard in patients with infected pancreatic necrosis. By delaying surgery up to the third or fourth week, sufficient debridement can be achieved, resulting in low mortality and morbidity rates. Early enteral feeding is preferred over total parenteral nutrition as it results in a reduced incidence of infection, length of hospital stay and mortality.

Besides full intensive treatment of acute pancreatitis there is a non changeable role of the surgical - operational treatment. Some indications for surgical treatment are no doubtful; some of them are the subject of discussion. The documented persistent infected necrosis and abscess is clear indication for the surgical treatment. Permanent acute abdomen, especially so called intra-abdominal compartment syndrome and persistent or increasing local complications (bleeding, ileus, bleeding of gastrointestinal tract, vascular ileus and others) are also the definite indication of the surgical intervention. Many authors consider the sterile necrosis, which causes the multi organ failure and which does not react to the maximal intensive treatment more than 72 hours, as an indicator of the surgical treatment (Götzinger, 2007).

The changes in the management of the patients with severe acute pancreatitis in the last decade contributed to the decrease of mortality. The aim of this study is to evaluate progress in the management of the patients with severe acute pancreatitis, comparing two clinical groups of patients.

2. Changes in the management of treatment in acute pancreatitis patients

Despite than mortality from severe acute pancreatitis has remarkably decreased (10-20%) during the last decades, many questions remain open about the treatment of this disease. Published literature on severe acute pancreatitis was reviewed and the decision to change the management of the treatment of severe acute pancreatitis has been made, at the First Department of Surgery, University Hospital in Košice, Slovakia. The management referred to the enteral nutrition, epidural analgesia, antibiotic prophylaxis, delay surgery to the later period in the case of infected necrosis.

2.1 Enteral nutrition

Enteral nutrition fed by the three-luminal tube applied by fibroscope, checking position by the contrast X-ray exam or by enteral nutrition through jejunostomy, in the case of already operated patient.

In 1997, McClave et al. demonstrated that nasojejunal feeding is a safe and beneficial method in mild and moderate pancreatitis (McClave et al., 1997). Later on, Nakad et al. found that nasojejunal feeding is feasible in severe acute pancreatitis, too (Nakad et al., 1998). Recently, some questioned whether nasojejunal feeding is the only proper route of enteral feeding in acute pancreatitis. The main disadvantage of nasojejunal feeding that it requires an endoscopist or radiologist to place the tube in, which may cause some delay in starting early enteral feeding (Spanier et al., 2011). Piciucchi et al. have found that enteral nutrition administered by nasogastric or nasojejunal tube seems to provide equal safety, tolerability and efficacy, even if more results are necessary to validate the routine use of nasogastric tubes in severe acute pancreatitis patients (Piciucchi et al., 2010).

One of the most common complications of enteral feeding is diarrhea, which can be detected in 20-30% of all patients. Diarrhea may deteriorate volume depletion and dehydration resulting in further weakening of the general condition of patients who are very sick anyway and usually need intensive care management. Wide-spectrum antibiotics, which are frequently used in severe acute pancreatitis, can contribute to the development of diarrhea as a significant additional factor (Whelan, 2007). It is possible that fiber enteral nutrition formulas have some preventive effect against diarrhea though (Elia et al., 2008). This observation was supported by a recently published study by Karakan et al. showed that prebiotic fiber supplementation reduced complication rate in acute pancreatitis in comparison to standard enteral solution (Karakan et al., 2007). A meta-analysis published by Petrov and Zagainov, which was based on six randomized control trials comparing enteral nutrition with parenteral nutrition, showed that enteral nutrition statistically significantly reduced the risk of hyperglycemia ($p=0.04$) as well as insulin requirement ($p=0.001$), so it is associated with better blood glucose control in severe acute pancreatitis patients (Petrov & Zagainov, 2007). The facts that enteral nutrition is most likely superior to parenteral nutrition in preventing septic complications of acute pancreatitis, it may also eliminate some complications of parenteral nutrition (catheter sepsis, pneumothorax, and thrombosis), and costs only 15% of the cost of total parenteral nutrition, make it an increasingly accepted treatment modality (Olah & Romics, 2010).

Composition of enteral formulas can be classified into three basic categories: polymeric, (semi)elemental, and immunoenhanced. While polymeric nutrient comprises non-hydrolyzed proteins, maltodextrins, oligofructosaccharides and long-chain triglycerides, (semi)elemental contains oligopeptides or amino-acids, maltodextrins, and medium and long-chain triglycerides. Theoretically, semi elemental nutrients stimulate pancreatic secretion in less extent, but enhance bowel absorption and those are tolerated better by patients than polymeric ones (Tiengou et al., 2006; Petrov et al., 2009b).

Immunoenhanced nutrients involve substrates which modulate the activity of the immune system. Various immunonutrition formulas felt in this category, such as glutamine, arginine, and omega-3 fatty acids as well as enteral nutrients supplemented by probiotics. Recently, a meta-analysis compared (semi)elemental and polymeric formulations indirectly, using 10 randomized controlled trials where parenteral nutrition was the reference treatment (Petrov et al., 2009a). The authors, however, could not demonstrate statistically significant difference with regard to tolerance of feeding, infectious complications, or mortality in between two enteral nutrition formulas ($p=0.611$). Enteral feeds with immune-enhancing ingredients such as glutamine, arginine, nucleotides, and omega-3 fatty acids that modulate the host immune and inflammatory response have recently attracted great interest (Bertolini et al., 2007). There are promising experimental studies, where supplementation of enteral feed with glutamine or omega-3 fatty acids could reduce the severity of experimental acute pancreatitis models (Foitzik et al., 2002; Rayes et al., 2009). Adding probiotics to enteral nutrients seemed to be a promising alternative for the future. In 10 of the 15 studies, probiotics significantly reduced bacterial infection rate compared to control groups. Two studies demonstrated a clear positive trend, but no statistical significance was detected (Olah & Romics, 2010). Sun et al., in a meta-analysis of four randomized controlled trials demonstrated that enteral feeding with probiotic could not reduce the infected necrosis (Sun et al., 2009). Eckerwall and Jacobson reported about timing when to resume oral feeding in patients with acute pancreatitis (Eckerwall et al., 2006; Jacobson et al., 2007). The usual criteria to initiate oral feeding are (1) absence of abdominal pain, (2) absence of nausea and vomiting, and return of appetite, and (3) absence of complications.

2.2 Antibiotics in acute pancreatitis

Infection of pancreatic necrosis by enteric bacteria is the most common cause of death in patients with necrotizing pancreatitis. Progress in the therapeutic management of this disease has led to a decrease in the mortality of patients without infection of pancreatic necrosis, which commonly is reported to range between 5% and 15% (Tenner et al., 1997). Nevertheless, mortality rates of 20%-30% are reported in patients with infected pancreatic necrosis (Büchler et al., 2000). The clinical importance of pancreatic infection has led to the idea that the prevention of infected necrosis could be a beneficial approach.
Antibiotics prophylaxis in severe acute pancreatitis has been a matter of discussion during the past years (Büchler et al., 2000; Slavin & Neoptolemos, 2001). Recent clinical studies seem to support the notion that early administration of broad-spectrum antibiotics is capable of reducing the incidence of infected pancreatic necrosis (Pederzoli et al., 1993; Golub et al., 1998; Sharma & Howden, 2001). Two randomized double-blind studies have addressed prophylactic antibiotics in patients with acute pancreatitis with prognostically severe and severe pancreatitis on imaging (Isenmann et al., 2004; Dellinger et al., 2007). These studies have failed to show any benefit from such drugs being routinely prescribed, no difference was found in the rate of pancreatic sepsis and mortality despite previous smaller non randomized studies suggesting a benefit. On the other hand, antibiotic overuse has been associated with up 30% of patients developing necrosis superinfection with Candida species which may confer a poorer prognosis (Büchler et al., 2000; Connor et al., 2004). If antimicrobials are prescribed, the duration should to be limited to 14 days.
Fourteen trials were included with a total of 841 patients in systematic review and meta-analysis of antibiotic prophylaxis in severe acute pancreatitis by Wittau et al. The authors have investigated that the use of antibiotic prophylaxis was not associated with a statistically significant reduction in mortality, in the incidence of infected pancreatic necrosis, in the incidence of non-pancreatic infections, and in surgical interventions (Wittau et al., 2011).

2.3 Epidural catheter

Severe acute pancreatitis is associated with the development of local complications, such as pancreatic and peripancreatic necrosis, abscesses or pseudocysts, and systemic complications, such as adult respiratory distress syndrome or renal failure with mortality rate is close to 15 % (Demirag et al., 2006). The pathophysiology of acute pancreatitis is incompletely understood but alteration in the pancreatic microcirculatory blood flow has been involved. Thus, a decrease in pancreatic blood flow occurs early in the course of acute pancreatitis and has been suggested to play a role in the conversion of edematous to necrotizing acute pancreatitis (Klar et al., 1994). The microcirculatory dysfunction includes arterial vasoconstriction with hypoperfusion, ischemia-reperfusion injury and obstruction of the venous outflow (Klar et al., 1991; Letko et al., 1994; Demirag et al., 2006).
Besides perfusion abnormalities, acute pancreatitis is also characterized by local and systemic inflammatory responses, including leukocyte activation as well as release of free radicals and cytokines (Frossard et al., 2001). Many therapeutic agents, such as dextran, heparin, procaine, L-arginine, antioxidants, or cytokine antagonists, have been tested experimentally and/or clinically to improve pancreatic tissue perfusion during acute pancreatitis, however, no significantly successful result has been achieved (Beger et al., 2001, Paszkowski et al., 2001). Epidural anesthesia that is used to induce analgesia in the

perioperative period might be an interesting treatment of the microcirculatory blood flow abnormalities (Demiraget al., 2006).

2.4 Type of surgical intervention

Severe acute pancreatitis is still related to high mortality rates. Over the past decades, management of severe acute pancreatitis changed from an early operative treatment to a more conservative approach. Surgical debridement is the gold standard in patients with infected pancreatic necrosis. However surgical intervention for sterile necrosis is only indicated in selected patients if aggressive intensive care is unsuccessful. Patients suspected to have infected pancreatic necrosis, should undergo computer tomography-guided or ultrasound-guided fine-needle aspiration for verification. By delaying surgery up to the third week, sufficient debridement can be achieved by a single operation, resulting in low mortality and morbidity rates.

2.4.1 Operative treatment of pancreatic necrosis

In patients with infected pancreatic necrosis, surgical necrosectomy is the established gold standard, whereas operative treatment of patients with sterile necroses is controversially discussed. Surgical debridement of infected pancreatic necrosis is based on two principles (Sahora et al., 2009). First, necrotic pancreatic tissue as well as pancreatic ascites is removed out of the peritoneal cavity and the lesser sac, to prevent absorption through the thoracic duct, which is accused to increase the incidence of systemic complications as development of single or multiple organ failure (Mayer et al., 1985). Second, as much as possible viable pancreatic tissue should be preserved to insure a good quality of life after recovery (Broome et al., 1996). Nowadays mortality in patients with infected pancreatic necrosis is about 10–30% in specialized centers as a result of right timing and patient selection (Büchler et al., 2000). Because of improvements in intensive care medicine, today more patients survive the first phase of acute pancreatitis, increasing the incidence of infected necrosis (Beger et al., 1986). Retroperitoneal gas or bacterial culture gained from fine-needle aspiration (ultrasound or computer tomography guided) is confirmation for infected pancreatic necrosis. Sterile necrosis, in general, is no indication for surgery. Multiple series have shown that patients with sterile necrosis can be managed by a conservative approach, but surgery might be indicated in case of late complications, disease progression or persistence. In these severely ill patients, who develop organ failure without signs of septic complications, the indication to surgery must be made individually (Sahora et al., 2009). As in patients with infected necrosis, early operation has shown high mortality rates and should also be delayed upon the third week (Büchler et al., 2000; Uhl et al., 2002; Hartwig et al., 2002a).

In the past, early surgical intervention was indicated for patients with severe acute pancreatitis, but was lead to mortality rates up to 65% (Smadja & Bismuth, 1986). The aim of this intervention was that patients would benefit from the initial removal of necrotic tissue, leading to the reduction of multisystemic complications related to enzymes and toxic substances (Fernandetz -Cruz et al., 1994). For evaluation of mortality rates, early surgical intervention was compared to a more conservative approach. In retrospective study performed by Hartwig et al., and in randomized control trial made by Mier et al., was found reduction of mortality rates in patients undergoing delayed surgery (Mier et al., 1997; Hartwig et al., 2002a).

At present, guidelines for the management of surgical treatment of severe acute pancreatitis agree that surgical intervention should be delayed as long as 3–4 weeks after onset (Uhl et al., 2002; Isaji et al., 2006). By deferring surgery a proper demarcation of pancreatic and peripancreatic necrosis can take place. The demarcation of necrotic masses from viable tissue enables an easier and safer debridement with a greater likelihood of sparing pancreatic tissue and leads to successful surgical control of pancreatic necrosis. Thus the risk of bleeding and the surgery-related loss of vital tissue that predisposes to surgery-induced endocrine and exocrine pancreatic insufficiency can be minimized by this approach (Hartwig et al., 2002b, Bober et al., 2003).

The aim of any intervention technique is to maximize debridement, preserve as much vital pancreatic parenchyma as possible and to secure postoperative drainage of debris and exudates (Götzinger et al., 2002). Resection procedures, as partial or total pancreatectomy, which also remove vital tissue, have been abandoned, because of impaired quality of life and higher mortality and morbidity (Nordback & Auvinen, 1985). Several open and minimal invasive techniques have been described, but an ideal method has not yet been defined. The surgical procedures including: open necrosectomy with closed continuous lavage, open necrosectomy with drainage and relaparotomy on demand, open necrosectomy with open packing and planned re-laparotomy. However morbidity (80%), including pancreatic, intestinal fistula, stomach outlet stenosis, local bleeding, and incisional hernia, is higher in patients undergoing multiple relaparotomies, which are mandatory in open packing procedure (Beger et al., 1982; Büchler et al., 2000; Fernandez-del Castilo et al.,1998).

The open approach for the surgical treatment of severe acute pancreatitis including blunt debridement is combined with laparostomy for drainage and access for revisions to further remove local debris. Operative access is gained by a way of a midline incision. Careful exploration is done to assess the extent of pancreatic and extrapancreatic necrosis, including a Kocher's mobilization of the second part of the duodenum. Furthermore the right and the left colon are mobilized. It is possible to approach the lesser sac through the gastrohepatic omentum or the gastrocolic omentum. If opening of the lesser sac is not possible because of a bounded inflammatory process, direct access from the infracolic compartment via the left transverse mesocolon is an alternative. The access through the mesocolon also allows drains to be placed in a more exact position once the debridement is completed. It is important to send fluid collection from the necrotic region for aerobic and anaerobic culture (Sahora, 2009). After sufficient debridement there remain cavities, which are often stiff and may bleed from the granulated surface. In these spaces is necessity to place 4–10 easy flow drains, which are brought out through left and or right side placed laparostomas. These drains are not removed unless the daily quantum of fluid loss is less than 20 ml. Another possibility is to stepwisely remove these drains that will result in a fistula due to a mature fistula tract. This fistula will close in a given period (Sahora et al. 2009).

Today several additional techniques to open surgical necrosectomy have been described. Percutaneous drainage, endoscopic techniques, and minimal invasive surgical procedures have been described as additive and alternative procedures. Percutaneous computer tomography-guided catheter debridement without surgery has been shown to be feasible in selected series in more than 50% of the included patients, with infected and sterile necrosis. Mortality rates of 12–30%, of patients treated by percutaneous drainage only, have been reported, using different access routes and a variety of catheter types (Bruennler et al., 2008;

Mortelé et al., 2009). The major reported complications were hemorrhage and injury to adjacent organs. The endoscopic drainage of sterile pancreatic necrosis using several transgastric and transduodenal catheters combined with a nasopancreatic catheter to lavage the necrotic cavity described Baron in 1996 (Baron et al., 1996). Using endoscopic drainage, many authors reported a high percentage of patients, who were treated without the need of surgery (Baron et al., 2002, Seifert et al., 2009, Seewald, 2005). Recently also minimally invasive necrosectomy techniques have been used with some promising results. Different approaches are described to access the necrotic mass. Some authors prefer a transabdominal access, which offers a good overview but harbors the risk of spreading intra-abdominal infection. As an alternative the necrotic focus can be reached through retroperitoneoscopy. Bücher et al. reported a group of 8 patients who underwent minimal invasive necrosectomy using a single large port, inserted over the percutaneous drainage channel. Complication rate was zero and despite one patient only a single session was needed (Bucher et al., 2008). Alternatively Parekh describes a laparoscopic hand-assisted method, using a transabdominal approach. In this series 19 patients, out of 23, were treated without the need of open laparotomy, zero postoperative complications, and a mortality of 10.5% (Perehk, 2006).

In conclusion, comparison of these minimal invasive procedures is almost impossible because of inhomogenity of patient selection. Today there are no randomized controlled trails comparing open surgery to one of the mentioned methods. Minimal invasive procedures may play a role in bridging the time to definite surgery in critically ill patients in some well-experienced clinical centers (Sahora et al., 2009).

2.4.2 Intra-abdominal hypertension

Intra-abdominal hypertension is increasingly reported in patients with severe acute pancreatitis, and is caused by several factors, including visceral edema and ascites associated with massive fluid resuscitation, paralytic ileus and retroperitoneal inflammation. There is a strong relation with early organ dysfunction and mortality in these patients, which makes intra-abdominal hypertension an attractive target for intervention. Several reports conclude that this phenomenon occurs within the first 5 days after admission, and that the kinetics of inta-abdominal hypertension is important: patients with persistent intra-abdominal hypertension seem to be at the highest risk for mortality. Several strategies to reduce intra-abdominal pressure have been developed, and given the pathophysiology, percutaneous drainage of ascites is a first logical step. However, if conservative measures fail to reduce intra-abdominal pressure in a setting with ongoing or worsening organ dysfunction, abdominal decompression is recommended. Intra-abdominal hypertension and intra-abdominal compartment syndrome have been described most often in patients with abdominal trauma or after emergency abdominal surgical procedures such as aortic aneurysm repair (De Waele, 2008). The intra-abdominal hypertension is defined as a sustained or repeated pathologic elevation of the intraabdominal pressure above 12mm Hg. The intra-abdominal compartment syndrome is described as the sustained elevation of intra-abdominal pressure above 20mmHg in combination with newly developed organ dysfunction (Malbrain et al., 2006).

It was shown that intra-abdominal hypertension is associated with higher mortality and morbidity rates, and prolonged intensive care unit stay, in comparison to other patients who had normal intra-abdominal pressure (Sugrue et al., 1999). Intra-abdominal hypertension has been recognized as a cause of organ dysfunction in critically ill patients, including those suffering from severe acute pancreatitis (Balogh et al., 2002). Placement of a urinary catheter for the monitoring of intra-abdominal pressure would be necessary in the severe acute pancreatitis patients. The symptoms caused by intra-abdominal hypertension in patients with acute pancreatitis are not very different from other conditions associated with intra-abdominal hypertension. Hemodynamic instability requiring vasoactive drugs, acute renal failure and respiratory failure are the most obvious clinical signs and symptoms that have been associated with intra-abdominal hypertension. The association between intra-abdominal hypertension and development of organ dysfunction in severe acute pancreatitis is well documented. De Waele et al. showed that there was a 95% incidence of respiratory failure, 91% cardiovascular and 86% acute renal failure rate in patients with intra-abdominal pressure of 15 mmHg or higher (De Waelle et al., 2005). The development of intra-abdominal hypertension in patients with severe acute pancreatitis is evidently an important problem, as it is associated with organ dysfunction and mortality. Therefore, intra-abdominal pressure should be measured routinely in patients admitted to the intensive care unit with severe acute pancreatitis, and intra-abdominal pressure should be considered a target for intervention in all patients.

Decompressive laparotomy has been shown to effectively reduce intra-abdominal pressure and reverse the symptoms typically associated with abdominal compartment syndrome (De Waelle et al., 2006; Dambrauskas et al., 2009). If decompression is needed more than 2-3 weeks after the onset of the disease and there is evidence of extensive necrosis on a computered tomography scan or established infection of peripancreatic necrosis, it is the feasible to perform a necrosectomy in conjunction with the decompressive laparotomy. In selected patients with extensive retroperitoneal fluid collections, a lumbotomy may provide access to the retroperitoneal space, and allow evacuation of pancreatic necrosis as well. The management of the open abdomen following decompression in severe acute pancreatitis is challenging. The best currently available technique is the utilization of the vacuum-assisted closure technique aiming for gradual closure of the abdominal wall. The use of a vacuum assisted closure system guarantees a perfect seal of the peritoneal cavity, avoiding possible superinfection of the pancreatic or peripancreatic necrosis.

Intra-abdominal hypertension seems to have a significant role in contributing to the early multi organ dysfunction syndrome, subsequent complications and mortality in severe acute pancreatitis. Intra-abdominal pressure monitoring is mandatory for all patients who develop organ dysfunction, and intra-abdominal pressure should be a target for intervention when intra-abdominal hypertension and organ dysfunction persist. Surgical decompression should be considered in all patients with persistent organ dysfunction after 3 days or later (Sugrue et al., 2007; De Waele, 2008).

3. Clinical group of patients and the methods

All patients who were hospitalized due to the acute pancreatitis symptoms in the period from January 2003 till December 2008 at the First Department of Surgery, University Hospital, in Kosice, were included to this study. Those patients, who were primarily hospitalized and treated at other workplaces and were moved to our institute during their disease, were excluded from this study.

The total number of the patients with acute pancreatitis during onset symptoms was 258 ones. All patients were hospitalized at the Intensive Care Unit, they received the standard intensive care (palliation of pain, nasal gastric tube, central vein catheter, urinary bladder catheter, intensive monitoring of the basic vital functions, intensive rehydratation treatment, giving the inhibitors of proton pump, low molecular weight heparin, giving the prophylactic antibiotic therapy). In the case of biliary acute pancreatitis, mainly joined with jaundice, cholangitis or ultrasound suspicion for the presence of the stones in common bile duct, the patients were underwent urgent endoscopic retrograde cholangio-pancreatography during the first 48 hours after onset acute pancreatitis. The distinguishing of the mild forms and severe forms of acute pancreatitis were carried out using Ranson criteria, APACHE score, the daily follow-up of level C-reactive protein and measurement of percentage of involvement of pancreatic tissue by computer tomography severity index (Balthazar computer tomography scoring system). The first computer tomography examination was carried out first time after 48 hours from the beginning of disease. The diagnosis of the infected necrosis we did according to the clinical finding, inflammatory markers (white blood cells, C-reactive protein, procalcitonin), and ultrasound and computer tomography finding (presence of gas bubbles).

Patients with multi organ failure were moved from the Intensive Care Unit to be hospitalized at the Department of Anesthesiology and Intensive Medicine of our institute.

The clinical group of hospitalized patients was divided into two subgroups. Group A included the patients hospitalized from January 2003 till December 2005. This group of patients was evaluated retrospectively. The second Group B included the patients hospitalized from January 2006 till December 2008. This group was studied prospectively, according to the clinical protocol prepared in advance, which reflected the changes in management of the patients with the severe acute pancreatitis after confirmation of necrosis. Fisher's exact and Pearson chi-square tests were used in data analysis. $P < 0.05$ was considered statistically significant.

3.1 Clinical protocol of changes in management of treatment acute pancreatitis patients

Enteral nutrition fed by the three-luminal tube applied by fibroscope, checking the position by the contrast X-rays exam or by enteral nutrition through jejunostomy, in the case of already operated patients. Enteral nutrition was applied if no signs of the cardiovascular instability were present. We used the enteral nutrition enriched of the glutamine, arginine and omega-3 fatty acids and fibres. The dose was gradually increased from 20ml/hour to 80ml/hour (maximum 1000ml/24 hours). The enteral nutrition was started at seven o´clock in the morning and takes 12.5 hours to half past seven in the evening. At night, the enteral nutrition was not administrated. The second change includes an application of the epidural catheter to palliate the pain and to recovery of intestinal peristaltic. The continual measurement of the intra-abdominal pressure with the catheter in urinary bladder was used. The changes in the prophylactic application of antibiotics include changing III.generation cephalosporin's which were administered in Group A for imipenem which were replaces in Group B. In both groups the prophylactic application lasted maximum 14 days. Necrosectomy was indicated and performed as late as possible; usually the surgical procedure was pushed to the third or fourth week of hospitalization.

3.2 Results

Basic characteristic of both subgroup A and B are documented in table 1. It follows less frequency in Group A, however the male/female ratio and occurrence of the severe acute pancreatitis was similar. The percentage of the patients with necrotic pancreas and the patients, who needed endoscopic retrograde cholangiography procedure, was similar as well.

	Group A	Group B
Number of patients	97	161
Male/Female	53 : 44	90 : 71
Mild acute pancreatitis	84 (86%)	132 (82%)
Severe acute pancreatitis	13 (14%)	29 (18%)
Number of patients + endoscopic retrograde cholangiopancreatography	34 (35%)	53 (33%)

Table 1. Groups of patients suffered from acute pancreatitis, group A (2003-2005), group B (2006-2008).

Further we will be concerned only with the patients with severe acute pancreatitis. More detailed characteristic of patients with severe acute pancreatitis is documented in table 2.

	Group A	Group B
Number of patients	13	29
Male/Female	8/5	16/13
Mean of age	38,5 year	42 year
Etiology of acute pancreatitis Alcohol Biliary disease Other	 7 (54%) 5 1	 14 (48%) 12 3
Ranson score	3,9 (3-9)	4,0 (2-9)
Number of patients with computer tomography scan necrosis more than 30%	12 (92%)	26 (90%)
Patients hospitalized at the Department of Anesthesiology et Intensive Medicine	6 (46%)	11 (37%)

Table 2. Group of patients suffered from severe acute pancreatitis

More detailed description of group of patients with severe acute pancreatitis is documented in table 2. In both groups of patients there is a dominance of male and the similar average age, Ranson score, as well as a number of patients with necrotic pancreas over than 30%. Alcoholic etiology occurred more often in Group A. Also we noticed the higher number of patients, who needed hospitalization at the Department of Anesthesiology and Intensive Medicine. During the hospitalization, mainly during the period from 72 hours to 7th day, we provided intensive treatment in both group of patients, however in some cases in spite of our intensive effort, the multi organ failure occurred. In the case of presence of abdominal compartment syndrome, we indicated the surgical intervention including intra abdominal decompression. Presence of the infected pancreatic necrosis or abscess was a clear indication for surgical intervention. Individual indications and the timing of the surgery are presented in table 3.

	Sterile necrosis + multi organ failure		Infected necrosis		Abscess		Together		Mortality	
Time	A	B	A	B	A	B	A	B	A	B
Till 72 hours	1	1					1	1	1	1
Till 7 days	3	2					3	2	3	1
After 7 days		1	1				1	1		
After 14 days			1	3			1	3	1	1
After 21 days			1	4		1	1	5		
Together	4	4	3	7		1	7	12	5 71%	3 25%

Table 3. Timing of surgery, surgical indication and mortality in group A and group B.

In Group A, it is shown more often indications to the surgical intervention in the first days and weeks of hospitalization period. Comparing Group B, mainly in the case of infected necrosis, the surgical operations were pushed to the third or fourth week. This was reflected also in the mortality of operated patients, when we recorded 71% mortality in Group A and 25% of mortality in Group B. The types of surgical procedures are documented in table 4. While during the first days we performed only the surgical revision and drainage, or open abdomen. In the case of infected necrosis we performed necrosectomy with closed continuous lavage. There are also documented the number of patients with reoperations in both groups of patients, which is less frequent in Group B.

	Primary surgery		Repeated surgery		Mortality	
Type of surgery	A	B	A	B	A	B
Revision, drainage, open abdomen, jejunostomy	2	1	0	0	2	0
Revision, drainage, jejunostomy	1	4	1	0	0	3
Necrosectomy, continuous lavage	4	7	2	4	3	0
Together	7	12	3 (43%)	4 (33%)	5	3

Table 4. Type of surgical procedures and mortality of patients in group of patients A and B.

The mortality in both groups of patients is presented in the Table 5. It shows less mortality in Group B (18%). Six patients were found with non infected necrosis 46% in Group A (2003-2005), but seventeen patients were documented with non infected necrosis 58% in Group B (2006-2008).

	Number of patients		Mortality	
	A	B	A	B
Acute pancreatitis patients	97	161	7 (7.2%)	5 (3.1%)
Severe acute pancreatitis patients	13	29	7 (53.8%)	5 (18%)
Severe acute pancreatitis patients after surgery	7	12	5	3
Severe acute pancreatitis patients with non infected necrosis	6	17	2	2

Table 5. Comparison of mortality of patients in group of patients A and B.

The comparison of the cause of the death in both groups is presented in table 6. There was statistically significant decrease in mortality in group of patients B (p=0.02).While only 2 patient's dead for the pancreatic sepsis with multi organ failure, the remainder 10 patient's dead for multi organ failure in first days after the admitting to hospital.

	Group of patients A (2003-2005)	Group of patients B (2006-2008)	P
Number of patients	13	29	-
Death	7 (54%)	5 (18%)	0.02
Multi organ failure	6 (85%)	4 (80%)	-
Pancreatic sepsis	1 (15%)	1 (20%)	-

Table 6. Cause of death in both groups of patients A and B.

4. Discussion

Despite of the lasting dissatisfaction with the mortality level of the patients with severe acute pancreatitis, nevertheless during last decades as a consequence of the positive shift in diagnostic methods and treatment of acute pancreatitis, we succeeded to decrease mortality of severe acute pancreatitis patients to 10%-20% (Del Campos et al., 1998). During the last 15 years a big step was done towards the understanding and development of acute pancreatitis and at the same time the great progress in the screening methods of pancreas (Uhl et al., 2002). In line with the other authors opinions (Bank et al., 2002), taking into account own experiences, we are convinced that the decrease of the mortality was causes by an early recognition of the severe acute severe and setting up the prompt and appropriate treatment, by the improvement of the nutritional support, early endoscopic retrograde cholangiopancreatography supplied to the accurately indicated patients, and using the effective antibiotic treatment.

The International Association of Pancreatology proposed for acute pancreatitis treatment eleven recommendations (Sarr, 2003; Uhl et al., 2002), which created the framework for contemporary management of acute pancreatitis. These recommendations are based on the principles of evidence based medicine. However, in many points, there is need of further comparative studies was observed.

Positive trend of the decreasing mortality in the cases of severe acute pancreatitis was visible also at our workplace. These results have been already published previously (Bober et al., 1995; Bober et al., 2002; Bober et al., 2003). During the period from 2003 to 2005 the results overall got worse, when the mortality level of severe acute pancreatitis increased to 53.8%. After in-depth analysis of the causes of this negative result, the decision to change management of the patients with acute pancreatitis was made. The new protocol was designed, which contained the change of the management.

The contemporary standard of management of acute pancreatitis is the intensive conservative treatment with possibility of the diagnosis of its complications in the course of the therapy (Huťan, 2006). Very important part of the acute treatment is early and adequate fluid resuscitation during the first hour after admission in the case of patients with cardiovascular instability. When diagnosis of acute pancreatitis is confirmed, the treatment in line with a new protocol was applied.

Many reports were published about the positive influence of the early enteral nutrition in the case of severe acute pancreatitis. Cao et al. published the results of meta-analysis, which compared the results achieved by the enteral nutrition and total parenteral nutrition in the case of severe acute pancreatitis. Patients with enteral nutrition have shown less risk of infection, less percentage of pancreatic and peripancreatic necrosis, as well as, less overall complications, less often multi organ failure and low mortality (Petrov et al., 2006; Cao et al., 2008). Application of the three-luminal tube with help of fibroscope was carried out in our Group B by own co-workers, who had enough experiences and own endoscopy certificate. The application of the gastric aspirate and the enteral nutrition was tolerated well by all patients. Some of them perceived the abdominal discomfort and the slight increasing of the intra abdominal pressure. In these cases we have temporarily reduced the volume of the enteral nutrition.

The aim of the prophylactic application of antibiotics is to protect the sterile necrotic tissue against the development of infection. In general, it is accepted, that 40%-70% necrosis is infected. With regard to the high percentage of this infection of pancreatic necrosis and with regard to the fact that mortality is higher in the case of infected necrosis than in the case of sterile ones, the preventive application of antibiotics prevention, which has to avoid the infection of the necrosis. The reason is except an unproved benefit from prevention also its possible risks (antibiotic resistance and development of mycotic super infection from antibiotics) (Dambraukas et al., 2007; Dellinger et al., 2007; Olejník & Brychta, 2008). At present, the routine application of the prophylactic antibiotics to the patients with proven necrosis, has many supporters (Xu & Cai, 2008; Rokke et al., 2007; Dambraukas et al., 2007; Otto et al., 2006; Uhl et al., 2002). The conclusions of their studies show that antibiotics prevention reduces the sepsis and mortality. The recommendation in International Association of Pancreatology reports that prophylactic application of broad-spectrum antibiotics reduces infection of computer tomography confirmed necrotic acute pancreatitis, but it does not improve survival rate. When choosing the antibiotics, it is pointed at the best results Imipenem or Meropenem (decrease of necrosis, less necessities to surgical treatment, lower mortality) (Carter et al., 2000). Comparing Imipenem and Meropenem, no differences in incidence of the septic complications were observed (Heinrich et al., 2006). Preventive antibiotics have to be administered during 7-14 days. Longer applications than 14 days is not recommended (Olejník & Brychta, 2008). Regarding the different opinions on the antibiotics prophylaxis, it is necessary to take into account the extent of necrosis of the pancreas. If the damage is less than 30% of pancreas parenchyma, the risk of infection is small (Olejník & Brychta, 2008). Despite of all contra version, many, also prestigious workplaces, at present administer the antibiotics prophylaxis in the case of severe acute pancreatitis, bearing the risk of contra productive effect. We assigned our workplace to this group.

In the cases of patients with severe acute pancreatitis, it is necessary from the beginning or during the treatment, in spite of the intensive conservative one, to consider the indication of the surgical treatment. During the initial phase after admission of patients with acute pancreatitis the situations appear, when in spite of the precise differential diagnostics (based on anamnesis, clinical examination, laboratory tests, ultrasound) these does not bring the clear breaking up and the indication of diagnostic exploration can be actual. Computer tomography examination can be very helpful in such situations and it can decrease these doubt to minimum. Despite of the risk of surgery, the published opinions say, that it is less probable, that the diagnostic exploration exacerbated local inflaming process, though it can increase the risk of infection of pancreatic necrosis. This risk should be reevaluated in situation, when there is no other alternative approach in treatment without surgical intervention (Dugernier et al., 2006).

The indications for surgery which are also now discussed are the patients with sterile pancreatic necrosis and multi organ failure, which are non-responsible to the intensive treatment more than 72 hours. In the literature, there is a published opinion, that patients with high extent of pancreatic necrosis with persistent multi organ failure, in spite of maximum intensive care, can have a benefit from surgery. The clinical status has to be revaluated daily, because the right timing of surgical intervention is very important. Intensive care is suitable until the indications for surgical solution are not fulfilled (Götzinger et al., 2002).

In our group of patients we indicated the surgical treatment for 7 patients in 7 days after admission to hospital. In this group of patients, we recorded 86% mortality (in Group A 100%, in Group B 67%). Some authors recommend surgical intervention to the patients with sterile necrosis, whose status is not improved during four weeks of intensive care (Hartwig et al., 2002b).

A right timing of necrosectomy is discussed up till now. Those, who propose an early surgery say, that patient benefits from the early removal of the tissue necrosis, as it results to the decreasing of the multisystem complications linked with the releasing of enzymes and toxic substations. In the past, an early surgical intervention was preferred especially in the cases of system functions damage, but it resulted to the high mortality (Götzinger, 2007).

Götzinger study pointed at the fact that a benefit from the delay of the surgical intervention is in the enclosure of demarcation process of dead tissue. This demarcation enables the safe and sufficient following debridement, which leads to be successful surgical control of pancreatic necrosis in one or more steps. The analysis of the timing showed, that necrosectomy performed after three weeks from the beginning of illness is linked with higher percentage of success of debridement of pancreatic necrosis, what results to the lower number of reoperation and lower mortality. Very early debridement (up to three weeks) means an oversize percentage of mortality (Götzinger, 2007).

In rare situation, also intra-abdominal hypertension is an indication to decompressive laparotomy (Šiller et al., 2007). Intra-abdominal hypertension is caused by paralytic ileus, by large inflammation of retroperitoneal tissue, increased vascular permeability and also by liquid collections in abdominal cavity. It can be caused also by aggressive liquid hyper resuscitation (Dugernier et al., 2006).

Intra-abdominal hypertension is typical at the beginning of illness and can lead to the intra-abdominal compartment syndrome (the intra-abdominal pressure is higher than 20mmHg), which can make worth organ dysfunctions (Malbrain et al., 2006).

At present some indications to surgical treatment are apparent and clear. The absolute indications to the urgent surgery are necrosis and pancreatic or peripancreatic abscess. Infected necrosis begins at 40-50% patients with necrotic acute pancreatitis (Hartwig et al., 2002b). Infected necrosis means the necrotic area with bacterial contamination in devitalized tissue. Necrosis of pancreas and peripancreatic tissue is the risky environment for bacterial contamination. The risk of pancreatic infection grows with the volume of devitalized tissue. It culminated in the third week from the beginning of the illness. But 25% of patients have the infection during first 7 days (Dugernier et al., 2006).

Although acute pancreatitis is at the beginning a sterile inflammatory disease, which leads to multi organ dysfunctional syndrome, so the clinical features are difficult to distinguish from severe sepsis. The confirmation of presence of infection is when gas bubbles are found on the computer tomography examination, also by the positive cultivation of specimen obtained from the necrosis by thin-needle technique. This technique is safe and 90% precise (Schmid et al., 1999).

Bacterial translocation from intestinal lumen (transmurally, by lymphatic and vascular way, by ascites) is the main mechanism of the infection transfer to the necrosis during the first weeks of the disease. The microbiological examination shows that the origin of infection of pancreas is first of all the intestinal infections. Later sources are nosocomial infections of staphylococcus and enterococcus, including the multiresistant microorganism and mycotic infections (Büchler et al., 2000). At present, the accepted opinion is that necrosectomy has to be done as soon as the evidence of the infected necrosis is confirmed (Huťan, 2008).

The approach of the surgical treatment of necrotic acute pancreatitis has been developed. Some of them are obsolete (resection methods), but various techniques of the necrosectomy of pancreatic and peripancreatic necrosis remain as dominant approach done by the classic open surgery, by laparoscopic retroperitoneal miniinvasive surgery or percutaneous necrosectomy.

Additional techniques (after necrosectomy) are based on knowledge, that during surgical intervention it is not possible to remove all necrosis, because demarcation is not complete and too radical removal of this necrosis causes rather damage than benefit. On the other hand the rest of the necrosis can be a source of the persistent sepsis.

From the range of additional techniques may be mentioned the conventional surgical drainage with closing of the abdominal cavity and with location of the gravity or suck tube drains, open abdomen techniques also called laparostomy and at last the closed continuous lavage. It is possible to combine to abovementioned additional techniques.

Own experiences with all additional technique have been published already (Bober et al., 2003). At present we use all of them, but we prefer the closed continuous lavage technique of bursa omentalis and retroperitoneum, as we published in 2003, accepting also results of comparative studies (Beger et al., 2002; Branum et al., 1998).

Delay of the necrosectomy to the third -fourth week of hospitalization with applying the closed continuous lavage we obtained very good results in number of postoperative local complications as well as in the need of reoperations and no mortality in this subgroup of patients.

During last year's many works were published about retroperitoneal necrosectomy (Connor et al., 2005; Van Santvoot et al., 2007) laparoscopic assisted percutaneous drainage of infected necrosis and peripancreatic abscess (Horvath et al., 2001), laparoscopic necrosectomy (Cushieri et al., 2002; Risse et al., 2004; Šutiak et al.,2008). Also other authors published the report about very positive results with percutaneous necrosectomy (Bruennler et al., 2008; Hartwig et al., 2002a). The benefit of percutaneous necrosectomy is mini invasive approach, which does not require total anesthesia, but the disadvantages are: longer time of hospitalization, higher doses of X-ray because of repetitive computer tomography controls and high percentage of cases, when patients had to perform of laparotomy due to the insufficiency of previous one.

Pancreatic abscess contrary to the infected necrosis is well demarcated collection of purulent liquid without solid necrotic material. It is a result of infection, which arises from accumulation of liquid collections or from the area of necrosis, which has liquidized in the meantime. Comparing with the infected necrosis, the pancreatic abscess appears later (more than four weeks from the beginning of a disease) and the prolonged process is typical for it (Fernandez Del Castilo et al., 1998). If the pancreatic abscess contains small, solids particles, very often it is not suitable to drain it in percutaneous or endoscopic way (Baril et al., 2000; Carter et al., 2000).

The other indication for surgery is the course of severe acute pancreatitis is bleeding. The intensive inflammation, large regional necrosis and secondary infection cause arouses of great vessels and cause a pseudoaneurysm, which rupture may cause massive hemorrhage to gastrointestinal tract, retroperitoneum or abdominal cavity.

The early diagnosis and following intervention radiology and surgical treatment are necessary for bleeding control. Debridement of the infected necrosis is the effective management for minimizing the risk of recurrent bleeding. Fortunately, the incidence of the hemorrhagic complications of severe acute pancreatitis decreases due to early recognition and intensive treatment of these patients (Huťan, 2008).

5. Conclusion

Despite the mortality of severe acute pancreatitis decreased after the implementation of new diagnostic and medical procedures in last two decade, many questions are still open. Recent studies of severe acute pancreatitis were reviewed and the decision to change the management of the treatment of severe acute pancreatitis has been made. The management referred to the enteral nutrition, epidural analgesia, antibiotic prophylaxis, delay surgery to the later period (three-four weeks after onset) in the case of infected necrosis.

Using enteral nutrition in preventing septic complications of acute pancreatitis seems to be better than parenteral nutrition. Epidural anesthesia is used to induce analgesia, to recovery of intestinal peristaltic and for improvement of the microcirculation blood flow. The continual measurement of the intra-abdominal pressure with the catheter in urinary bladder was used. After confirmation of necrosis, the prophylactic application of antibiotics including imipenem was used for severe acute pancreatitis patients. The prophylactic

application lasted maximum 14 days. By deferring surgery a proper demarcation of pancreatic and peripancreatic necrosis can take place. The demarcation of necrotic masses from viable tissue enables as easier and safer debridement with a great likelihood of sparing pancreatic tissue and leads to successful surgical control of pancreatic necrosis.
Applying the change of the management of treatment of the patients with the complicated form of acute pancreatitis, there were found an interesting results, which could recommended to use this management for patients suffered from severe acute pancreatitis.

6. References

Balogh, Z.; McKinley, BA.; Cocanour, CS.; Kozar, RA.;Holcomb, JB.; Ware, DN. & Moore, FA. (2002). Secondary abdominal compartment syndrome is an elusive early complication of traumatic shock resuscitation. In: *American Journal of Surgery*, Vol.184, No.6, (December 2002), pp. 538-543, ISSN 002-9610

Bank, S.; Singh, P.; Pooran, N. & Stark, B. (2002). Evaluation of factors that have reduced mortality from acute pancreatitis over the past 20 years. In: *Journal of Clinical Gastroenterology*, Vol.35, No.1, (July 2002), pp. 50-60, ISSN 0192-0790

Baril, NB.; Ralls, PW.; Wren, SM.; Selby, RR.; Radin,R.; Parekh,D.; Jabbour,N. & Stain,SC. (2000). Does an infected peripancreatic fluid collection or abscess mandate operation? In: *Annals of Surgery*, Vol.231, No.3, (March 2000), pp. 361-367, ISSN 0003-4932

Baron, TH.; Morgan, DE. & Stanley RJ. (1996). Endoscopic therapy for organized pancreatic necrosis. In: *Gastroenterology*, Vol.111, No.3, (September 1996), p.755–764, ISSN 0002-9270

Baron, TH.; Gavin, CH.; Desiree, EM. &Munford, RY.(2002). Outcome differences after endoscopic drainage of pancreatic necrosis, acute pancreatic pseudocysts, and chronic pancreatic pseudocysts. In: *Gastrointestinal Endoscopy*, Vol.56, No.1, (July 2002), pp.7–17, ISSN 0016-5107

Beger, HG.; Block, S.; Krautzberger, W. & Bittner, R. (1982). Necrotizing pancreatitis. Surgical indications and results in 118 patients. In: *Chirurg*, Vol.53, No.12, (December 1982), pp.784–789, ISSN 0009-4722

Beger HG.; Bittner,R.; Block, S. & Büchler M. (1986). Bacterial contamination of pancreatic necrosis. A prospective clinical study. In: *Gastroenterology*, Vol.91, No.2, (August 1986), pp. 433-438, ISSN 0016-5085

Beger, HG.; Rau, B.; Mayer, J. & Pralle, U. (1997). Natural course of acute pancreatitis. In: *World Journal of Surgery*, Vol.21, No.2, (February 1997), pp. 130-135, ISSN 0364-2313

Beger, HG.; Rau, B. & Isenmann, R. (2001). Prevention of severe change in acute pancreatitis: prediction and prevention. In: *Journal of Hepato-Biliary-Pancreatic Surgery*, Vol.8, No.2, (April 2001), pp. 140-147, ISSN 1868-6974

Beger, HG. & Isenmann, R. (2002). Acute pancreatitis: who needs an operation? In: *Journal of Hepato-Biliary-Pancreatic Surgery*, Vol.9, No.4, (October 2002), pp. 436-444, ISSN 1868-6974

Bertolini, G.; Luciani, D. & Biolo, G. (2007). Immunonutrition in septic patients: a philisophical view of the current situation. In: *Clinical Nutrition*, Vol.26, No.1, (February 2007), pp. 25-29, ISSN 0261-5614

Bober, J.; Kraus, L.; Mathernyová, E.; Harbul'ák, P.; Chymčák, I. & Závacký, P. (1995). Laparostomy in the treatment of severe hemorrhagic-necrotic pancreatitis. In: *Bratislavské lekárske listy,* Vol.96, No.9, (September 1995), pp. 493-495, ISSN 0006-9248

Bober, J.; Firment, J.; Grochová, M.; Steranková, M. & Harbuľák, P. (2002). Treatment algorithm for severe necrotic pancreatitis from the point of view of interdisciplinary collaboration. In: *Anesteziologie a Intenzívní Medicína,* Vol.13, No.5, (November 2002), pp. 227-230, ISSN 1214-2158

Bober, J. & Harbuľák, P. (2003). Continuous lavage in the treatment of severe necrotizing pancreatitis. In: *Rozhledy v Chirurgii,* Vol.82, No.5, (May 2003), pp. 245-249, ISSN 0035-9351

Branum, G.; Galloway, J.; Hirchowitz, W.; Fendley, M. & Hunter, J. (1998). Pancreatis necrosis. Results of necrosectomy, packing and ultimate closure over drains. In: *Annals of Surgery,* Vol.227, No.6, (June 1998), pp. 870-877, ISSN 0003-4932

Broome, AH.; Eisen, GM.; Harland, RC.; Collins,BH.; Meyers, WC. & Pappaset TN. (1996). Quality of life after treatment for pancreatitis. In: *Annals of Surgery,* Vol.223, No.6, (June 1996), pp. 665-670, ISSN 0003-4932

Bruennler, T.; Langgartner, J.; Lang, S.; Zorger, N.; Herold,T.; Salzberger, B.; Feuerbach, S.; Schoelmerich, J. & Hamer, OW. (2008). Percutaneous necrosectomy in patients with acute necrotizing pancreatitis. In: *European Radiology,* Vol.18, No.8, (August 2008), pp. 604–610, ISSN 0938- 7994

Büchler, MW.; Gloor, B.; Müller, CA.; Friess, H.; Seiler, CA. & Uhl, W. (2000). Acute necrotizing pancreatitis: treatment strategy according to the status of infection. In: *Annals of Surgery,* Vol.232, No.5, (November 2000), pp. 619-626, ISSN 0003-4932

Bucher, P.; Pugin, F. & Morel, P. (2008). Minimally invasive necrosectomy for infected necrotizing pancreatitis. In: *Pancreas,* Vol.36, No.2, (February 2008), pp. 113-119, ISSN 0885-3177

Carter, CR.; McKay, CJ. & Imrie, CW. (2000). Percutaneous necrosectomy and sinus tract endoscopy in the management of infected pancreatic necrosis: An initial experience. In: *Annals of Surgery,* Vol.232, No.2, (August 2000), pp. 175-180, ISSN 0003-4932

Cao, Y.; Xu, Y.; Tingna, L.; Gao, F. & Zegnan, M. (2008). Meta- analysis of enteral nutrition versus total parenteral nutrition in patients with severe acute pancreatitis. In: *Annals of Nutrition and Metabolism,* Vol.53, No.3-4, (February 2009), pp. 268-275, ISSN 0250-6807

Connor, S.; Alexakis, N.; Neal, T.; Raraty, M.; Ghaneh, P.; Evans, J.; Hughes, M.; Rowlands, P.; Garvey, CJ.; Sutton, R. & Neoptolemos, JP. (2004). Fungal infection but not type of bacteral infection is associated with a high mortality in primary and secondary infected pancreatic necrosis. In: *Digestive Surgery,* Vol.21, No.4, (October 2004), pp. 297-304, ISSN 0253-4886

Connor, S.; Raraty, MG.; Howes, N.; Evans, J.; Ghaneh, P.; Sutton, R. & Neoptolemos, JP. (2005). Surgery in the treatment of acute pancreatitis - Minimal access pancreatic necrosectomy. In: *Scandinavian Journal of Surgery,* Vol.94, No.2, (April 2005), pp. 135-142, ISSN 0036-5521

Cushieri, A. (2002). Pancreatis necrosis: pathogenesis and endoscopic management. In: *Seminars in Laparoscopic Surgery,* Vol.9, No.1, (March 2002), pp. 54-63, ISSN 1071-5517

Dambrauskas, Z.; Gulbinas, A.; Pundzius, J. & Barauskas, G. (2007). Meta-analysis of prophylactic parenteral antibiotic use in acute necrotizing pancreatitis. In: *Medicina,* Vol.43, No.4, (April 2007), pp. 291-300, ISSN 1010-660X

Dambrauskas, Z.; Parseliunas, A.; Gulbinas, A.; Pundzius, J. & Barauskas, G. (2009). Early recognition of abdominal campartment syndrome in patients with acute pancreatitis. In: *World Journal of Gastronterology,* Vol.15, No.6, (February 2009), pp. 717-721, ISSN 1007-9327

De Campos, T.; Braga, CF.; Kuryura, L.; Hebara, D.; Assef, JC. & Rasslan, S. (2008). Changes in the management of patients with severe acute pancreatitis. In: *Arquivos de Gastroenterologia,* Vol.45, No.3, (July/September 2008), pp. 181-185, ISSN 0004-2803

Dellinger, EP.; Tellado, JM.; Soto, NE.; Ashley, SW.; Barie, PS.; Dugernier, T.; Imrie, CW.; Johnson, CD.; Knaebel, HP.; Laterre, PF.; Maravi-Poma, E.; Kissler, JJ.; Sanchez-Garcia, M. & Utzolino, S. (2007). Early antibiotic treatment for severe acute necrotizing pancreatitis: a randomized, double-blind, placebo-controlled study. In: *Annals of Surgery,* Vol.245, No.5, (May 2007), pp. 674-683, ISSN 0003-4932

Demirag, A.; Pastor, CM.; Morel, P.; Jean-Christophe, C.; Sielenkämper, AW.; Güvener,N.; Mai, G.; Berney, T.; Frossard, JL. & Bühler, LH. (2006). Epidural anaesthesia restores pancreatic microcirculation and decreases the severity of acute pancreatitis. In: *World Journal of Gastroenterology,* Vol.12, No.6, (February 2006), pp. 915-920, ISSN 1007-9327

De Waele, J.; Hoste, E.; Blot, SI.; Decruyenaere, J. & Colardyn, F. (2005). Intraabdominal hypertension in patients with severe acute pancreatitis. In: *Critical Care,* Vol.9, No.4, (August 2005), pp. 452-457, ISSN 1364-8535

De Waele, J.; Pletinckx, P.; Blot, S. & Hoste, E. (2006). Saline volume in transvesical intra-abdominal pressure measurement: enough is enough. In: *Intensive Care Medicine,* Vol.32, No.3, (March 2006), pp. 455-459, ISSN 0342-4642

De Waele, J. (2008). Abdominal Compartment Syndrome in Severe Acute Pancreatitis – When to Decompress? In: *European Journal of Trauma and Emergency Surgery,* Vol.34, No.1, (February 2008), pp. 11-16, ISSN 1863-9933

Dugernier, TH.; Dewaelw, J. & Laterre, PF. (2006). Current surgical management of acute pancreatitis. In: *Acta Chirurgica Belgica,* Vol.106, No.2, (April 2006), pp. 165-171, ISSN 0001-5458

Eckerwall, GE.; Axelsson, JB. & Andersson, RG. (2006). Early nasogastric feeding in predicted severe acute pancreatitis: a clinical, randomized study. In: *Annals of Surgery,* Vol.244, No.6, (December 2006), pp. 959–965, ISSN 0003-4932

Elia, M.; Engfer, MB.; Green, CJ. & Silk, DB. (2008). Systematic review and meta-analysis: the clinical and physiological effects of fibre-containing enteral formulae. In: *Alimentary Pharmacology & Therapeutics,* Vol.27, No.1, (January 2008), pp. 120–145, ISSN 1365-2036

Fernandez-Cruz L.; Navarro, S.; Valderrama, R.; Sáenz, A.; Guarner, L.; Aparisi, L.; Espi, A.; Jaurietta, E.; Marruecos, L. & Gener, J. (1994). Acute necrotizing pancreatitis:

a multicenter study. In: *Hepatogastroenterology,* Vol.41, No.2, (April 1994), pp.185–189, ISSN 0172-6390

Fernandez-del Castillo, C.; Rattner, RD.; Makary, MA.; Mostafavi, A.; McGrath, D. & Warshaw, AL. (1998). Debridement and closed packing for the treatment of necrotizing pancreatitis. In: *Annals of Surgery,* Vol.228, No.5, (November 1998), pp. 676–684, ISSN 0003-4932

Foitzik, T.; Eibl, G.; Schneider, P.; Wenger, FA.; Jacobi, CA. & Buhr, HJ. (2002). Omega-3 fatty acid supplementation increases antiinflammatory cytokines and attenuates systemic disease sequelae in experimental pancreatitis. In: *Journal of Parenteral and Enteral Nutrition,* Vol.26, No.6, (November 2002), pp.351–356, ISSN 0148-6071

Frossard, JL.; Hadengue, A. & Pastor, CM. (2001). New serum markers for the detection of severe acute pancreatitis in humans. In: *American Journal of Respiratory and Critical Care Medicine,* Vol.164, No.1, (July 2001), pp. 162-170, ISSN 1073-449X

Golub, R.; Siddiqi, F. & Pohl, D. (1998). Role of antibiotics in acute pancreatitis: a meta-analysis. In: *Journal of Gastrointestinal Surgery,* Vol.2, No.6, (December 1998), pp. 496-502, ISSN 1091-255X

Götzinger, P.; Sautner, T.; Kriwanek, S.; Beckerhinn, P. & Barlan, M. (2002). Surgical treatment for severe acute pancreatitis: extent and surgical control of necrosis determine outcome. In: *World Journal of Surgery,* Vol.26, No.4, (April 2002), pp.474-478, ISSN 0364-2313

Götzinger, P. (2007). Operative treatment of severe acute pancreatitis, In: *European Surgery,* Vol.39, No.6, (December 2007), pp. 325-329, ISSN 1682-8631

Hartwig, W.; Werner, J.; Müller, CA., Uhl, M. & Büchler, MW. (2002a). Surgical management of severe pancreatitis including sterile necrosis. In: *Journal of Hepato-Biliary-Pancreatic Surgery,* Vol.9, No.4, (October 2002), pp. 429-435, ISSN 1868-6974

Hartwig, W.; Werner, J.; Uhl, M. & Büchler, MW. (2002b). Management of infection in acute pancreatitis. In: *Journal of Hepato-Biliary-Pancreatic Surgery,* Vol.9, No.4, (October 2002), pp. 423-428, ISSN 1868-6974

Heinrich, S.; Schäfer, M.; Rousson, V. & Clavien, PA. (2006) Evidence-based treatment of acute pancreatitis: A look at established paradigms. In: *Annals of Surgery,* Vol.243, No.2, (February 2006), pp. 154-168, ISSN 0003-4932

Horvath, KD.; Kao, LS.; Wherry, KL.; Pellegrini, CA. & Sinanan, MN. (2001). A technique for laparoscopic-assisted percutaneous drainage of infected pancreatic necrosis and pancreatic abscess. In: *Surgical Endoscopy,* Vol.15, No.10, (October 2001), pp. 1221-1225, ISSN 0930-2794

Huťan, M. (2006). *Staging a Chirurgická Liečba Akútnej Pankreatitídy,* (1. Edition), X print s.r.o., ISBN 80-969462-3-4, Bratislava, Slovakia.

Isaji, S.; Takada, T.; Kawarada, Y.; Hirata, K.; Mayumi, T.; Yoshida, M.; Sekimoto, M.; Hirota, M.; Kimura, Y.; Takeda, K.; Koizumi, M.; Otsuki, M. & Matsuno, S. (2006). JPN Guidelines for the management of acute pancreatitis: surgical management. In: *Journal of Hepato-Biliary-Pancreatic Surgery,* Vol.13, No.1, (January 2006), pp. 48-55, ISSN 1868-6974

Isenmann, R.; Rünzi, M.; Kron, M.; Kahl, S.; Kraus, D.; Jung, N.; Maier, L.; Malfertheiner, P.; Goebell, H. & Beger, HG. Prophylactic antibiotic treatment in patients with predicted severe acute pancreatitis: a placebo-controlled, double-blind trial. In: *Gastroenterology,* Vol.126, No.4, (April 2004), pp. 997-1004, ISSN 0016-5085

Jacobson, BC.; Vander Vliet, MB.; Hughes, MD.; Maurer, R.; McManus, K. & Banks, PA. (2007). A prospective, randomized trial of clear liquids versus low-fat solid diet as the initial meal in mild acute pancreatitis. In: *Clinical Gastroenterology and Hepatology,* Vol.5, No.8, (August 2007), pp. 946–951, ISSN 1542-3565

Karakan, T.; Ergun, M.; Dogan, I.; Cindoruk, M. & Unal, S. (2007). Comparison of early enteral nutrition in severe acute pancreatitis with prebiotic fiber supplementation versus standard enteral solution: a prospective randomized double-blind study. In: *World Journal of Gastroenterology,* Vol.13, No.19, (May 2007), pp. 2733-2737, ISSN 1007-9327

Klar, E.; Rattner, DW.; Compton, C.; Stanford, G.; Chernow, B. & Warshaw AL. (1991). Adverse effect of therapeutic vasoconstrictors in experimental acute pancreatitis. In: *Annals of Surgery,* Vol.214, No.2, (August 1991), pp. 168-174, ISSN 0003-4932

Klar, E.; Schratt, W.; Foitzik, T.; Buhr, H.; Herfarth, C. & Messmer, K. (1994). Impact of microcirculatory flow pattern changes on the development of acute edematous and necrotizing pancreatitis in rabbit pancreas. In: *Digestive Diseases and Sciences,* Vol.39, No.12, (December 1994), pp. 2639-2644, ISSN 0163-2116

Letko, G.; Nosofsky, T.; Lessel, W. & Siech M. (1991). Transition of rat pancreatic juice edema into acute pancreatitis by single ethanol administration. In: *Pathology Research and Practice,* Vol.187, No.2-3, (March 1991), pp. 247-250, ISSN 0344-0338

Malbrain, ML.; Cheatham, ML.; Kirkpatrick, A.; Sugrue, M.; Parr, M.; De Waele, J.; Balogh, Z.; Leppaniemi, A.; Olvera, C.; Ivatury, R.; D'Amours, S.; Wendon, J.; Hillman, K.; Johansson, K.; Kolkman, K. & Wilmer, A. (2006). Results from the international conference of experts on intraabdominal hypertension and abdominal compartment syndrome. I. Definitions. In: *Intensive Care Med*icine, Vol.32, No.11, (November 2006), pp. 1722–32, ISSN 0342-4642

Mayer, AD.; Airey, M.; Hodgson, J. & McMahon, MJ. (1985). Enzyme transfer from pancreas to plasma during acute pancreatitis. The contribution of ascitic fluid and lymphatic drainage of the pancreas. In: *Gut,* Vol.26, No.9, (Septembet 1985), pp. 876–881, ISSN 0017-5749

McClave, SA.; Snider, H.; Owens, N. & Sexton, LK. (1997). Clinical nutrition in pancreatitis. In: *Digestive Diseases and Sciences,* Vol.42, No.10, (October 1997), pp. 2035–2044, ISSN 0163-2116

Mier, J.; Luque-de León, E.; Armando Castillo, F.; Robledo, F. & Blanco, R. (1997). Early versus late necrosectomy in severe necrotizing pancreatitis. In: *American Journal of Surgery,* Vol.173, No.2, (February 1997), pp.71–5, ISSN 002-9610

Mortelé, KJ.; Girshman, J.; Szejnfeld, D.; Ashley, SW.; Erturk, SM.; Banks, PA. & Silverman, SG. (2009). CT-guided percutaneous catheter drainage of acute necrotizing pancreatitis: clinical experience and observations in patients with sterile and infected necrosis. In: *American Journal of Roentgenology,* Vol.192, No.1, (January 2009), pp.110–116, ISSN 0361-803X

Nakad, A.; Piessevaux, H.; Marot, JC.; Hoang, P.; Geubel, A.; Van Steenbergen, W. & Reynaert, M. (1998). Is early enteral nutrition in acute pancreatitis dangerous?

About 20 patients fed by an endoscopically placed nasogastrojejunal tube. In: *Pancreas,* Vol.17, No.2, (August 1998), pp. 187–193, ISSN 0885-3177

Nordback, IH. & Auvinen, OA. (1985). Long-term results after pancreas resection for acute necrotizing pancreatitis. In: *British Journal of Surgery,* Vol.72, No.9, (September 1985), pp. 687-789, ISSN 1365-2168

Oláh, A. & Romics, L. (2010). Evidence-based use of enteral nutrition in acute pancreatitis. In: *Langenbeck's Archives of Surgery,* Vol.395, No.4, (April 2010), pp. 309-316, ISSN 1435-2443

Olejník, J. & Brychta I. (2008). Aktuálny antimikrobiálny management ťažkej akútnej pankreatitídy. In: *Slovenská Chirurgia,* Vol.5, No.3, (September 2008), pp. 16-21, ISSN 1336-5975

Otto, W.; Komorzycki, K. & Krawczyk, M. (2006). Efficacy of antibiotic penetration into pancreatic necrosis. In: *HPB,* Vol.8, No.1, (January 2006), pp. 43-48, ISSN 1477-2574

Parekh, D. (2006). Laparoscopic-assisted pancreatic necrosectomy: a new surgical option for treatment of severe necrotizing pancreatitis. In: *Archives of Surgery,* Vol.141, No.9, (September 2006), pp. 895-902, ISSN 0003-0010

Paszkowski, AS.; Rau, B.; Mayer, JM.; Moller, P. & Beger, HG. (2002). Therapeutic application of caspase 1/interleukin-1beta-converting enzyme inhibitor decreases the death rate in severe acute experimental pancreatitis. In: *Annals of Surgery,* Vol.235, No.1, (January 2002), pp. 68-76, ISSN 0003-4932

Pederzoli, P.; Bassi, C.; Vesentini, S. & Camedelli, A. (1993). A randomized multicenter clinical trial of antibiotic prophylaxis of septic complications in acute necrotizing pancreatitis with imipenem. In: *Surgery, Gynecology and Obstetrics,* Vol.176, No.5, (May 1993), pp. 480-483, ISSN 0039-6087

Petrov, MS.; Kukush, MV. & Emelyanov NV. (2006). A randomized controlled trial of enteral versus parenteral feeding in patients with predicted severe acute pancreatitis shows a significant reduction in mortality and in infected pancreatic complications with total enteral nutrition. In: *Digestive Surgery,* Vol.23, No.5-6, (February 2007), pp. 336-344, ISSN 0253-4886

Petrov, MS. & Zagainov, VE. (2007). Influence of enteral versus parenteral nutrition on blood glucose control in acute pancreatitis: a systemic review. In: *Clinical Nutrition,* Vol.26, No.5, (October 2007), pp. 514–523, ISSN 0261-5614

Petrov, MS.; Pylypchuk, RD. & Uchugina, AF. (2009a). A systematic review on the timing of artificial nutrition in acute pancreatitis. In: *British Journal of Nutrition,* Vol.101, No.6, (March 2009), pp. 787-789, ISSN 0007-1145

Petrov, MS.; Loveday, PB.; Pylypchuk, RD.; McIlroy, K.; Phillips, ARJ. & Windsor, JA. (2009b). Systematic review and meta-analysis of enteral nutrition formulations in acute pancreatitis. In: *British Journal of Surgery,* Vol.96, No.11, (November 2009), pp. 1243–1252, ISSN 1365-2168

Piciucchi, M.; Merola, E; Marignani, M.; Signoretti, M.; Valente, R.; Cocomello, L.; Baccini, F.; Panzuto, F.; Capurso, G. & Delle Fave, G. (2010). Nasogastric or nasointestinal feeding in severe acute pancreatitis. In: *World Journal of Gastroenterology,* Vol. 16, No. 29, (August 2010), pp. 3692-3696, ISSN 1007-9327

Rayes, N.; Seehofer, D. & Neuhaus, P. (2009). Prebiotics, probiotics, synbiotics in surgery—are they only trend, truly effective or even dangerous? In: *Langenbeck´s Archives of Surgery*, Vol.394, No.3, (May 2009), pp. 547–555, ISSN 1435-2443

Risse, O.; Auguste, T.; Delannoy, P.; Cardin, N.; Bricault, I. & Létoublon, C. (2004). Percutaneous video-assisted necrosectomy for infected pancreatic necrosis. In: *Gastroenterologie Clinique et Biologique*, Vol.28, No.10, (October 2004), pp. 868-871, ISSN 0399-8320

Rokke, O.; Harbitz, TB.; Liljedal, J.; Pettersen, T.; Fetvedt, T.; Heen, LO.; Skreden, K. & Viste, A. (2007). Early treatment of severe pancreatitis with imipenem: A prospective randomized clinical trial. In: *Scandinavian Journal of Gastroenterology*, Vol.42, No.6, (June 2007), pp. 771-776, ISSN 0036-5521

Sarr, MG. (2003). IAP guidelines in acute pancreatitis - So what? In: *Digestive Surgery*, Vol.20, No.1, (January 2003), pp. 1-2, ISSN 0253-4886

Sahora, K.; Jakesz, R. & Götzinger, P. (2009). The role of surgery in severe acute pancreatitis. In: *European Surgery*, Vol.41, No.6, (October 2009), pp. 280-285, ISSN 1682-8631

Schmid, SW.; Uhl, W.; Friess, H.; Malfertheiner, P. & Büchler, MW. (1999). The role of infection in acute pancreatitis. In: *Gut*, Vol.45, No.2, (August 1999), pp. 311-316, ISSN 0017-5749

Seifert, H.; Biermer, M.; Schmitt, W.; Jürgensen, C.; Will, U.; Gerlach, R.; Kreitmair, C.; Meining, A.; Wehrmann, T. & Rösch, T. (2009). Transluminal endoscopic necrosectomy after acute pancreatitis: a multicenter study with long-term follow-up (the GEPARD study). In: *Gut*, Vol.58, No.9, (September 2009), pp.1260–1266, ISSN 0017-5749

Seewald, S.; Groth, S.; Omar, S.; Imazu, H.; Seitz, U.; de Weerth, A.; Soetikno, R.; Zhong, Y.; Sriram, PV.; Ponnudurai, R.; Sikka, S.; Thonke, F. & Soehendra, N. (2005). Aggressive endoscopic therapy for pancreatic necrosis and pancreatic abscess: a new safe and effective treatment algorithm. In: *Gastrointestinal Endoscopy*, Vol.62, No.1, (July 2005), pp.92–100, ISSN 0016-5107

Sharma, VK. & Howden, CW. (2001). Prophylactic antibiotic administration reduces sepsis and mortality in acute necrotizing pancreatitis: A meta-analysis. In: *Pancreas*, Vol.22, No.1, (January 2001), pp. 28-31, ISSN 0885-3177

Sielenkämper, AW.; Eicker, K. & Van Aken, H. (2000). Thoracic epidural anesthesia increases mucosal perfusion in ileum of rats. In: *Anesthesiology*, Vol.93, No.3, (September 2000), pp. 844-851, ISSN 0003-3022

Šiller, J.; Daněk, T.; Turnovský, P. & Havlíček, K. (2007). Význam měření intraabdominálního tlaku v prevenci vzniku abdominálního kompartmentového syndromu u pacientů hospitalizovaných na chirurgické jednotce intenzivní péče, In: *Slovenská Chirurgia*, Vol.4, No.4, (October 2007), pp. 7-26, ISSN 1336-5975

Slavin, J. & Neoptolemos, JP. (2001).Antibiotic prophylaxis in severe acute pancreatitis - what are the facts? In: *Langenbeck´s Archives of Surgery* , Vol.386, No.2, (April 2001), pp. 155-159, ISSN 1435-2443

Smadja, C. & Bismuth H. (1986). Pancreatic debridement in acute necrotizing pancreatitis: an obsolete procedure? In: *British Journal of Surgery*, Vol.73, No.5, (May 1986), pp. 408-410, ISSN 1365-2168

Spanier, BW.; Bruno, MJ. & Mathus-Vliegen, EM. (2011). Enteral nutrition and acute pancreatitis: a review. In: *Gastroenterology Research and Practice,* Vol.2011, 9 pp, ISSN 1687-6121, Available from: http://www.hindawi.com/journals

Sugrue, M.; Jones, F.; Deane, SA.; Bishop, G.; Bauman, A. & Hillman, K. (1999). Intra-abdominal hypertension is an independent cause of postoperative renal impairment. In: *Archives of Surgery,* Vol.134, No.10, (October 1999), pp. 1082-1085, ISSN 0004-0010

Sugrue, M.; D'Amours, SK. & Kolkman, KA. (2007). Temporary abdominal closure. In: *Acta Clinica Belgica,* Vol.2, No.1 Suppl., (January 2007), pp. 210-214, ISSN 00015458

Sun, S.; Yang, K.; He, X.; Tian, J.; Ma, B. & Jiang, L. (2009). Probiotics in patients with severe acute pancreatitis: a meta-analysis. In: *Langenbeck´s Archives of Surgery* , Vol.394, No.1, (January 2009), pp.171–177, ISSN 1435-2443

Šutiak, L.; Janík, J.; Mikolajčík, A.; Strelka, L. & Mištuna, D. (2008). Použitie laparoskopie pri liečbe ťažkej akútnej pankreatitídy. In: *Slovenská Chirurgia,* Vol.5, No.4, (July 2008), pp. 21-27, ISSN 1336-5975

Tenner, S.; Sica, G.; Highes, M.; Noordhoek, E.; Feng, S.; Zinner, M. & Banks, PA. (1997). Relationship of necrosis to organ failure in severe acute pancreatitis. In: *Gastroenterology,* Vol.113, No.3, (September 1997), pp. 899-903, ISSN 0016-5085

Tiengou, LE.; Gloro, J.; Pouzoulet, J.; Bouhier,K.; Read,MH.; Arnaud-Battandier, F.; Plaze,JM.; Blaizot,X.; Dao, T. & Piquet, MA. (2006). Semi-elemental formula or polymeric formula: is there a better choice for enteral nutrition in acute pancreatitis? Randomized comparative study. In: *Journal of Parenteral and Enteral Nutrition,* Vol.30, No.1, (February 2006), pp. 1–5, ISSN 0148-6071

Uhl, W.; Warshaw, A.; Imrie, C.; Bassi, C.; McKay, CJ.; Lankisch, PG.; Carter, R. & Büchler, MW. (2002). IAP guidelines for the surgical management of acute pancreatitis. In: *Pancreatology,* Vol.2, No.6, (November 2002), pp.565-573, ISSN 1424-3903

Van Santvoort, HC.; Besselink, MG.; Bollen, TL.; Buskens, E.; Van Ramshorst, B. & Gooszen, HG. (2007). Case-matched comparison of the retroperitoneal approach with laparotomy for necrotizing pancreatitis. In: *World Journal of Surgery,* Vol.31, No.8, (August 2007), pp. 1635-1642, ISSN 0364-2313

Whelan, K. (2007). Enteral-tube-feeding diarrhoea: manipulating the colonic microbiota with probiotics and prebiotics. In: *Proceedings of the Nutrition Society,* Vol.66, No.3, (March 2007), pp. 299-306, ISSN 0029-6651

Wittau, M.; Mayer, B.; Scheele, J.; Henne-Bruns, D.; Dellinger, EP. & Isenmann, R. (2011). Systematic review and meta-analysis of antibiotic prophylaxis in severe acute pancreatitis. In: *Scandinavian Journal of Gastroenterology,* Vol. 46, No. 3, (March 2011), pp. 261-270, ISSN 0036-5521

Xu, T. & Cai, Q. (2008). Prophylactic antibiotic treatment in acute necrotizing pancreatitis: Results from a meta-analysis. In: *Scandinavian Journal of Gastroenterology,* Vol.43, No.10, (Oktober 2008), pp. 1249-1258, ISSN 0038-5521

16

Hypertriglyceride Induced Acute Pancreatitis

Joshua Lebenson and Thomas Oliver
Uniformed Services University of the Health Sciences, United States

1. Introduction

Pancreatitis is a common clinical entitiy with multiple contributing etiologies[1]. Triglyceride (TG) levels greater than 1000 mg/dL are seen in a small but significant number of cases of acute pancreatitis (AP), with estimates ranging between 1-7% of all cases and perhaps slightly higher in patients who present during pregnancy[2-4]. The clinical presentation of hypertriglyceridemic pancreatitis (HTGP) is similar to other causes of acute pancreatitis, but some evidence suggests that there may be an increased severity and risk of complications[5,6]. Multiple etiologies of highly elevated TG levels have been implicated, including congenital disorders, metabolic perturbations and certain medications but a definitive treatment regimen for profoundly elevated serum TG in association with acute, and often severe, pancreatitis has yet to be demonstrated[7-10].

Dietary restriction is the cornerstone of therapy. Additional treatment modalities have included insulin and heparin to stimulate the synthesis, release and activation of lipoprotein lipase (LPL) from capillary endothelial cells to promote TG degradation into free fatty acids for further metabolism or storage[11]. We present a case of HGTP managed with insulin, heparin and octreotide with dramatic results; a logarithmic decrease in serum TGL magnitude and a significant reduction in the time to resolution as compared with previous reports of treatment with insulin and heparin alone. Recent advances in the management of HGTP, including proposed mechanisms, will be reviewed. Adjunctive therapies, including plasmapheresis and more chronic therapy with lipid lowering agents and dietary modification will be discussed.

2. Case report

A 51-year-old Hispanic man presented to the emergency department with 2 days of epigastric pain radiating to the back. The patient reported one episode of emesis but denied fever, chills, dyspnea, diarrhea, or constipation. His past medical history was significant for asthma and gastroesophageal reflux disease. Medications included omeprazole daily and as needed acetaminophen, ibuprofen, and albuterol. Social history was significant for tobacco use, one pack per month, and ethanol use, two cans of beer daily.

Temperature was 97.6°F. Blood pressure was 117/72 mm Hg, heart rate 80 min, regular, and respiratory rate was 18/min. Examination of the cardiopulmonary and nervous system was unremarkable. The abdomen was diffusely tender without rebound, guarding or discoloration. No xanthelasmas, eruptions, arcus, or xanthomas were noted. Relevant laboratory measurements from lipemic serum are listed in Table 1. The urine toxicology screen was positive for barbiturates. Cardiac screening (enzymes, electrocardiogram) was negative and ultrasound imaging revealed no abnormalities of the gall bladder, common bile duct, or pancreas. A CT scan performed on the second hospital day was remarkable for peripancreatic fat stranding without necrosis or hemorrhage.

Analyte	**Reference Range**	**Admission**	**24 h**	**48 h**
Amylase	25-125 U/L	80	126	141
Lipase	23-203 U/L	179	166	96
Glucose	74-118 mg/dL	100	83	93
Triglycerides	30-190 mg/dL	20891	1423	355
Cholesterol	60-160 mg/dL	862	997	594
Sodium	136-144 mmol/L	111	121	140
AST	<40 IU/L	737	186	74
ALT	<33 IU/L	227	135	39

Table 1. Laboratory Values at Presentation and While Hospitalized

The patient was diagnosed with HTGP and initial management included elimination of enteral intake, aggressive fluid repletion, and opiate analgesia. Subsequent therapy included a continuous insulin infusion, a 10% dextrose infusion titrated to maintain euglycemia, 60 U/kg unfractionated heparin intravenous (IV) bolus every 4 hours, and 100μg octreotide bolus subcutaneously every 8 hours. TG fell by 2 orders of magnitude in 2 days, falling from 21,000 to 355 mg/dL, the rest of the laboratory values were improved (Table 1), and the lipemia resolved. The clinical course was uncomplicated and the patient was discharged after 4 days.

3. Clinical presentation of hypertriglyceridemic pancreatitis

The clinical features of acute HTGP are similar to that of other causes of pancreatitis[12]. Patients may present with sudden and severe epigastric abdominal pain often accompanied by anorexia and profound nausea lasting hours to days[13]. Other less common findings, more indicative of chronic hyperlipidemia, include the presence of eruptive xanthomas over the extensor surfaces, lipemia retinalis, arcus and hepatospenomeglay due to fatty infiltration of the liver.[14] Frequently, those presenting with significant TG elevations and pancreatitis have an underlying metabolic abnormality in lipid metabolism[15,16]. Patient presentations where HTGP is encountered include poorly controlled diabetics with or without a history of HTG, alcoholics with hypertriglyceridemia or lactescent serum on admission, non-diabetic, non-obese patients with drug or diet-induced HTG and patients presenting with AP without secondary risk factors; the first three of these comprise the majority of clinical presentations of HTGP[12,17,18].

Following the onset of HTGP, TGL tend to fall rapidly over 72 hours in the fasting state as a result of decreased supply and absorption of chylomicrons[19]. In addition, VLDL secretion from the liver is reduced secondary to the administration of hypocaloric intravenous fluids, thus leading to a direct reduction in TGL[20].

4. Lipid physiology

Lipoproteins are macromolecules containing both organic proteins and bound lipids that are found in plasma in varying proportions and can be separated by density via ultracentrifugation. In increasing order of density, these separate into layers of chylomicrons, very low density lipoprotein (VLDL), intermediate density lipoprotein (IDL), low density proteins (LDL) and high density lipoprotein (HDL)[21].

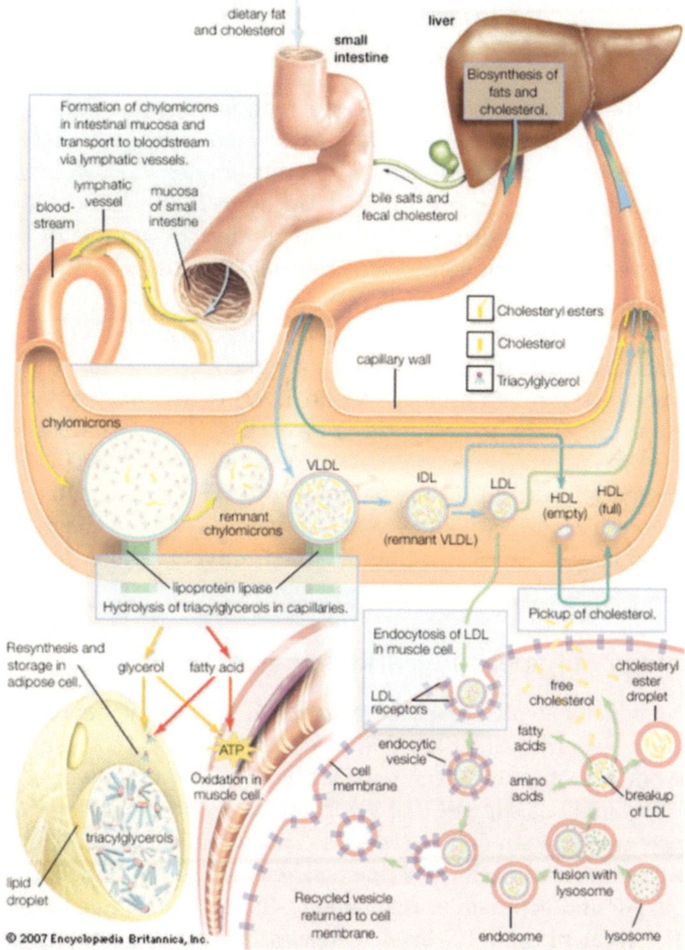

Fig. 1. Fat metabolism
http://www.britannica.com/bps/media-view/92255/0/0/0

TG are a major lipid constituent of chylomicrons and VLDL. The former contains Apo B-48 and is derived from dietary sources while the latter contains Apo B-100 and is liver generated[22,23]. Cholesterol is the primary component of IDL and LDL[24].

Dietary TG are absorbed through the brush border of intestinal enterocytes, incorporated into chylomicrons and pass through the basolateral aspect where they enter the lymphatics before entering the venous circulation via the thoracic duct, ultimately acquiring apolipoprotein C-II, a critical cofactor for lipoprotein lipase (LPL)[25].

Both chylomicrons and VLDL are transported to muscle and adipose tissue where they are metabolized by LPL to meet energy demands or stored for future use[26,27]. LPL is secreted into the venous circulation by parenchymal cells in many tissues, migrates through the vasculature and anchors to the capillary endothelium via a heparan sulfate chain. Upon activation, it facilitates lipoprotein binding and TG degradation[28]. This process results in the release of fatty acids and acylglycerols which can then be utilized directly by myocytes to meet metabolic demands or be reincorporated into triglyceride for storage in adipocytes[29].

5. Diagnosis and laboratory evaluation

The clinical presentation and course of HTG pancreatitis does not differ greatly from other causes of AP[30]. Lipemic serum, frequently associated with an underlying metabolic abnormality or compromising medications, is the single most reliable clue that the pancreatitis is associated with or precipitated by hyperlipidemia[31]. Although the serum triglyceride threshold for considering HTGP is generally considered to be in the range of 1000 mg/dL, the severity, clinical course and complication rate do not correlate with lipid levels. In a study of 43 patients with HTGP, no correlation was observed between admission HTG and APACHE II score, nor was there a relation between TG level and pancreatic inflammatory complications or ultimate patient outcome[32].

Historically, clinicians have relied on increases in levels of serum amylase, and/or lipase to secure the diagnosis of acute pancreatitis. Newer diagnostic modalities, such as urine trypsinogen, procarboxypeptidase A and carboxypeptidase A, are becoming more available and may become more relevant[33-35]. Some patients with HTG pancreatitis and lipemic serum present with spurious laboratory values that can complicate the diagnosis[36] but a serum lipase sensitivity and specificity of 67% and 97% respectively, argue that this test remains a valuable diagnostic tool[37].

6. Pathophysiology of hypertriglyceridemic pancreatitis

The mechanism by which elevated levels of plasma TG lead to the development of AP is not fully understood. It is generally accepted that levels greater than 1000 mg/dL are required to precipitate an episode of pancreatitis, but such levels of TG do not always cause HTGP.[38] The most recent ATP III guidelines suggest that a normal TG level is considered to be less than 150 mg/dl, while those greater than 500 mg/dl are considered very high[39]. Pancreatic lipase, a digestive enzyme concentrated in the exocrine pancreas which participates in TG degradation, may be liberated in AP and act in an unregulated fashion to contribute to tissue breakdown[40]. Additionally, if the local plasma TG level increases beyond the enzymatic capacity of the pancreas, free fatty acids begin to accumulate and can lead to injury of pancreatic acinar cells and surrounding tissues[41,42]. Altered pancreatic blood flow, perhaps aggravated by the hyperviscosity of chylomicronemia, may also create a more acidic environment in which free fatty acids become more toxic to the surrounding tissue[43-46]. The resultant cellular injury leads to further pancreatic inflammation, injury and destruction.

7. Causes of hypertriglyceridemia

Primary Causes: Primary causes of HTG consist of a series of genetic disorders leading to abnormalities in lipid metabolism and patients presenting with HTG or lipemic serum should be evaluated for Frederickson classification dyslipidemias types I, IV and V as they are strongly associated with highly elevated serum TG[47,48].

Secondary Causes:

Diabetes – Poorly controlled, or uncontrolled, diabetes is a common cause of HTGP[49]. In type 1 diabetes mellitus, the paucity of insulin reduces LPL synthesis and thus compromises effective TG hydrolysis and release of free fatty acids. The latter are already accumulating in the absence of insulin-facilitated storage[50,51]. Similarly, in type 2 diabetes mellitus, increased insulin resistance leads to enhanced production and reduced clearance of TGs[52]. The causal role of diabetic ketoacidosis (DKA) in HTG was evaluated in a prospective study of 100 patients with DKA, 11 of whom had AP, and of these, HTG was the only attributable cause in 4 cases[53]. Serum TG levels normalized in these patients after control of the acidosis.

Primary HTG *Genetic:* Frederickson type I, IV, V
Secondary HTG *Diet:* alcohol excess, weight gain/obesity *Drugs:* exogenous estrogens, tamoxifen, retinoids, thiazides, beta blockers, protease inhibitors, propofol, parenteral lipid infusions *Disorders of Metabolism:* Diabetes, pregnancy, chronic renal failure, hypothyroidism, porphyria *Adapted from Ref [12]

Table 2. Common Etiologies of HTG

Alcohol – Ethanol compromises fuel and energy metabolism, thereby resulting in decreased serum glucose levels with elevated levels of lipids due to increased production and decreased utilization of energy sources. Alcohol can aggravate HTG and the liberated free fatty acid esters can promote calcium influx which leads to calcium-mediated pancreatic necrosis[57]. Nutritional deficiencies, including hypoglycemia, activated counterregulatory mechanisms and reduced cofactor availability reduce or inhibit insulin secretion, thus further compromising energy metabolism and exacerbating hyperlipidemia[58].

Medications- Several medications are known to increase plasma TG levels, including isotretinoin[59], propofol[60], protease inhibitors[61] and furosemide[62]. Estrogens and Tamoxifen are two well studied drugs in which the tendency to promote HTG and steatohepatitis is well described[63].

Estrogen – Exogenous estrogens increase serum TG and fatty acids primarily by reducing levels of lipoprotein and hepatic lipases which subsequently decreases clearance and aggravates insulin resistance, perhaps by as much as 40%[64-66]. Goldenberg et al., evaluated 56 female patients at a Cholesterol Center because of TG >400 mg/dl and/or HTGP, and/or failure of TG-lowering therapy. Of that cohort, 17 females (30%) had a history of AP and of those, 9 (53%) had taken, or were concurrently taking exogenous steroid hormones[67]. The authors concluded that hormone therapy remain relatively contraindicated with plasma TG>300mg/dl and strictly contraindicated when TG greater than >500 mg/dl in order to avoid an episode of pancreatitis.

Tamoxifen – Tamoxifen is a non-steroidal anti-estrogen commonly used in the treatment of patients with breast cancer and has shown the ability to decrease LDL and total cholesterol levels. There is frequently an increase in VLDL synthesis and subsequent rise in plasma TG levels due to reductions in lipoprotein lipase activity[68,69]. Elisaf, et al., reported 12 patients with serum TG >1000 mg/dl who were observed after administration of 20mg/day of tamoxifen[70]. Four of these patients, two of whom had a personal or family history of hyperlipidemia, developed HTGP. This led them to the conclusion that, like synthetic estrogens, the tamoxifen-mediated rise in TGs may be either contributory or causative in the development of AP.

Pregnancy - Gestational AP is an uncommon condition, with studies ranging incidence between 1 in 3,500-4,000 pregnancies[71]. Most cases of AP during pregnancy are mild and are most often attributable to biliary disease, while severe AP most commonly results from hypertriglyceridemia and tends to occur in the second and third trimesters[72]. During pregnancy there is a physiologic increase in plasma lipids. Cholesterol and TG increase due to an increased production of VLDL and the decreased actions of LPL and hepatic lipase[73]. HTGP tends to develop in women with an underlying disorder in lipid metabolism, such as LPL[74] or apolipoprotein C-II deficiency[75]. Maternal mortality in cases complicated by HGTP is estimated to be near 20% and cause of death has been linked to the pancreatitis itself, or, rarely, has been associated with HELLP syndrome.[76] The mainstay of treatment, as in the non-pregnant state, is early recognition and intervention[77,78]. A major difference in long term management is that the use of HMG-CoA reductase inhibitors (statins) is contraindicated in pregnancy as they are a teratogenic category X pharmaceutical[79].

	Type I	**Type IV**	**Type V**
Elevated lipoproteins	Chylomicrons	VLDL	VLDL Chylomicrons
Cholesterol	Normal	Normal or Increased	Normal
Triglycerides	+++	++	+++
Plasma appearance †	Clear plasma, creamy supernatant	Turbid	Turbid plasma, creamy supernatant
Genotype	LPL deficiency Apo C-II deficiency	FCH Sporadic HTG	Familial HTG
Age of onset (primary form)	Infancy or childhood	Usually adulthood	Usually adulthood
Xanthomas ‡	Eruptive or tuberous	None usually	Eruptive or tuberoeruptive
Other clinical features	Recurrent abdominal pain Pancreatitis Lipemia retinalis Hepatosplenomegaly	Premature CAD Pancreatitis Obesity Glucose intolerance Arthritic symptoms Gall bladder disease Hyperuricemia	Recurrent abdominal pain Pancreatitis Lipemia retinalis Hepatosplenomegaly Peripheral paresthesis Glucose intolerance Hyperuricemia

*Adapted from Reference 12
† Plasma obtained after 12 hours of fasting, left undisturbed in refrigerator overnight
‡Seen only in a minority of patients, frequency increases as plasma lipid levels rise
LPL, lipoprotein lipase; HTG, hypertriglyceridemia; Apo C-II, apolipoprotein CII; CAD, coronary artery disease; FCH, familial combined hyperlipidemia.

Table 3. Familial Hyperlipidemias*

Hypothyroidism – HTG is common in hypothyroidism, having been reported in up to 35% of cases[80]. Decreased free thyroid hormone increases the synthesis of LPL and decreases hepatic lipase activity with a net tendency toward increased plasma TG levels, perhaps further complicated by the down-regulation of LDL receptors[81-84]. One patient with central hypothyroidism secondary to a craniopharyngioma developed HTG with a level of (3,300 mg/dL) which precipitated an episode of AP[85].

8. Treatment

Initial Management – Initial management of patients presenting with HTGP mirrors that of other causes of AP[86]. Patients should be placed on bowel rest, receive nothing by mouth and undergo aggressive fluid resuscitation due to third space losses[87]. Adequate pain control is essential, often through the use of opioid narcotics[88-90]. Some controversy still remains about the potential for medication-induced sphincter of Oddi dysfunction aggravating the clinical picture although low dose transdermal fentanyl patches appear do not to compromise sphincteric function[91,92]. Meperidine has been used as an alternative analgesic to treat pain in those suffering from acute pancreatitis, but concern for the production of toxic metabolites has altered prescribing practices[93-95]. Enteral nutrition should be resumed as soon as is practical, recognizing that the reintroduction of fats, the building blocks of chylomicrons, may be deleterious[96-100]. Assessment of exocrine function prior to refeeding may be prudent, given that pancreatic destruction has the potential to compromise secretion of digestive enzymes[101].

Beyond initial management, HTGP therapy must include measures to reduce serum TG, both acutely and following the episode to minimize the risk of recurrence[102]. Laboratory tests including liver function tests, glucose, renal function, thyroid stimulating hormone and urine protein should be obtained to rule out secondary causes of HTG[103]. Specific tests documenting LPL or Apo C-II deficiency should be obtained if type I hyperlipidemia is suspected[104-107]. No standard treatment guidelines yet exist in the specific treatment of HTGP although a rational treatment strategy should include rapidly lowering serum TG, blocking the induction of pro-inflammatory mediators that lead to pancreatic destruction and reducing the likelihood of recurrence by eliminating offending agents, as is possible, and through the use of antihyperlipidemic medications[108-111].

Insulin – Intravenous insulin administration is an effective therapy for patients diagnosed with HTG induced pancreatitis, including those with and without diabetes mellitus[112,113]. VLDL is a triglyceride-rich lipid moiety and the use of insulin decreases hepatic production of apolipoprotein B-100 rich VLDL1 and intestinal production of VLDL2, rich in apoprotein B-48 while also increasing hydrolysis of TG by LPL[114,115]. Insulin promotes storage of both glucose and fatty acids, thus a continuous infusion of insulin should reduce serum levels of both of these fuels[116,117]. Intravenous (IV) insulin may be considered more effective and easier to titrate than subcutaneous (SQ) administration based upon absorption and delivery kinetics, although both have been used with some success[104,118,119]. Insulin has been used alone, but is commonly used in conjunction with other TG lowering modalities[120,121]. Mikhail et al. reported lowering TG from 7,700 mg/dL to 246 mg/dL in one patient using only intravenous insulin at 3-9 units per hour for 4 days while maintaining euglycemia[122]. In the same report, a second patient treated in a similar fashion saw TG levels drop from 10,500 mg/dL to 656 mg/dL over 4 days using 4 units SQ insulin (Lispro) every four hours.

Although no standard protocol for insulin administration in the context of HTGP has been defined, the authors have achieved success with insulin doses titrated from an initial rate of

0.1-0.4 units/kg per hour. Once an effective insulin infusion dose has been achieved, we have kept this constant while the dextrose infusion is titrated to maintain euglycemia, contrary to what is usually done when insulin is infused.

Heparin - Heparin is an effective treatment in the management of elevated TG in the presence of HTGP[123]. LPL, the enzyme which hydrolyzes TG rich lipoproteins, is normally bound by a heparan sulfate proteoglycan chain to the capillary endothelium[124]. Heparin, when administered in a bolus dose, has a stronger affinity for the LPL binding site than does the heparan sulfate, leading it to dissociate from the endothelium tissue into the plasma as a heparan-LPL complex.[125] This surge of "free" LPL is then able to bind and metabolize lipoproteins at an accelerated rate, thus lowering serum TG levels[126]. Although there is an initial rise in available LPL, there is also a peaking of activity, after which, LPL activity begins to wane as the enzyme is transported and degraded in the liver[127]. This heparin-stimulated increase and then reduction in LPL activity can be minimized by the use of intermittent heparin dosing and results in an initial drop in serum TGs, but then followed by a gradual increase[128,129]. This phenomenon tends to be more pronounced with the use of LMW heparin, versus un-fractionated heparin, although studies have shown both preparations capable of lowering severely elevated TG in the setting of HTGP.[130]

Heparin has been used as successful monotherapy in treatment of profound HTG in previous studies[131-133]; however, more dramatic results have been achieved when used in combination with other modalities (Table 4). At present, no studies have been conducted as to the best route of administration (IV or SQ) or dosage in the treatment of HTGP. It is the opinion of the authors that bolus dosing of IV heparin 18 units/kg[134] dosed every 4-6 hours is more effective than continuous administration.

Patient	**Trig Level (mg/dL) at Admission**	**IV Insulin U/h: IV Heparin Units; SC Octreotide μg**	**Triglyceride Results**
41-year-old female ETOH abuse	7037	Insulin 1-5 U/h for 5d; heparin 500-900 U/h for 3d	5111 mg/dL by day 3
51-year-old male ETOH abuse	7900	Insulin 12 U/h; heparin 5000 U b.i.d	670 mg/dL by day 4
31-year-old female at 30 wk gestation	4445	Insulin 20 U/h; heparin 10,000 U/24h	880 mg/dL by day 3
51-year-old* ETOH abuse	21,000	Insulin 2 U/h minimum; heparin 60 U/kg every 4h; octreotide 100 μg subcutaneously every 8 h	355 mg/dL in 48 hr

*Our patient.
Adapted from Ref 122

Table 4. Published Reports of Management of Hypertriglyceridemia With IV Insulin and Heparin: Comparison to Case Patient

Octreotide™ - Somatostatins, also called somatotropin release inhibitory factors (SRIFs) are cyclic peptide hormones which exist in 2 forms, SRIF14 (14 amino acids) and SRIF28 (28 amino acids)[135], and are synthesized in several sites within the body, including the central nervous system, pituitary, gastrointestinal (GI) tract, liver, pancreas, and urogenital system[135,136]. SRIFs bind to 6 subpopulations of somatostatin receptors (sstrs) (1, 2_A, 2_B, 3, 4, 5) located both peripherally and centrally[137]. The sstr 2_B receptor has been demonstrated in rodents but not unequivocally in humans[138]. Binding of somatostatins to each of these receptors leads to the inhibition of adenylate cyclase via a pertussis toxin sensitive G-protein$_{(G\alpha i)}$ and, at agonist concentrations greater than 1-nM, there is stimulation of phospholipase C which increases calcium ion mobilization[139]. In neuroendocrine cells, sstrs 2,3,4 and 5 bind to inward rectifying potassium channels[140].

SRIFs inhibit the secretion of several GI tract hormones including insulin, glucagon, gastrin, cholecystokinin, vasoactive intestinal peptide and secretin and also inhibit exocrine gastric acid, pepsin, pancreatic enzymes, bile and intestinal fluid secretions [141]. The pancreas expresses sstrs on both acinar cells (sstr4, sstr5)[142] and islet cells (sstr1 > sstr5 > sstr2 > sstr3 > sstr4)[143]. In rodents, sstr2 in the dorsal vagal complex exerts some control of pancreatic exocrine secretion[144].

Octreotide, a somatostatin analog, has particular affinity for types 2_A, 2_B and somewhat for sstr5[145]. Octreotide has been used in the treatment of pancreatitis with varying degrees of success[146]. The evidence that pancreatic sstrs are down-regulated in acute pancreatitis suggests that the mechanisms of action of octreotide therapy may include both receptor and non-receptor mediated mechanisms[147]. Secretion of insulin and glucagon are inhibited by agonists of sstr2, sstr5, and sstr1[148]. Inhibition of glucagon secretion with octreotide therapy may potentiate the fatty acid storing action of insulin and lead to a greater reduction of serum TG[149]. Octreotide's effect on the hypoglycemic counter regulatory system, notably the hyperglycemic actions of glucagon, necessitates the co-administration of dextrose and frequent monitoring of glucose levels to maintain euglycemia.

Study	No. of patients	No. of patients with complete recovery (%)	Mortality (%)
Yeh et al.	17	13(76.5)	2 (11.8)
Kyriakidis et al.	10	9 (90)	1 (10)
Kadikoylu et al.	7	7 (100)	0
Lennertz et al.	5	5 (100)	0

* Adapated from Ref 5

Table 5. Apheresis in hypertriglyceridemic pancreatitis *

Plasmapheresis – Although the primary methods of treating HTGP are dietary fat restriction and lipid lowering medications, these treatments may be inadequate in the setting of severe acute HTGP[150,151]. Plasmapheresis has been used with some measure of success and is thought to work through two mechanisms: the removal of serum TG from the patient's serum and the supplementation of LPL and apolipoprotein found in the fresh frozen plasma of the donor plasma[152,153]. Yeh, et. al found that a single exchange removed 66.3% of TG, while a second exchange removed 83.3% of serum TG[154]. The number of sessions, however, did not correlate with clinical outcome. Syed et al., evaluated patients with HTGP receiving plasmapheresis and observed an average reduction in TG levels of 89.3% with the first treatment, but found no clear relationship between APACHE II scores or length of hospital stay[155].

Plasmapheresis is not without risk, and at this time its use in HTGP remains undefined. Potential complications or adverse reactions include allergic reaction and transfusion related infections. One patient undergoing plasmapheresis was reported to develop anaphylactoid shock[154,156]. At present the American Society for Apheresis Guidelines of 2007 places apheresis in its role for HTGP as a category three due to limited data and conflicting reports[157].

Apheresis Recommendations*

Category	Recommendation
I	First line therapy
II	Second line therapy
III	Specific role not determined
IV	Not recommended

*Journal of Clinical Apheresis, Special Issue(Vol 25, 2010)

9. Long-term management

Diet and General Precautions -Primary causes of hyperlipidemia often require medications but, where possible, reducing the impact of secondary causes with therapeutic lifestyle changes such as reducing alcohol intake, weight reduction, improved diabetic control and discontinuing precipitating medications are all vital steps[158]. Dietary advice should be obtained through a certified nutritionist, but fat consumption should be reduced to 7% of total caloric intake, cholesterol limited to 200mg and trans fatty acid intake should be limited[159]. Medium chain TG are an improved source of fat calories as they are absorbed directly into portal circulation and do not require chylomicrons for hepatic uptake and lower TG levels at the cost of a slightly elevated cholesterol level[160]. A meta-analysis performed by Dattilo and Kris-Etherson observed a strong correlation between weight loss and decrease in plasma TG levels.[161]

Medications:

Fibrates - Fibric acid derivatives are a class of medications which bind to peroxisome proliferator alpha (PPARα) receptors and are capable of increasing serum HDL while simultaneously lowering TG and are an effective adjunct in treating patients with HTGP who cannot be managed with diet alone[162]. They are typically used in treating primary HTG and include drugs such as gemfibrozil, bezafibrate and fenofibrate[163]. Fibrates lower serum TG by increasing the levels of LPL and hepatic lipase, reducing levels of Apo CIII, which down-regulates LPL activity, and by increasing fatty acid uptake by the liver[164,165]. Toxicities include elevated liver enzyme levels, cholelithithiasis, myalgias and rhabdomyolysis; the last two of these are more common when used in patients with impaired renal function[166]. Two cases have been reported where patients developed pancreatitis while taking fibrate or fibrate-statin combinations.[167, 168] It is unclear whether the cause of the pancreatitis was directly related to the drug itself, a failure of treatment or possibly through the formation of biliary sludge or gallstone formation.

Niacin - Niacin, a B vitamin somewhat less potent than the fibric acids, decreases TG levels by reducing hepatic secretion of VLDL and TG while raising HDL and lowering LDL levels,

an overall positive impact on the lipid profile[169]. When used as doses of 1,500mg/day, no adverse impact on glucose metabolism is seen but significant prostaglandin D2-mediated flushing limits the clinical utility of this drug[170].
Statins - HMG-CoA reductase inhibitors (statins) are not the preferred method for lowering serum TG as their role in lipid management remains in prevention (primary and secondary) of coronary artery disease in the presence of elevated cholesterol, but only mild to moderate triglyceride elevations[171]. Statins are not suitable monotherapy for long-term management of HTG, however, they may have some synergistic benefit when combined with fibrates[172,173].
Omega 3 Fatty Acids - Fish oils and omega-3 fatty acids are effective adjuncts to other drug therapy as they lead other drug therapy as they lead to a decrease in VLDL and lower endogenously derived TG-rich lipoproteins[174,175]. Active TG lowering molecules in these supplements include eicosapentaenoic acid (EPA) and docosahexaenoic acid (DHA)[176]. Omega-3 fatty acids were studied in a prospective, double-blinded trial and were able to lower TG levels, ranging from 500-2,000 mg/dL, by an average of 45%[177]. The minimum effective dose is approximately 1 g/d; however, a dose of 3 to 4 g/d has shown to reduce serum TG by 30-50% in hyperlipidemic patients[178].

10. Conclusion

HTG is a significant cause of AP, with most estimates ranging from 1-7% of all cases. Presentation is often similar to other forms of AP, with lipemic serum usually the only distinguishing initial sign. Clinicians should routinely test TG levels in patients with suspected or confirmed AP, especially those who have a history of diabetes, alcoholism, obesity, are taking a known precipitating medication, are pregnant or display normal amylase in the presence of elevated lipase.
To date, there are no official guidelines for the treatment of HTGP, although a number of different treatment modalities have been employed to rapidly lower the serum TG, including insulin, heparin, fibric acids and omega 3 fatty acids. Plasmapheresis can also rapidly lower serum TG levels, but significant potential side effects and lack of rigorous proof of efficacy have yet to clarify its role in treatment of HTGP. Long term management with diet modification and anti-hyperlipidemic medications such as statins, niacin and omega-3 fatty acids are excellent adjuncts in controlling TGs in patients with HTGP and preventing potential recurrences.
We have achieved dramatic effects with the combination of insulin, heparin and octreotide, a reduction in TG levels of two orders of magnitude in 48 hours, results unprecedented in the literature. These results, while impressive, have yet to be reproduced and one must remain appropriately circumspect when interpreting this case report. It is also important to note that the positive barbiturate level may have unmasked an inducible porphyria and that rapid resolution of HTGP was aided by the removal of this compound from the metabolic milieu. No clear treatment algorithm exists for the management of HTGP and well-designed, controlled, prospective studies are needed to clearly delineate the ideal regimen.

11. Disclaimer

The views expressed in this manuscript are those of the authors and do not reflect the official policy or position of the Department of the Armed Forces, Department of Defense, or the U.S. Government

12. References

[1] Brisinda G, Vanella S, Crocco A, et al. Severe acute pancreatitis: advances and insights in assessment of severity and management. Eur J Gastroenterol Hepatol 2011;23:541-51.

[2] Khan AS, Latif SU, Eloubeidi MA. Controversies in the etiologies of acute pancreatitis. JOP 2010;11:545-52.

[3] Kayatas SE, Eser M, Cam C, Cogendez E, Guzin K. Acute pancreatitis associated with hypertriglyceridemia: a life-threatening complication. Arch Gynecol Obstet 2010;281:427-9.

[4] Gubensek J, Buturovic-Ponikvar J, Marn-Pernat A, et al. Treatment of hyperlipidemic acute pancreatitis with plasma exchange: a single-center experience. Ther Apher Dial 2009;13:314-7.

[5] Tsuang W, Navaneethan U, Ruiz L, Palascak JB, Gelrud A. Hypertriglyceridemic pancreatitis: presentation and management. Am J Gastroenterol 2009;104:984-91.

[6] Ewald N, Hardt PD, Kloer HU. Severe hypertriglyceridemia and pancreatitis: presentation and management. Curr Opin Lipidol 2009;20:497-504.

[7] Thrower EC, Gorelick FS, Husain SZ. Molecular and cellular mechanisms of pancreatic injury. Curr Opin Gastroenterol 2010;26:484-9.

[8] Cornett DD, Spier BJ, Eggert AA, Pfau PR. The Causes and Outcome of Acute Pancreatitis Associated with Serum Lipase >10,000 U/L. Dig Dis Sci 2011.

[9] Anderson F, Mbatha SZ, Thomson SR. The early management of pancreatitis associated with hypertriglyceridaemia. S Afr J Surg 2011;49:82-4.

[10] Lee KM, Paik CN, Chung WC, Yang JM. Association between acute pancreatitis and peptic ulcer disease. World J Gastroenterol 2011;17:1058-62.

[11] Jain D, Zimmerschied J. Heparin and insulin for hypertriglyceridemia-induced pancreatitis: case report. ScientificWorldJournal 2009;9:1230-2.

[12] Yadav D, Pitchumoni CS. Issues in hyperlipidemic pancreatitis. J Clin Gastroenterol 2003;36:54-62.

[13] Bae JH, Baek SH, Choi HS, et al. Acute pancreatitis due to hypertriglyceridemia: report of 2 cases. Korean J Gastroenterol 2005;46:475-80.

[14] Durrington P. Dyslipidaemia. Lancet 2003;362:717-31.

[15] Whitcomb DC. Genetic aspects of pancreatitis. Annu Rev Med 2010;61:413-24.

[16] Fujita K, Maeda N, Kozawa J, et al. A case of adolescent hyperlipoproteinemia with xanthoma and acute pancreatitis, associated with decreased activities of lipoprotein lipase and hepatic triglyceride lipase. Intern Med 2010;49:2467-72.

[17] Kyriakidis AV, Raitsiou B, Sakagianni A, et al. Management of acute severe hyperlipidemic pancreatitis. Digestion 2006;73:259-64.

[18] Tremblay K, Methot J, Brisson D, Gaudet D. Etiology and risk of lactescent plasma and severe hypertriglyceridemia. J Clin Lipidol 2011;5:37-44.

[19] Dominguez-Munoz JE, Malfertheiner P, Ditschuneit HH, et al. Hyperlipidemia in acute pancreatitis. Relationship with etiology, onset, and severity of the disease. Int J Pancreatol 1991;10:261-7.

[20] Chait A, Brunzell JD. Chylomicronemia syndrome. Adv Intern Med 1992;37:249-73.

[21] Ellington AA, Kullo IJ. Atherogenic lipoprotein subprofiling. Adv Clin Chem 2008;46:295-317.

[22] van Greevenbroek MM, de Bruin TW. Chylomicron synthesis by intestinal cells in vitro and in vivo. Atherosclerosis 1998;141 Suppl 1:S9-16.
[23] Olofsson SO, Boren J. Apolipoprotein B: a clinically important apolipoprotein which assembles atherogenic lipoproteins and promotes the development of atherosclerosis. J Intern Med 2005;258:395-410.
[24] Packard CJ, Shepherd J. Lipoprotein heterogeneity and apolipoprotein B metabolism. Arterioscler Thromb Vasc Biol 1997;17:3542-56.
[25] Iqbal J, Hussain MM. Intestinal lipid absorption. Am J Physiol Endocrinol Metab 2009;296:E1183-94.
[26] Cianflone K, Paglialunga S, Roy C. Intestinally derived lipids: metabolic regulation and consequences--an overview. Atheroscler Suppl 2008;9:63-8.
[27] Dallinga-Thie GM, Franssen R, Mooij HL, et al. The metabolism of triglyceride-rich lipoproteins revisited: new players, new insight. Atherosclerosis 2010;211:1-8.
[28] Takahashi S, Sakai J, Fujino T, et al. The very low-density lipoprotein (VLDL) receptor: characterization and functions as a peripheral lipoprotein receptor. J Atheroscler Thromb 2004;11:200-8.
[29] Nasstrom B, Olivecrona G, Olivecrona T, Stegmayr BG. Lipoprotein lipase during continuous heparin infusion: tissue stores become partially depleted. J Lab Clin Med 2001;138:206-13.
[30] Andersson R, Sward A, Tingstedt B, Akerberg D. Treatment of acute pancreatitis: focus on medical care. Drugs 2009;69:505-14.
[31] Michalakis K, Basiakou E, Xanthos T, Ziakas P. Lipemic serum in hyperlipidemic pancreatitis. Cases J 2009;2:198.
[32] Balachandra S, Virlos IT, King NK, Siriwardana HP, France MW, Siriwardena AK. Hyperlipidaemia and outcome in acute pancreatitis. Int J Clin Pract 2006;60:156-9.
[33] Abraham P. Point-of-care urine trypsinogen-2 test for diagnosis of acute pancreatitis. J Assoc Physicians India 2011;59:231-2.
[34] Kemik O, Kemik AS, Sumer A, et al. Serum procarboxypeptidase a and carboxypeptidase a levels in pancreatic disease. Hum Exp Toxicol 2011.
[35] Yadav D, Agarwal N, Pitchumoni CS. A critical evaluation of laboratory tests in acute pancreatitis. Am J Gastroenterol 2002;97:1309-18.
[36] Brooks AM, Paisey RB, Waterson MJ, Smith JC. Diagnostic difficulties with a lipaemic blood sample. BMJ 2010;340:b5530.
[37] Treacy J, Williams A, Bais R, et al. Evaluation of amylase and lipase in the diagnosis of acute pancreatitis. ANZ J Surg 2001;71:577-82.
[38] Athyros VG, Giouleme OI, Nikolaidis NL, et al. Long-term follow-up of patients with acute hypertriglyceridemia-induced pancreatitis. J Clin Gastroenterol 2002;34:472-5.
[39] Executive Summary of The Third Report of The National Cholesterol Education Program (NCEP) Expert Panel on Detection, Evaluation, And Treatment of High Blood Cholesterol In Adults (Adult Treatment Panel III). JAMA 2001;285:2486-97.
[40] Wilde PJ, Chu BS. Interfacial & colloidal aspects of lipid digestion. Adv Colloid Interface Sci 2011;165:14-22.
[41] Petersen OH, Sutton R, Criddle DN. Failure of calcium microdomain generation and pathological consequences. Cell Calcium 2006;40:593-600.
[42] Criddle DN, Raraty MG, Neoptolemos JP, Tepikin AV, Petersen OH, Sutton R. Ethanol toxicity in pancreatic acinar cells: mediation by nonoxidative fatty acid metabolites. Proc Natl Acad Sci U S A 2004;101:10738-43.

[43] Zhang WZ, Xie JX, Shen J, Lin F. Hypertriglyceridemic acute pancreatitis in a patient with Sheehan's syndrome. Hepatobiliary Pancreat Dis Int 2006;5:468-70.
[44] Sakorafas GH, Tsiotou AG. Etiology and pathogenesis of acute pancreatitis: current concepts. J Clin Gastroenterol 2000;30:343-56.
[45] Piolot A, Nadler F, Cavallero E, Coquard JL, Jacotot B. Prevention of recurrent acute pancreatitis in patients with severe hypertriglyceridemia: value of regular plasmapheresis. Pancreas 1996;13:96-9.
[46] Kimura W, Mossner J. Role of hypertriglyceridemia in the pathogenesis of experimental acute pancreatitis in rats. Int J Pancreatol 1996;20:177-84.
[47] Kolovou GD, Anagnostopoulou KK, Kostakou PM, Bilianou H, Mikhailidis DP. Primary and secondary hypertriglyceridaemia. Curr Drug Targets 2009;10:336-43.
[48] Bildirici I, Esinler I, Deren O, Durukan T, Kabay B, Onderoglu L. Hyperlipidemic pancreatitis during pregnancy. Acta Obstet Gynecol Scand 2002;81:468-70.
[49] Fortson MR, Freedman SN, Webster PD, 3rd. Clinical assessment of hyperlipidemic pancreatitis. Am J Gastroenterol 1995;90:2134-9.
[50] Karabatas L, Oliva ME, Dascal E, et al. Is Lipotoxicity presents in the early stages of an experimental model of autoimmune diabetes? Further studies in the multiple low dose of streptozotocin model. Islets 2010;2:190-9.
[51] Poupeau A, Postic C. Cross-regulation of hepatic glucose metabolism via ChREBP and nuclear receptors. Biochim Biophys Acta 2011;1812:995-1006.
[52] Rivellese AA, De Natale C, Di Marino L, et al. Exogenous and endogenous postprandial lipid abnormalities in type 2 diabetic patients with optimal blood glucose control and optimal fasting triglyceride levels. J Clin Endocrinol Metab 2004;89:2153-9.
[53] Nair S, Yadav D, Pitchumoni CS. Association of diabetic ketoacidosis and acute pancreatitis: observations in 100 consecutive episodes of DKA. Am J Gastroenterol 2000;95:2795-800.
[54] Apte MV, Wilson JS. Alcohol-induced pancreatic injury. Best Pract Res Clin Gastroenterol 2003;17:593-612.
[55] Begriche K, Massart J, Robin MA, Borgne-Sanchez A, Fromenty B. Drug-induced toxicity on mitochondria and lipid metabolism: mechanistic diversity and deleterious consequences for the liver. J Hepatol 2011;54:773-94.
[56] Lapolla A, Tessari P, Duner E, et al. Hormonal and metabolic profiles in patients with alcohol-induced, mixed hypertriglyceridemia before and after abstinence from ethanol and before and after a lipid-lowering diet. Atherosclerosis 1986;60:151-9.
[57] Criddle DN, Sutton R, Petersen OH. Role of Ca2+ in pancreatic cell death induced by alcohol metabolites. J Gastroenterol Hepatol 2006;21 Suppl 3:S14-7.
[58] Ngatchu T, Sangwaiya A, Dabiri A, Dhar A, McNeil I, Arnold JD. Alcoholic ketoacidosis with multiple complications: a case report. Emerg Med J 2007;24:776-7.
[59] Greene JP. An adolescent with abdominal pain taking isotretinoin for severe acne. South Med J 2006;99:992-4.
[60] Mirtallo JM, Dasta JF, Kleinschmidt KC, Varon J. State of the art review: Intravenous fat emulsions: Current applications, safety profile, and clinical implications. Ann Pharmacother 2010;44:688-700.
[61] Durval A, Zamidei L, Bettocchi D, Luzzio MG, Consales G. Hyperlipidemic acute pancreatitis: a possible role of antiretroviral therapy with entecavir. Minerva Anestesiol 2011.

[62] Juang P, Page RL, 2nd, Zolty R. Probable loop diuretic-induced pancreatitis in a sulfonamide-allergic patient. Ann Pharmacother 2006;40:128-34.
[63] Farrell GC. Drugs and steatohepatitis. Semin Liver Dis 2002;22:185-94.
[64] Perseghin G, Scifo P, Pagliato E, et al. Gender factors affect fatty acids-induced insulin resistance in nonobese humans: effects of oral steroidal contraception. J Clin Endocrinol Metab 2001;86:3188-96.
[65] Glueck CJ, Lang J, Hamer T, Tracy T. Severe hypertriglyceridemia and pancreatitis when estrogen replacement therapy is given to hypertriglyceridemic women. J Lab Clin Med 1994;123:59-64.
[66] Brinton EA. Oral estrogen replacement therapy in postmenopausal women selectively raises levels and production rates of lipoprotein A-I and lowers hepatic lipase activity without lowering the fractional catabolic rate. Arterioscler Thromb Vasc Biol 1996;16:431-40.
[67] Goldenberg NM, Wang P, Glueck CJ. An observational study of severe hypertriglyceridemia, hypertriglyceridemic acute pancreatitis, and failure of triglyceride-lowering therapy when estrogens are given to women with and without familial hypertriglyceridemia. Clin Chim Acta 2003;332:11-9.
[68] Esteva FJ, Hortobagyi GN. Comparative assessment of lipid effects of endocrine therapy for breast cancer: implications for cardiovascular disease prevention in postmenopausal women. Breast 2006;15:301-12.
[69] Hozumi Y, Kawano M, Saito T, Miyata M. Effect of tamoxifen on serum lipid metabolism. J Clin Endocrinol Metab 1998;83:1633-5.
[70] Elisaf MS, Nakou K, Liamis G, Pavlidis NA. Tamoxifen-induced severe hypertriglyceridemia and pancreatitis. Ann Oncol 2000;11:1067-9.
[71] Croucher C, Wilson J. Idiopathic acute pancreatitis in pregnancy. J Obstet Gynaecol 1997;17:588-9.
[72] Sun L, Li W, Geng Y, Shen B, Li J. Acute pancreatitis in pregnancy. Acta Obstet Gynecol Scand 2011;90:671-6.
[73] Winkler K, Wetzka B, Hoffmann MM, et al. Low density lipoprotein (LDL) subfractions during pregnancy: accumulation of buoyant LDL with advancing gestation. J Clin Endocrinol Metab 2000;85:4543-50.
[74] Hieronimus S, Benlian P, Bayer P, Bongain A, Fredenrich A. Combination of apolipoprotein E2 and lipoprotein lipase heterozygosity causes severe hypertriglyceridemia during pregnancy. Diabetes Metab 2005;31:295-7.
[75] Coca-Prieto I, Valdivielso P, Olivecrona G, et al. Lipoprotein lipase activity and mass, apolipoprotein C-II mass and polymorphisms of apolipoproteins E and A5 in subjects with prior acute hypertriglyceridaemic pancreatitis. BMC Gastroenterol 2009;9:46.
[76] Gursoy A, Kulaksizoglu M, Sahin M, et al. Severe hypertriglyceridemia-induced pancreatitis during pregnancy. J Natl Med Assoc 2006;98:655-7.
[77] Hsia SH, Connelly PW, Hegele RA. Successful outcome in severe pregnancy-associated hyperlipemia: a case report and literature review. Am J Med Sci 1995;309:213-8.
[78] Eskandar O, Eckford S, Roberts TL. Severe, gestational, non-familial, non-genetic hypertriglyceridemia. J Obstet Gynaecol Res 2007;33:186-9.
[79] Uhl K, Kennedy DL, Kweder SL. Risk management strategies in the Physicians' Desk Reference product labels for pregnancy category X drugs. Drug Saf 2002;25:885-92.
[80] Regmi A, Shah B, Rai BR, Pandeya A. Serum lipid profile in patients with thyroid disorders in central Nepal. Nepal Med Coll J 2010;12:253-6.

[81] Brenta G, Berg G, Arias P, et al. Lipoprotein alterations, hepatic lipase activity, and insulin sensitivity in subclinical hypothyroidism: response to L-T(4) treatment. Thyroid 2007;17:453-60.
[82] Velkoska Nakova V, Krstevska B, Bosevski M, Dimitrovski C, Serafimoski V. Dyslipidaemia and hypertension in patients with subclinical hypothyroidism. Prilozi 2009;30:93-102.
[83] Kern PA, Ranganathan G, Yukht A, Ong JM, Davis RC. Translational regulation of lipoprotein lipase by thyroid hormone is via a cytoplasmic repressor that interacts with the 3' untranslated region. J Lipid Res 1996;37:2332-40.
[84] Duntas LH. Thyroid disease and lipids. Thyroid 2002;12:287-93.
[85] Gan SI, Edwards AL, Symonds CJ, Beck PL. Hypertriglyceridemia-induced pancreatitis: A case-based review. World J Gastroenterol 2006;12:7197-202.
[86] Martinez DP, Diaz JO, Bobes CM. Eruptive xanthomas and acute pancreatitis in a patient with hypertriglyceridemia. Int Arch Med 2008;1:6.
[87] Talukdar R, Swaroop Vege S. Early management of severe acute pancreatitis. Curr Gastroenterol Rep 2011;13:123-30.
[88] Munsell MA, Buscaglia JM. Acute pancreatitis. J Hosp Med 2010;5:241-50.
[89] Pezzilli R, Zerbi A, Di Carlo V, Bassi C, Delle Fave GF. Practical guidelines for acute pancreatitis. Pancreatology 2010;10:523-35.
[90] Cruciani RA, Jain S. Pancreatic pain: a mini review. Pancreatology 2008;8:230-5.
[91] Toouli J. Sphincter of Oddi: Function, dysfunction, and its management. J Gastroenterol Hepatol 2009;24 Suppl 3:S57-62.
[92] Koo HC, Moon JH, Choi HJ, et al. Effect of transdermal fentanyl patches on the motility of the sphincter of oddi. Gut Liver 2010;4:368-72.
[93] Spiegel B. Meperidine or morphine in acute pancreatitis? Am Fam Physician 2001;64:219-20.
[94] Thompson DR. Narcotic analgesic effects on the sphincter of Oddi: a review of the data and therapeutic implications in treating pancreatitis. Am J Gastroenterol 2001;96:1266-72.
[95] Munoz A, Katerndahl DA. Diagnosis and management of acute pancreatitis. Am Fam Physician 2000;62:164-74.
[96] Gianotti L, Meier R, Lobo DN, et al. ESPEN Guidelines on Parenteral Nutrition: pancreas. Clin Nutr 2009;28:428-35.
[97] Gramlich L, Taft AK. Acute pancreatitis: practical considerations in nutrition support. Curr Gastroenterol Rep 2007;9:323-8.
[98] Marik PE. What is the best way to feed patients with pancreatitis? Curr Opin Crit Care 2009;15:131-8.
[99] Mayerle J, Hlouschek V, Lerch MM. Current management of acute pancreatitis. Nat Clin Pract Gastroenterol Hepatol 2005;2:473-83.
[100] Heinrich S, Schafer M, Rousson V, Clavien PA. Evidence-based treatment of acute pancreatitis: a look at established paradigms. Ann Surg 2006;243:154-68.
[101] Pezzilli R, Simoni P, Casadei R, Morselli-Labate AM. Exocrine pancreatic function during the early recovery phase of acute pancreatitis. Hepatobiliary Pancreat Dis Int 2009;8:316-9.
[102] Kadikoylu G, Yukselen V, Yavasoglu I, Coskun A, Karaoglu AO, Bolaman Z. Emergent therapy with therapeutic plasma exchange in acute recurrent pancreatitis due to severe hypertriglyceridemia. Transfus Apher Sci 2010;43:285-9.

[103] Leaf DA. Chylomicronemia and the chylomicronemia syndrome: a practical approach to management. Am J Med 2008;121:10-2.

[104] Triay JM, Day A, Singhal P. Safe and rapid resolution of severe hypertriglyceridaemia in two patients with intravenous insulin. Diabet Med 2010;27:1080-3.

[105] Peterfy M, Ben-Zeev O, Mao HZ, et al. Mutations in LMF1 cause combined lipase deficiency and severe hypertriglyceridemia. Nat Genet 2007;39:1483-7.

[106] Okubo M, Horinishi A, Saito M, et al. A novel complex deletion-insertion mutation mediated by Alu repetitive elements leads to lipoprotein lipase deficiency. Mol Genet Metab 2007;92:229-33.

[107] Nauck MS, Nissen H, Hoffmann MM, et al. Detection of mutations in the apolipoprotein CII gene by denaturing gradient gel electrophoresis. Identification of the splice site variant apolipoprotein CII-Hamburg in a patient with severe hypertriglyceridemia. Clin Chem 1998;44:1388-96.

[108] Kumar AN, Schwartz DE, Lim KG. Propofol-induced pancreatitis: recurrence of pancreatitis after rechallenge. Chest 1999;115:1198-9.

[109] Steinberg W, Tenner S. Acute pancreatitis. N Engl J Med 1994;330:1198-210.

[110] Matern D, Seydewitz H, Niederhoff H, Wiebusch H, Brandis M. Dyslipidaemia in a boy with recurrent abdominal pain, hypersalivation and decreased lipoprotein lipase activity. Eur J Pediatr 1996;155:660-4.

[111] Butman M, Taylor D, Bostrom K, Quinones M, Nicholas SB. Hypertriglyceridemia and Recurrent Pancreatitis following Splenectomy. Case Rep Gastroenterol 2007;1:96-102.

[112] Kawanishi M, Okamoto S, Nishimura Y, Yoshikawa M, Kajiyama G. A case of acute pancreatitis with hyperlipemia and hyperglycemia induced by alcohol abuse. Hiroshima J Med Sci 1994;43:31-6.

[113] Lawson EB, Gottschalk M, Schiff DE. Insulin infusion to treat severe hypertriglyceridemia associated with pegaspargase therapy: a case report. J Pediatr Hematol Oncol 2011;33:e83-6.

[114] Pavlic M, Xiao C, Szeto L, Patterson BW, Lewis GF. Insulin acutely inhibits intestinal lipoprotein secretion in humans in part by suppressing plasma free fatty acids. Diabetes 2010;59:580-7.

[115] Wang H, Eckel RH. Lipoprotein lipase: from gene to obesity. Am J Physiol Endocrinol Metab 2009;297:E271-88.

[116] Hua Q. Insulin: a small protein with a long journey. Protein Cell 2010;1:537-51.

[117] Vihma V, Tikkanen MJ. Fatty acid esters of steroids: synthesis and metabolism in lipoproteins and adipose tissue. J Steroid Biochem Mol Biol 2011;124:65-76.

[118] Hahn SJ, Park JH, Lee JH, Lee JK, Kim KA. Severe hypertriglyceridemia in diabetic ketoacidosis accompanied by acute pancreatitis: case report. J Korean Med Sci 2010;25:1375-8.

[119] Jabbar MA, Zuhri-Yafi MI, Larrea J. Insulin therapy for a non-diabetic patient with severe hypertriglyceridemia. J Am Coll Nutr 1998;17:458-61.

[120] Jain P, Rai RR, Udawat H, Nijhawan S, Mathur A. Insulin and heparin in treatment of hypertriglyceridemia-induced pancreatitis. World J Gastroenterol 2007;13:2642-3.

[121] Monga A, Arora A, Makkar RP, Gupta AK. Hypertriglyceridemia-induced acute pancreatitis--treatment with heparin and insulin. Indian J Gastroenterol 2003;22:102-3.

[122] Mikhail N, Trivedi K, Page C, Wali S, Cope D. Treatment of severe hypertriglyceridemia in nondiabetic patients with insulin. Am J Emerg Med 2005;23:415-7.
[123] Cole RP. Heparin treatment for severe hypertriglyceridemia in diabetic ketoacidosis. Arch Intern Med 2009;169:1439-41.
[124] Mead JR, Irvine SA, Ramji DP. Lipoprotein lipase: structure, function, regulation, and role in disease. J Mol Med (Berl) 2002;80:753-69.
[125] Alagozlu H, Cindoruk M, Karakan T, Unal S. Heparin and insulin in the treatment of hypertriglyceridemia-induced severe acute pancreatitis. Dig Dis Sci 2006;51:931-3.
[126] Malmstrom R, Packard CJ, Caslake M, et al. Effect of heparin-stimulated plasma lipolytic activity on VLDL APO B subclass metabolism in normal subjects. Atherosclerosis 1999;146:381-90.
[127] Neuger L, Vilaro S, Lopez-Iglesias C, Gupta J, Olivecrona T, Olivecrona G. Effects of heparin on the uptake of lipoprotein lipase in rat liver. BMC Physiol 2004;4:13.
[128] Chevreuil O, Hultin M, Ostergaard P, Olivecrona T. Depletion of lipoprotein lipase after heparin administration. Arterioscler Thromb 1993;13:1391-6.
[129] Chevreuil O, Hultin M, Ostergaard P, Olivecrona T. Biphasic effects of low-molecular-weight and conventional heparins on chylomicron clearance in rats. Arterioscler Thromb 1993;13:1397-403.
[130] Nasstrom B, Stegmayr BG, Olivecrona G, Olivecrona T. Lower plasma levels of lipoprotein lipase after infusion of low molecular weight heparin than after administration of conventional heparin indicate more rapid catabolism of the enzyme. J Lab Clin Med 2003;142:90-9.
[131] Loo CC, Tan JY. Decreasing the plasma triglyceride level in hypertriglyceridemia-induced pancreatitis in pregnancy: a case report. Am J Obstet Gynecol 2002;187:241-2.
[132] Sharma P, Lim S, James D, Orchard RT, Horne M, Seymour CA. Pancreatitis may occur with a normal amylase concentration in hypertriglyceridaemia. BMJ 1996;313:1265.
[133] Sleth JC, Lafforgue E, Servais R, et al. [A case of hypertriglycideremia-induced pancreatitis in pregnancy: value of heparin]. Ann Fr Anesth Reanim 2004;23:835-7.
[134] Santamarina-Fojo S. The familial chylomicronemia syndrome. Endocrinol Metab Clin North Am 1998;27:551-67, viii.
[135] Patel YC. Somatostatin and its receptor family. Front Neuroendocrinol 1999;20:157-98.
[136] Epelbaum J, Dournaud P, Fodor M, Viollet C. The neurobiology of somatostatin. Crit Rev Neurobiol 1994;8:25-44.
[137] Ben-Shlomo A, Melmed S. Pituitary somatostatin receptor signaling. Trends Endocrinol Metab 2010;21:123-33.
[138] Cole SL, Schindler M. Characterisation of somatostatin sst2 receptor splice variants. J Physiol Paris 2000;94:217-37.
[139] Meyerhof W. The elucidation of somatostatin receptor functions: a current view. Rev Physiol Biochem Pharmacol 1998;133:55-108.
[140] Kreienkamp HJ, Honck HH, Richter D. Coupling of rat somatostatin receptor subtypes to a G-protein gated inwardly rectifying potassium channel (GIRK1). FEBS Lett 1997;419:92-4.
[141] Weckbecker G, Lewis I, Albert R, Schmid HA, Hoyer D, Bruns C. Opportunities in somatostatin research: biological, chemical and therapeutic aspects. Nat Rev Drug Discov 2003;2:999-1017.

[142] Taniyama Y, Suzuki T, Mikami Y, Moriya T, Satomi S, Sasano H. Systemic distribution of somatostatin receptor subtypes in human: an immunohistochemical study. Endocr J 2005;52:605-11.
[143] Pilichowska M, Kimura N, Schindler M, Kobari M. Somatostatin type 2A receptor immunoreactivity in human pancreatic adenocarcinomas. Endocr Pathol 2001;12:147-55.
[144] Liao Z, Li ZS, Lu Y, Wang WZ. Microinjection of exogenous somatostatin in the dorsal vagal complex inhibits pancreatic secretion via somatostatin receptor-2 in rats. Am J Physiol Gastrointest Liver Physiol 2007;292:G746-52.
[145] Ben-Shlomo A, Melmed S. Somatostatin agonists for treatment of acromegaly. Mol Cell Endocrinol 2008;286:192-8.
[146] Bang UC, Semb S, Nojgaard C, Bendtsen F. Pharmacological approach to acute pancreatitis. World J Gastroenterol 2008;14:2968-76.
[147] Wu JX, Yuan YZ, Xu JY, et al. Changes in somatostatin receptor expression of the pancreas and effectiveness of octreotide in rats with acute necrotizing pancreatitis. Chin J Dig Dis 2004;5:35-9.
[148] Singh V, Brendel MD, Zacharias S, et al. Characterization of somatostatin receptor subtype-specific regulation of insulin and glucagon secretion: an in vitro study on isolated human pancreatic islets. J Clin Endocrinol Metab 2007;92:673-80.
[149] Bertelli E, Bendayan M. Association between endocrine pancreas and ductal system. More than an epiphenomenon of endocrine differentiation and development? J Histochem Cytochem 2005;53:1071-86.
[150] Takaishi K, Miyoshi J, Matsumura T, Honda R, Ohba T, Katabuchi H. Hypertriglyceridemic acute pancreatitis during pregnancy: prevention with diet therapy and omega-3 fatty acids in the following pregnancy. Nutrition 2009;25:1094-7.
[151] Roth EM, Bays HE, Forker AD, et al. Prescription omega-3 fatty acid as an adjunct to fenofibrate therapy in hypertriglyceridemic subjects. J Cardiovasc Pharmacol 2009;54:196-203.
[152] Stefanutti C, Di Giacomo S, Vivenzio A, et al. Therapeutic plasma exchange in patients with severe hypertriglyceridemia: a multicenter study. Artif Organs 2009;33:1096-102.
[153] Ewald N, Kloer HU. Severe hypertriglyceridemia: an indication for apheresis? Atheroscler Suppl 2009;10:49-52.
[154] Yeh JH, Chen JH, Chiu HC. Plasmapheresis for hyperlipidemic pancreatitis. J Clin Apher 2003;18:181-5.
[155] Syed H, Bilusic M, Rhondla C, Tavaria A. Plasmapheresis in the treatment of hypertriglyceridemia-induced pancreatitis: A community hospital's experience. J Clin Apher 2010;25:229-34.
[156] Dodd RY. The risk of transfusion-transmitted infection. N Engl J Med 1992;327:419-21.
[157] Szczepiorkowski ZM, Bandarenko N, Kim HC, et al. Guidelines on the use of therapeutic apheresis in clinical practice: evidence-based approach from the Apheresis Applications Committee of the American Society for Apheresis. J Clin Apher 2007;22:106-75.
[158] Pejic RN, Lee DT. Hypertriglyceridemia. J Am Board Fam Med 2006;19:310-6.
[159] Carson JA. Nutrition therapy for dyslipidemia. Curr Diab Rep 2003;3:397-403.

[160] Asakura L, Lottenberg AM, Neves MQ, et al. Dietary medium-chain triacylglycerol prevents the postprandial rise of plasma triacylglycerols but induces hypercholesterolemia in primary hypertriglyceridemic subjects. Am J Clin Nutr 2000;71:701-5.
[161] Kris-Etherton PM, Pearson TA, Wan Y, et al. High-monounsaturated fatty acid diets lower both plasma cholesterol and triacylglycerol concentrations. Am J Clin Nutr 1999;70:1009-15.
[162] Shah A, Rader DJ, Millar JS. The effect of PPAR-alpha agonism on apolipoprotein metabolism in humans. Atherosclerosis 2010;210:35-40.
[163] Abourbih S, Filion KB, Joseph L, et al. Effect of fibrates on lipid profiles and cardiovascular outcomes: a systematic review. Am J Med 2009;122:962 e1-8.
[164] Kolovou GD, Kostakou PM, Anagnostopoulou KK, Cokkinos DV. Therapeutic effects of fibrates in postprandial lipemia. Am J Cardiovasc Drugs 2008;8:243-55.
[165] Staels B, Dallongeville J, Auwerx J, Schoonjans K, Leitersdorf E, Fruchart JC. Mechanism of action of fibrates on lipid and lipoprotein metabolism. Circulation 1998;98:2088-93.
[166] Goldenberg I, Benderly M, Goldbourt U. Update on the use of fibrates: focus on bezafibrate. Vasc Health Risk Manag 2008;4:131-41.
[167] Gang N, Langevitz P, Livneh A. Relapsing acute pancreatitis induced by re-exposure to the cholesterol lowering agent bezafibrate. Am J Gastroenterol 1999;94:3626-8.
[168] Abdul-Ghaffar NU, el-Sonbaty MR. Pancreatitis and rhabdomyolysis associated with lovastatin-gemfibrozil therapy. J Clin Gastroenterol 1995;21:340-1.
[169] Gouni-Berthold I, Krone W. Hypertriglyceridemia-why, when and how should it be treated? Z Kardiol 2005;94:731-9.
[170] Kamanna VS, Kashyap ML. Mechanism of action of niacin. Am J Cardiol 2008;101:20B-6B.
[171] Grundy SM, Cleeman JI, Merz CN, et al. Implications of recent clinical trials for the National Cholesterol Education Program Adult Treatment Panel III guidelines. Circulation 2004;110:227-39.
[172] Roth EM, McKenney JM, Kelly MT, et al. Efficacy and safety of rosuvastatin and fenofibric acid combination therapy versus simvastatin monotherapy in patients with hypercholesterolemia and hypertriglyceridemia: a randomized, double-blind study. Am J Cardiovasc Drugs 2010;10:175-86.
[173] Watts GF, Karpe F. Triglycerides and atherogenic dyslipidaemia: extending treatment beyond statins in the high-risk cardiovascular patient. Heart 2011;97:350-6.
[174] Bays HE, McKenney J, Maki KC, Doyle RT, Carter RN, Stein E. Effects of prescription omega-3-acid ethyl esters on non--high-density lipoprotein cholesterol when coadministered with escalating doses of atorvastatin. Mayo Clin Proc 2010;85:122-8.
[175] Jacobson TA. Role of n-3 fatty acids in the treatment of hypertriglyceridemia and cardiovascular disease. Am J Clin Nutr 2008;87:1981S-90S.
[176] Skulas-Ray AC, Kris-Etherton PM, Harris WS, Vanden Heuvel JP, Wagner PR, West SG. Dose-response effects of omega-3 fatty acids on triglycerides, inflammation, and endothelial function in healthy persons with moderate hypertriglyceridemia. Am J Clin Nutr 2011;93:243-52.
[177] Harris WS, Ginsberg HN, Arunakul N, et al. Safety and efficacy of Omacor in severe hypertriglyceridemia. J Cardiovasc Risk 1997;4:385-91.
[178] Harris WS. n-3 fatty acids and serum lipoproteins: human studies. Am J Clin Nutr 1997;65:1645S-54S.

17

The Role of Percutaneous Drainage in the Treatment of Severe Acute Pancreatitis on the Basis of the Modified Atlanta Classification

Zsolt Szentkereszty, Róbert Kotán and Péter Sápy
University of Debrecen, Medical Health Science Center, Institute of Surgery, Hungary

1. Introduction

According to the Atlanta Classification in many cases of acute pancreatitis there are three well-defined fluid collections: acute peripancreatic fluid collection (APFC), the so-called postnecrotic pancreatic/peripancreatic fluid collection which develops in the region of liquified pancreatic necrosis, and the pseudocyst that develops in the late phase of the illness.

In many cases, these anatomic entities can be succesfully treated with radiological interventional methods.

It is difficult to correctly interpret the articles that review the treatment of numerous patients because the nomenclature is unclear. The aim of this article is to analyse the indications, limits and results of the listed complications treated by percutaneous drainage (PD) which aggravate acute pancreatitis on the basis of the literature.

2. What to drain?

2.1 Acute peripancreatic fluid collection (APFC)

According to the Atlanta Classification peripancreatic fluid collection develops in the early phase of acute pancreatitis in about 40% of cases. The acute fluid collection usually develops around the pancreas but sometimes emerges in the glandular area and does not contain a high quantity of necrosis. Not rarely, it spreads into the chest, mediastinum and/or into the pararenal area. Several fluid collections can develop at the same time and can shuttle together. The rich pancreatic enzyme content of the fluid can indicate communication with the pancreatic duct or indicate parenchymal necrosis. They do not have definite walls, and are limited by the walls of the surrounding organs. In a significant number of cases (about 30-50%), spontaneous resolution occurs without surgical or other intervention. If they do not show tendency towards resolution, they can become of significant size and cause clinical symptoms or complications [5,6,33,44].

The most frequent complaints caused by a big, 8-15 cm size acute fluid collection are pain, tension, and increasing abdominal pressure which can significantly worsen the efficiency of breathing [1,9]. In other cases they can cause compression symptoms (jaundice, duodenal obstruction) or bleeding can develop inside of them. Another frequent complication is the superinfection of the fluid that can be confirmed by fine needle aspiration (FNA) [1,2,11,19,25,33,37,40,44].

The APFC can be visualized by CT scan or ultrasound examination as well. The number of acute fluid collections correlate to the severity of the pancreatitis, the length of hospitalization and mortality [19].

Even today the treatment of acute peripancreatic fluid collections is not totally clear. In a small sized fluid collection, conservative treatment (naso-jejunal feeding, the resting of pancreas) is usually effective. Fluid evacuation is advisable when it causes severe symptoms. In the past only surgical intervention was available. The authors do not recommend surgical treatment in the early phase of the illness because of the high morbidity and mortality rates. With the development of interventional radiology and manipulative laparo-endoscopy there are other possibilities to evacuate these fluid collections without operation [1,6,11,14,21,25,35,40,44].

For the treatment of sterile fluid collection percutaneous puncture and drainage are widely applied. It is disputed whether repeated punctures or drainage is the most suitable for the treatment of fluid collections. There are some who are satisfied with the clearing of the fluid collection with only one or repeated punctures in sterile cases. However, this is succesful only in a few cases and drainage or surgical intervention follows [6,28,40,44].

According to those who are pro drainage in the treatment of sterile acute peripancreatic fluid collections, drainage can be applied effectively [1,3,4,14,21,25,34,35,40,44]. Acute compartment syndrome caused by massive acute peripancreatic fliud collection can be treated effectively with PD [9]. In the randomized controlled trial of Zerem et al. they commit themselves to drainage treatment [44].

Those who are against drainage treatment claim that it is the treatment itself which causes the dreadful complication, the infection of the fluid. According to the literature the rate of iatrogenous infection is about 8-27% [12,25,28,40]. Walser, Zerem et al. report a very high, 50% rate of infection which is, in our opinion, the result of the irrigation 2-3 times a day [40,44]. To determine the correct rate of iatregenous infections treated without drainage or puncture a prospective randomized trial should be performed which is not available at this time.

With regard to the management of infected acute peripancreatic fluid collections, views are not as varied in these cases: percutaneous drainage is suggested [1,5,8,18,21,22,25,33,34].

Surgery can often be avoided by drainage treatment, and in other cases the intervention is suitable for delaying operative treatment. In such cases, when drainage is not effective, operation is suggested [5,6,8,18,21,22,25,34,35,44].

2.2 Post-necrotic Pancreatic Fluid Collection (PNPFC), Walled-off Pancreatic Necrosis (WOPN)

Necrosis can liquify and can be accompanied by the development of different sizes of fluid collections. These cases are equivalent to the pathological entity accepted in the modified Atlanta Classification as postnecrotic peripancreatic/pancreatic fluid collection and walled-off pancreatic necrosis. WOPN can be misdiagnosed by contrast-enhanced CT for pseudocyst but MRI, abdominal or endoscopic ultrasound can help with differential diagnosis for these are suitable for proving the significant quantity of necrosis in the fluid. This differentiation is very important because treatment, especially the minimally invasive one, is different because in cases of WOPN the necrotized tissues should be removed. PNPFC cases can be sterile and infected as well [5,12,18,22,24,33,34,43].

In cases of PNFC puncture and/or drainage is usually not enough, the evacuation of necrotic tissues are also necessary and for this reason some authors are explicitely against drainage treatment [3,6,22]. According to other authors the evacuation of necrosis and fluid collection is possible with the help of irrigation through 14-30 F bore drains. Necrosectomy can be performed by using dormia basket. For such treatment more catheters should be placed in the cavity [5,10,11,12,18,21,26,29,33,36,38,43]. Bruennel et al. did not find a relation between the thickness, or the number of the drains and the effectiveness. With so-called 'sinus tract endoscopy' necrectomy can be performed effectively following the dilatation of the drain's channel [23,36,43]. Horvath et al. performed necrosectomy via the channels of the drains with a supplementary incision using laparoscopy [16,17].
More than 20% of the patients treated with the minimal invasive method recovered without operation. An alternative method for the treatment of WOPN is the endoscopic transmural necrosectomy and drainage [13,15,27,30,31,41]. Necrosectomy during operation is the suitable method in cases of unsuccessfully treated patients [3,6,10,11,12,22,24,26,28, 33,34,36,43].

2.3 Acute pseudocyst

The acute pseudocyst appears on CT scan as a walled, oval or circle shaped fluid. It often develops in the area of an earlier acute fluid collection which did not show any tendency to resolution. The frequency of this is about 30-50%. The wall of the pseudocyst contains inflammatory tissues but is not covered by epithelium. It develops most frequently in the environment of the pancreas but mediastinal or pelvic appearances are also known. About 4 weeks are needed for the development of the mutation from the beginning of the disease. Its content is usually sterile but sometimes bacteria can be detected without any clinical manifestation, in other cases it contains pus [5].
Almost 50% of acute pseudocysts do not cause any clinical symptoms and show spontaneous absorbing susceptibility. Especially smaller pseudocysts that are not bigger than 4-6 cm, recover with conservative treatment (eg: naso-jejunal feeding) [18,33,37]. Bigger pseudocysts can cause explicit clinical complaints. Compressive symptoms and pain are the most frequent among them. As a complication the content can become infected. Air bubbles can be seen in it on CT examination. In its cavity pseudoaneurysm can develop which can cause fatal bleeding [2,6,11,14,28,33,37].
In those cases where compressive or respiratory complications or pain develop, surgery or less burdensome percutaneous drainage gives an opportunity for treatment, allowing for the descent of the fluid as well as its bacterological examination [3,4,6,8,11,18,24,33,35]. More drains can be placed in cases of multiple pseudocysts [11,18,35]
Operation can be avoided in cases treated this way and drainage can lead to complete recovery, in other cases it is suitable for delaying the time of operation [3,4,6,8,11,18,37,43]. In those cases where the cyst cavity communicates with the Wirsung ductal system, external drainage is not effective. For this reason, the anatomical conditions of the pseudocyst must be cleared by ERCP prior to external drainage [18]. In cases when communication is detected between the pancreatic duct and the necroma as a well accepted method internal endoscopic transluminal drainage (NOTES) and lavage, with endoscopic necrosectomy is indicated [13,30].
The infected pseudocyst appears as a pancreatic abscess in the late phase of severe acute pancreatitis, at least 4 weeks after the beginning of the disease and needs radiologic

intervention or surgery in each case. It does not contain a considerable quantity of necrotic tissue mass in opposition to the infected liquified necrosis (Post-necrotic Pancreatic Fluid Collection, Walled-off Pancreatic Necrosis). On CT scan gas bubbles can be observed [1,2,5,6,18,20,29,37,43].

Surgery in these cases involves a lower rate of morbidity and mortality than those performed in the early phase of pancreatitis. The results are good [20,37]. Percutaneous drainage treatment can be applied in cases of pancreatic abscess with good results and it can be suggested as the first intervention [4,5,6,8,18,20,29,33,37,38,43]. Drainage can be also applied in cases of numerous abscesses. It is important to carry out bacterological analysis from each abscess one by one because different types of bacteria can be cultured from them. The management must be supplemented with antibiotics [1,4,5,18,20,26].

PD has an effectiveness of 31-94% in the treatment of pancreatic abscesses [1,4,5, 8,18,20,26,33,37,43].

3. How to drain?

For drainage a pig-tail catheter is well accepted. The insertion of the drain can be guided by CT or ultrasound and fluoroscopy or without it [5,6,8,10,11,12,18,21,28,32,39,42,44]. The catheter with the main wire is led into the fluid collection and following verification of its placement the wire is removed (Figure 1-2). The indication of the location and function is that a proper quantity of fluid appears. Depending on the quality of the fluid, different size of drains should be used. If there is an abscess, the thicker (14-30F), otherwise the thinner (8-10F), pig-tail catheter is to be used [1,6,8,10,11,12,21,32,36,39]. The drained fluid shlould be sent for bacterological analysis in each case. More drains can be inserted at a time if necessary [5,8,10,11,12,18,21,32,33,35,39,42,44].

The drain is usually placed without active suction. The daily quantity and quality of the fluid must be measured and examined. If the sterile fluid becomes thickened or purulent, it signifies bacterial infection. If pus appears or the fluid is dense, the irrigation of the cavity is also possible [1,10,11,21,42,44].

Ultrasound examination is the most suitable for the observation of the size of the fluid collection. It is also inexpensive and can also be performed bedside (Figure 3). The cavity filled with contrast material can be well demonstrated and is apt for showing fistulae [1,6,10,11,42,44].

The drain can be removed if the fluid has cleared up, has become „sterile", the quantity of the drained fluid is less than 10-30 ml per day and the cavity has deflated on imaging examinations [1,6,10,12,44].

More than 20% of patients (20-50%) recover without surgery, by drainage treatment. If the drained cavity does not decrease during drainage or the septic state does not show a tendency towards resolution, surgical treatment is indicated. In such cases with the application of drainage early operation can be avoided [1,4,6,8,10,11,12,21,26,32,35,39,42]. Others suggest transluminal endoscopic (NOTES) procedure if percuteanous drainage is failed [7,13,15,27,30,31,41] Some authors suggest the combination of external and internal drainage with endoscpopic necrosectomy [27,30,].

Complications related to percutaneous drainage are rare. In an experienced hand the rate of iatrogenic injuries are negligible, less than 2%, generally the injury of the surrounding organs, bleeding can be noticed [1,4,11,12,21,32,35,39,44,]. Sometimes the drain can get clogged or slip out, then its replacement is required [8,35,42,44].

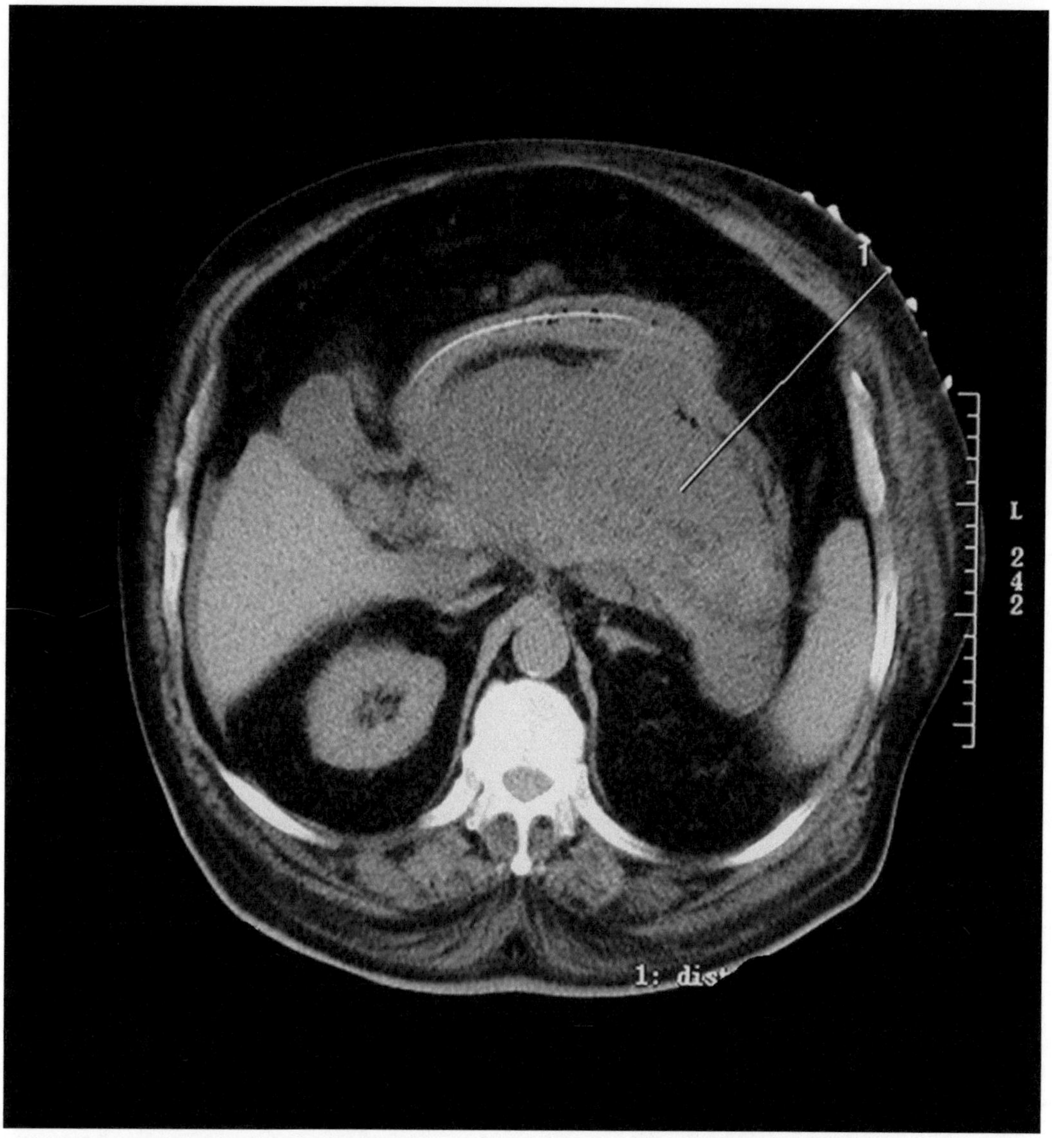

Fig. 1. Percutaneous CT guided puncture of acute peripancreatic fluid collection

A late complication of PD is the development of pancreatic fistulae, which may be in relation with the skin or gastrointestinal tract and most close spontaneously. The facts that influence the effectiveness of PD of infected fluid collections positively are the presence of a single fluid collection, the lack of necrosis, the low APACHE-II and Ransome points and the lack of failure [8,35,42,44].

In this chapter the authors suggest reviewing the transmural endoscopic (NOTES) necrosectomy as a minimal invasive method. More and more authors in selected patients use this method for necrosectomy with a successful rate of 73-92% [2,7,13,15,27,30,31,41]. The necrotic cavity can be drained to the stomach or the duodenum. The effectiveness of this method can be enhanced with the use of endoscopic ultrasound (ES) [7,13,15,27,30,31,41].

After dilating the puncture chanel to 8-20 mm the necrectomy can be performed with the use of baskets, snares, transparent scope caps, nets and/or water jet [7,13,27,30,31,41]. This procedure must be repeated till the complete emptying of the necroma [7,13,27,30,31]. After the necrectomy it is essential to drain the cavity with pigtail catheters, or stents [13,41]. The endoscopic drainage of WOPN decreases the length of hospitalization, the duration of external drainage, the number of CT scans [15]. This method is a possible therapy before or instead of surgery [2,7,13,27,30,31,41].

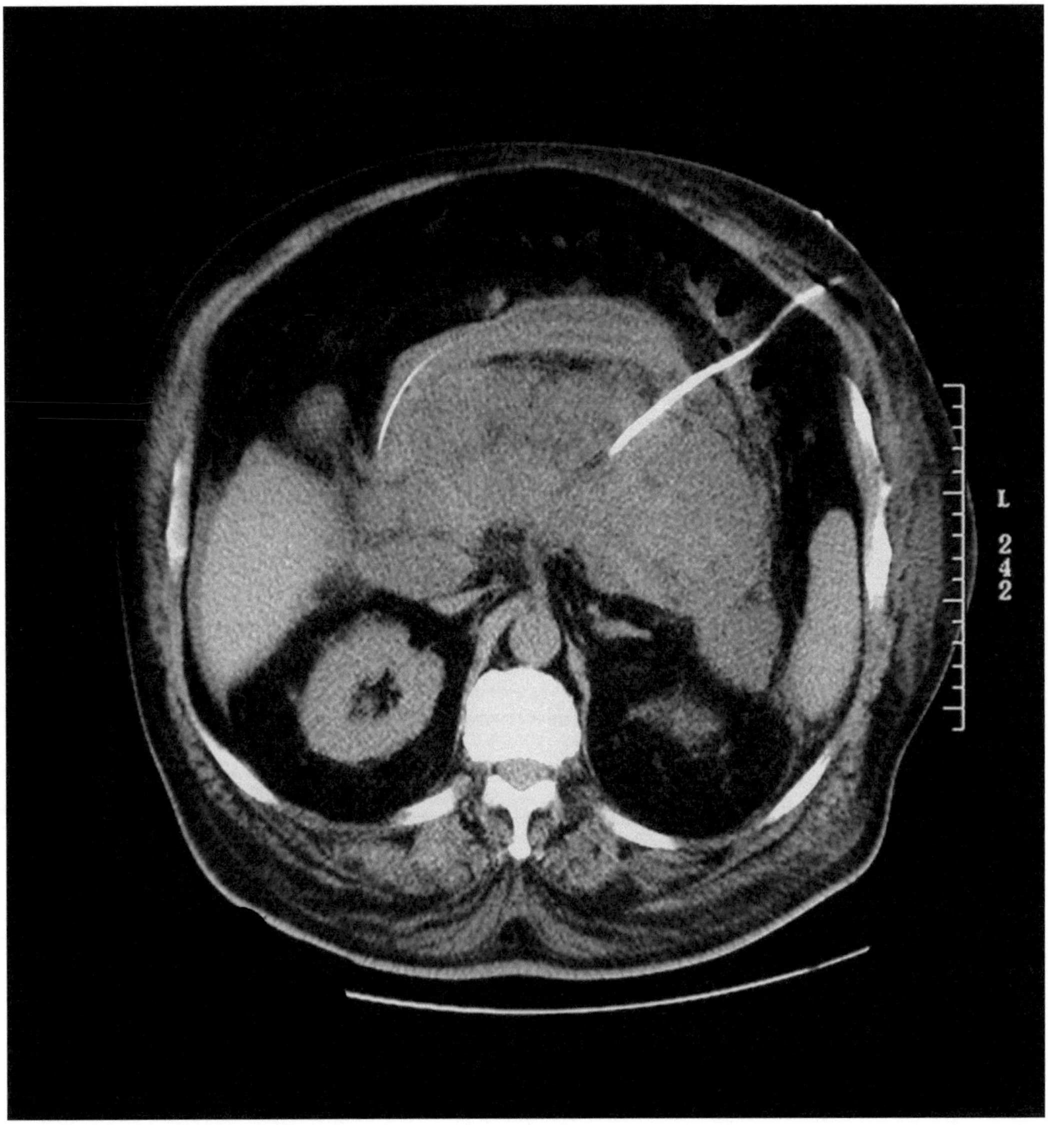

Fig. 2. Percutaneous CT-guided drainage of acute peripancreatic fluid collection

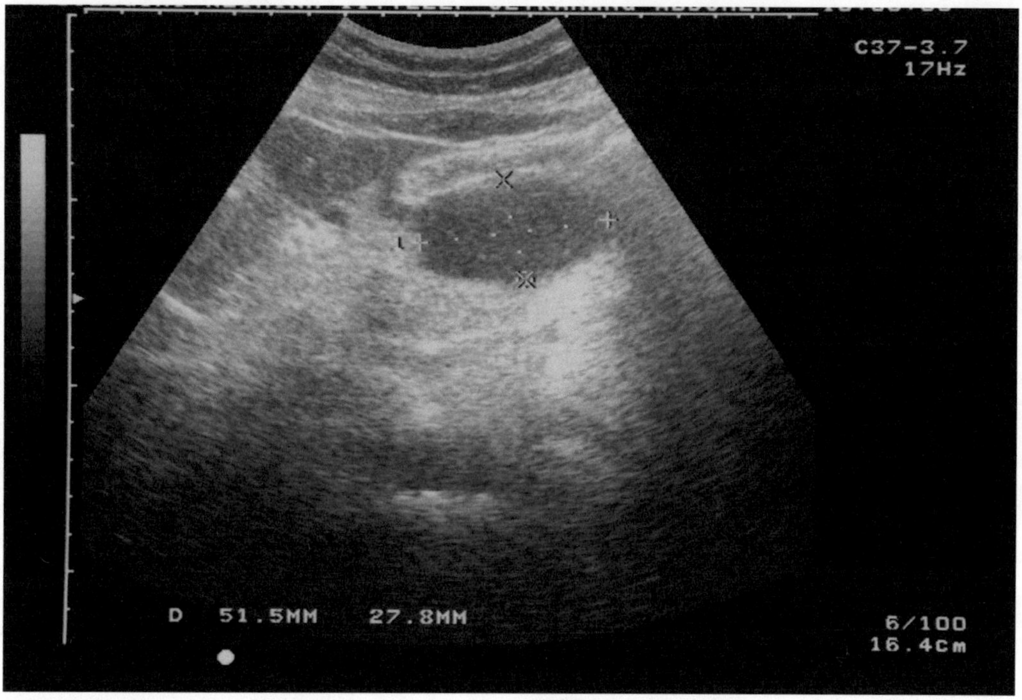

Fig. 3. Ultrasound wiew of drainaged acute peripancreatic fluid collection

In conclusion percutaneous drainage plays an important role in the treatment of concomitant sterile ad septic fluid collections (APFC, PNPFC, WOPN, acute pseudocyst) in severe acute pancreatitis. In well selected cases percutaneous drainage with appropriate caliber drains and supplementary therapy in the greater part of cases leads to complete recovery. In other cases PD is useful to delay surgery or to avoid early operation.

4. Abbreviations

APFC: Acute Peripancreatic Fluid Collection
PD: Percutaneous Drainage
FNA: Fine Needle Aspiration
CT: Computed Tomography
PNPFC: Post-necrotic Pancreatic Fluid Collection
WOPN: Walled-off Pancreatic Necrosis
MRI: Magnetic Resonance Image
ERCP: Endoscopic Retrograde Cholangio-Panreatographia
ES: Endoscopic Ultrasound
NOTES: Natural Orifice Transluminal Endoscopic Surgery

5. References

[1] Ai X, Qian X, Pan W, Xu J, Hu W, Terai T, Sato N, Watanabe S: Ultrasound-guided percutaneous drainage may decrease the mortality of severe acute pancreatitis. J Gastroenterol 2010, 45, 77-85.

[2] Amano H, Takada T, Isaji S, Takeyama Y, Hirata K, et al.: Therapeutic intervention and surgery of acute pancreatitis. J Hepatobiliary Pancreat Sci 2010, 17, 53-9.
[3] Aultman DF, Bilton BD, Zibari GB, McMillan RW, McDonalds JC: Nonoperative therapy for acute necrotizing pancreatitis. Am Surg 1997, 63, 1114-1117.
[4] Baril NB, Ralls SM, Selby RR, Radin R., Parekh D, Jabbour N, et al.: Does infected peripancreatic fluid collection or abscess mandate operation? Ann Surg 2000, 231, 361-367.
[5] Bruennler T, Langgartner J, Lang S, Wrede CE, Klebl F, Zierhut S, et al.: Outcome of patients with acute, necrotizing pancreatitis requiring drainage-does drainage size matter? W J Gastroenterol 2008, 14, 725-730.
[6] Chalmers AG: The role of imaging in acute pancreatitis. Eur. J. Gastro. Hepatol 1997, 9, 106-116.
[7] Charnley RM, Lochan R, Gray H, O'Sullivan CB, Scott J, et al.: Endoscopic necrosectomy as primary therapy in the management of infected pancreatic necrosis. Endoscopy 2006, 38, 925-8.
[8] Chen YF, Chiang HJ, Chang JH.: Abdominal fluid collection secondary to acute pancreatitis: treated with percutaneous cathater drainage. Chin Med J 1997, 60, 265-72.
[9] Dambrauskas Z, Parseliūnas A, Maleckas A, Gulbinas A, Barauskas G, Pundzius J: Interventional and surgical management of abdominal compartment syndrome in severe acute pancreatitis. Medicina (Kaunas) 2010, 46, 249-255.
[10] Echenique AM, Sleeman D, Yrizzary J, et al.: Percutaneous catheter-directed debridement of infected pancreatic necrosis: Results in 20 patients. J Vasc Interv Radiol 1998, 9, 565-571.
[11] Fotoohi M, D'Agostino HB, Wollman B, Chon K, Shahrokni S, van Sonnenberg E: Persistent pancreatocutaneous fistula after percutaneous drainage of pancreatic fluid collections: role of cause and severity of pancreatitis. Radiology 1999, 213, 573-578.
[12] Freeny PC, Hauptmann E, Althaus SJ, Traverso LW, Sinanan M: Percutaneous CT-guided catheter drainage of infected acute necrotizing pancreatitis: techniques and results. Am J Roengennol 1998, 170, 969-975.
[13] Friedland S, Kaltenbach T, Sugimoto M, Soetikno R.: Endoscopic necrosectomy of organized pancreatic necrosis: a currently practiced NOTES procedure. J Hepatobiliary Pancreat Surg 2009, 16, 266-9.
[14] Gambiez LP, Denimal FA, Porte HL, Saudemont A, Chambon J-PM, Quandalle PA: Retroperitoneal approach and endoscopic management of peripancreatic necrosis collections. Arch Surg 1998, 133, 66-72.
[15] Gluck M, Ross A, Irani S, Lin O, Hauptmann E, Siegal J, Fotoohi M, Crane R, Robinson D, Kozarek RA.: Endoscopic and percutaneous drainage of symptomatic walled-off pancreatic necrosis reduces hospital stay and radiographic resources. Clin Gastroenterol Hepatol 2010, 8, 1083-8.
[16] Horvath KD, Kao LS, Ali A, Wherry K.L, Pellegrini CA, Sinanan MN: Laparoscopic assisted percutaneous drainage of infected pancreatic necrosis. Surg Endosc 2001, 15, 677-682.

[17] Horvath KD, Kao LS, Wherry KL, Pellegrini CA, Sinanan MN: A technique for laparoscopic-assisted percutaneous drainage of infected pancreatic necrosis and abscess. Surg Endosc 2001, 15, 1221-1225.
[18] Loveday BP, Mittal A, Phillips A, Windsor JA: Minimally invasive management of pancreatic abscess, pseudocyst, and necrosis: A systematic review of current guidlines. W J Surg 2008, 32, 2383-2394.
[19] Luo Y, Yuan CX, Peng YL, Wei PL, Zhang ZD, Jiang JM, et al.: Can ultrasound predict severity of acute pancreatitis early by observing acute fluid collection. World J Gastroenterol 2001, 7, 293-295.
[20] Mithöfer K., Mueller P.R., Warshaw A.L.: Interventional and surgical treatment of pancreatic abscess. World J Surg 1997, 21, 162-168.
[21] Mortelé KJ, Girshman J, Szejnfeld D, Ashley SW, Erturk SM, Banks PA, Silverman SG: CT-guided percutaneous catheter drainage of acute necrotizing pancreatitis: clinical experience and observations in patients with sterile and infected necrosis. AJR Am J Roentgenol 2009, 192, 110-6.
[22] Mueller PR.: Percutaneous drainage of pancreatic necrosis: Is it ecstasy or agony? Am J Roengennol 1998, 170, 976-977.
[23] Mui LM, Wong SK, Ng EK, Chan AC, Chung SC: Combined sinus tract endoscopy and endoscopic retrograde cholangiopancreatography in management of pancreatic necrosis and abscess. Surg Endosc 2005, 19, 393-397.
[24] Navalho M, Pires F, Duarte A, Gonçalves A, Alexandrino P, Távora I: Percutaneous drainage of infected pancreatic fluid collections in critically ill patients: Correlation with C-reactive protein values. J Clin Imaging 2006, 30, 114-119.
[25] Nealon WH, Bawduniak J, Walser EM.: Appropriate timing of cholecystectomy in patients who present with moderate to severe gallstone-associated acute panreatitis with peripancreatic fluid collections. Ann Surg 2004, 239, 741-749.
[26] Oláh A, Balágyi T, Bartek P, Pohárnok L, Romics L jr: Alternative treatment modalities of infected pancreatic necrosis. Hepato-Gastroenterol 2006, 53, 603-607.
[27] Papachristou GI, Takahashi N, Chahal P, Sarr MG, Baron TH.: Peroral endoscopic drainage/debridement of walled-off pancreatic necrosis. Ann Surg 2007, 245, 943-51.
[28] Paye F, Rotman N, Radier C, Nouira R, Fagniez PL: Percutaneous aspiration for bacteriological studies in patients with necrotizing pancreatitis. Br J Surg 1998, 85, 755-759.
[29] Pezzilli R, Zerbi A, Di Carlo V, Bassi C, Delle Fave GF; Working Group of the Italian Association for the Study of the Pancreas on Acute Pancreatitis.: Practical guidelines for acute pancreatitis. Pancreatology 2010, 10, 523-35.
[30] Ross A, Gluck M, Irani S, Hauptmann E, Fotoohi M, et al.: Combined endoscopic and percutaneous drainage of organized pancreatic necrosis. Gastrointest Endosc 2010, 71, 79-84.
[31] Seewald S, Groth S, Omar S, Imazu H, Seitz U, et al.: Aggressive endoscopic therapy for pancreatic necrosis and pancreatic abscess: a new safe and effective treatment algorithm (videos). Gastrointest Endosc 2005, 62, 92-100.
[32] Segal D, Mortele KJ, Banks PA, Silverman SG.: Acute necrotizing pancreatitis: role of CT-guided percutaneous catheter drainage. Abdom Imaging 2007, 32, 351-361.

[33] Shankar S, vanSonnenberg E, Silverman SG, Tuncali K, Banks PA: Imaging and percutaneous management of acute complicated pancreatitis. Cardiovasc Intervent Radiol 2004, 27, 567-580.

[34] Stamatakos M, Stefanaki C, Kontzoglou K, Stergiopoulos S, Giannopoulos G, et al: Walled-off pancreatic necrosis. World J Gastroenterol 2010, 14, 1707-1712.

[35] Szentkereszty Zs, Kerekes L, Hallay J, Czako D, Sápy: CT guided percutaneous peripancreatic drainage: a possible therapy in acute necrotizing pancreatitis. Hepato-Gastroenterol 2002, 49, 1696-1698.

[36] Tang LJ, Wang T, Cui JF, Zhang BY, Li S, Li DX, Zhou S: Percutaneous catheter drainage in combination with choledochoscope-guided debridement in treatment of peripancreatic infection. World J Gastroenterol 2010, 16, 513-517.

[37] Tsiotos GG, Sarr MG.: Management of fluid collections nad necrosis in acute pancreatitis. Curr Gastroenterol Rep 1999, 1, 87-88.

[38] Uomo G.: Classical, minimally invasive necrosectomy or percutaneous drainage in acute necrotizing pancreatitis. Does changing the order of the factors change the result? JOP 2010, 11, 415-417.

[39] van Baal MC, van Santvoort HC, Bollen TL, Bakker OJ, Besselink MG, Gooszen HG; Dutch Pancreatitis Study Group.: Systematic review of percutaneous catheter drainage as primary treatment for necrotizing pancreatitis Br J Surg 2011, 98, 18-27.

[40] Walser EM, Nealon WH, Marroquin S, Raza S, Hernandez JA, Vasek J: Sterile fluid collections in scute pancreatitis: Catheter drainage versus simple aspiration. Cardiovasc. Intervent Radiol, 2006, 29, 102-107.

[41] Wehrmann T, Martchenko K, Riphaus A.: Dual access endoscopic necrosectomy of infected pancreatic necrosis: a case report. Eur J Gastroenterol Hepatol 2010, 22, 237-40.

[42] Wig JD, Gupta V, Kocchar R, Doley RP, Yadav TD, Poornachandra K S, et al.: The role of non-operative strategies in the management of severe acute pancreatitis. JOP 2010, 11, 553-559.

[43] Wysocki AP, McKay CJ, Carter CR: Infected pancreatic necrosis: minimizing the cut. ANZ J Surg 2010, 80, 58-70.

[44] Zerem E, Imamovic G, Omerović S, Imširović B.: Randomized controlled trial on sterile fluid collections management in acute pancreatitis: Should they removed? Surg Endosc 2009, May 15. [Epub ahead of print]